The Complete

Reflexology Tutor

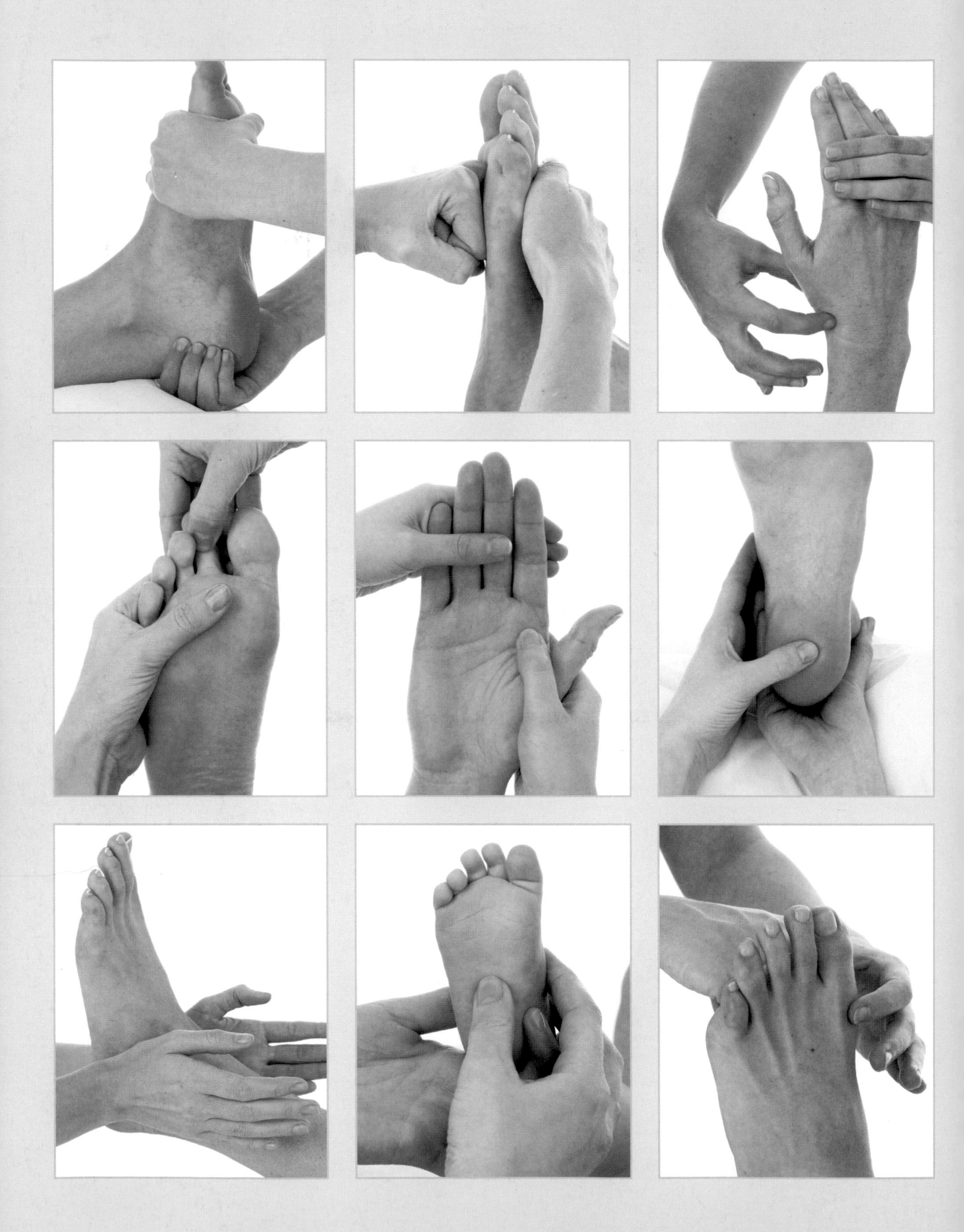

The Complete Reflexology Tutor

Everything you need to achieve professional expertise

Ann Gillanders

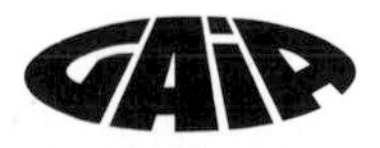

To my brother Anthony Porter (ART), who encouraged me to train in reflexology some 30 years ago and who has given me much support over the years.

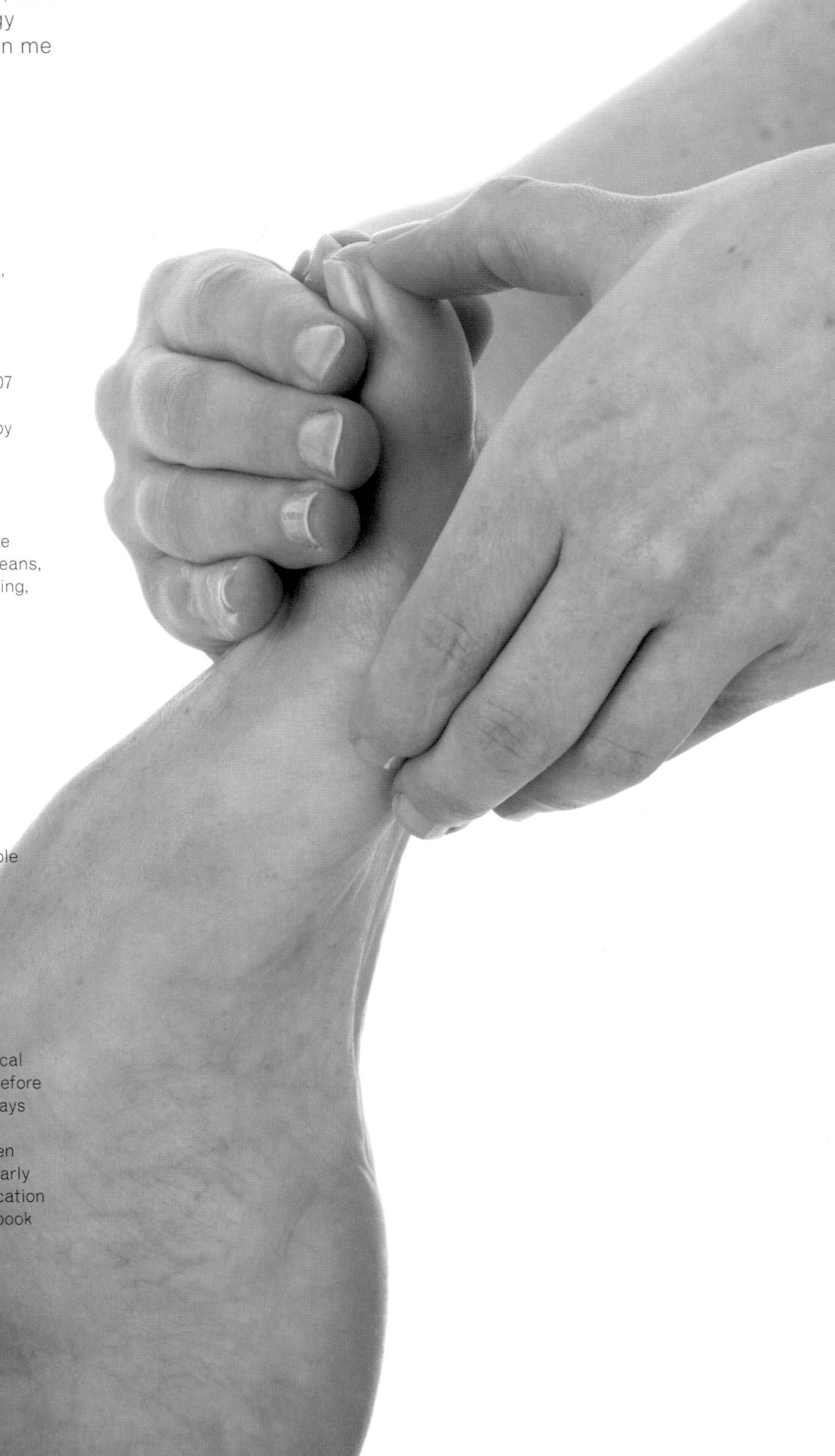

An Hachette Livre UK Company

First published in Great Britain in 2007 by Gaia,
a division of Octopus Publishing Group Ltd
2–4 Heron Quays, London E14 4JP
www.octopusbooks.co.uk

Distributed in the United States and Canada by
Sterling Publishing Co., Inc.,
387 Park Avenue South,
New York, NY 10016–8810

ISBN-13: 978-1-85675-283-1

ISBN-10: 1-85675-283-6

A CIP catalogue record for this book is available from the British Library.

Printed and bound in China

10 9 8 7 6 5 4 3 2 1

Contents

Introduction

This book has been written as a comprehensive guide for trainee reflexologists, and also as a quick reference for qualified practitioners, who may need to look up specific information during a consultation when treating individual medical conditions.

Reflexology is a holistic treatment, centuries old, and the aim of the reflexologist is to treat the whole person – body, mind and spirit – to induce a state of relaxation, balance and harmony, which will encourage the natural ability of the body to heal itself. Reflexology is of benefit to young and old, male and female, and there is an increasing interest in this form of natural healing. Many patients turn to reflexology when all else has failed. They have consulted their doctors, taken drugs, maybe even had surgery, and still their condition persists. Reflexology can be a revelation in these circumstances, bringing relief from the physical and mental stress of long-term illness, giving maximum support to patients and providing a feeling of wellbeing that may be new to them.

The professional advice offered in this book will give practitioners the comprehensive information they need to set up a practice. However, reflexology can never be learned solely from reading a book and examining a coloured foot chart. Trainee reflexologists must also seek training from an expert who has worked as a practitioner and who has plenty of teaching experience.

Practice makes perfect

When learning the practical skills, you should practise on as many different people as possible to get a sense of the way different feet respond. Reflexes are just the size of a pinhead and sensitivities can be easy to miss. As you relax in an armchair in the evening, practise developing the slow, forward creeping movement you will need, working with your thumb and index finger on the arm of the chair. It takes time to develop the strength you will need in your hands.

Always make sure you hold and support the feet in the way recommended in this book. It is essential to support the feet accurately and to use the correct thumb/finger technique in order to give a professional treatment. The way in which you sit and use your hands will also help to minimize the stresses and strains on you, the practitioner.

You might have to treat patients with a wide range of severe illnesses during your time as a reflexology practitioner, so it is crucial that you understand how the body works and are clear about the function, position and reflexes of each organ and system. While you are training, get a friend or family member to quiz you on anatomy and physiology in order to help you with your studies.

The guidelines on foot charts in this book will help you to find your way around the feet. Take a note of whether the reflexes lie above, below or on the inside or outside of the guidelines. It is vital that you identify the position of the reflexes accurately when giving a treatment, so that you can work on the part of the body that needs it.

During your training, you should get into the habit of taking notes during and after each practice session, making a record of each sensitivity found. Note whether the sensitivities decrease with

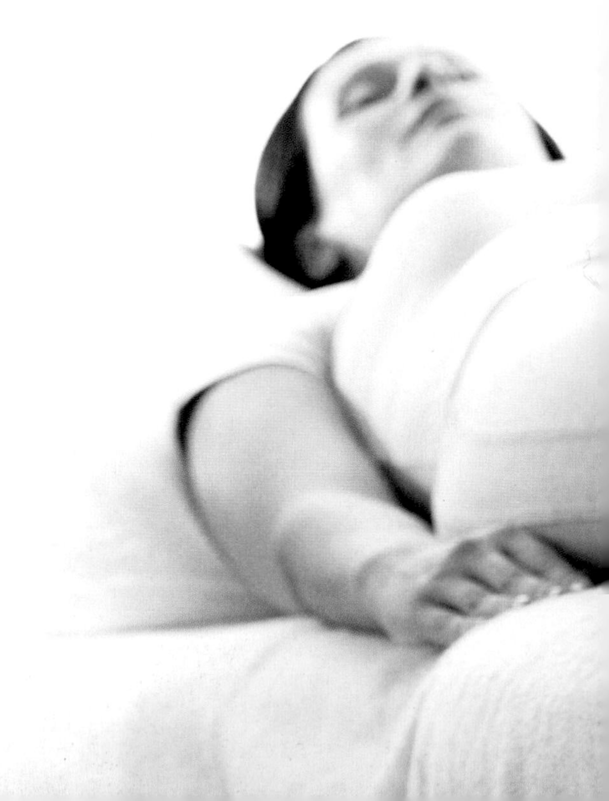

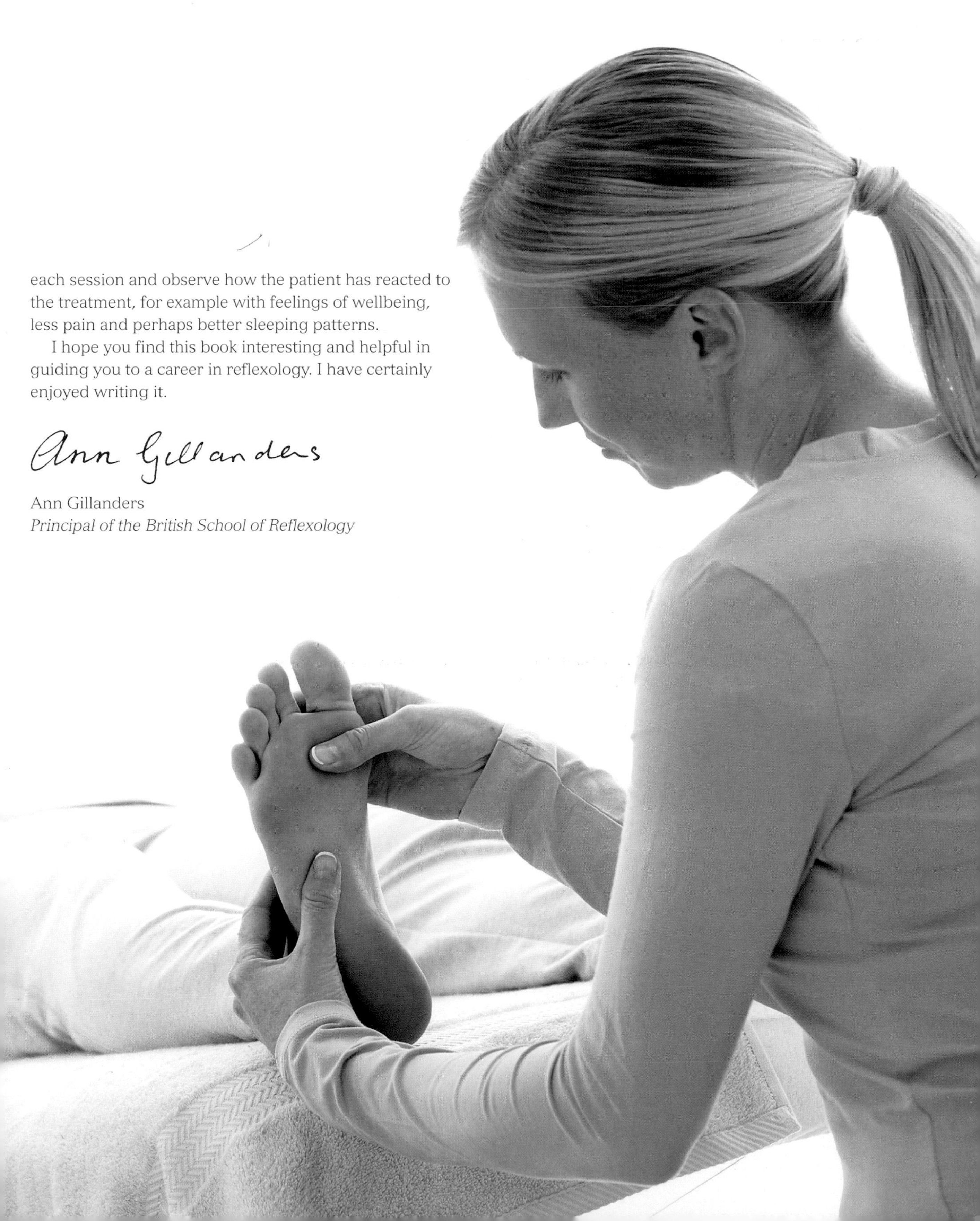

each session and observe how the patient has reacted to the treatment, for example with feelings of wellbeing, less pain and perhaps better sleeping patterns.

I hope you find this book interesting and helpful in guiding you to a career in reflexology. I have certainly enjoyed writing it.

Ann Gillanders

Ann Gillanders
Principal of the British School of Reflexology

How to use this book

Trainees should work comprehensively through each chapter, while experienced practitioners can use the index to find the specific advice they need when treating patients.

The first chapter of this book, 'The origins of reflexology' (pages 10–23) gives some background information about the development of reflexology over the centuries, and explores the holistic nature of the therapy's healing power. It also looks at the clinical evidence for the effectiveness of reflexology.

'How does reflexology work?' (pages 24–37) explains the zones and guidelines of the feet, and on pages 32–37 you will find detailed foot charts showing this information visually. Over time these will become as familiar to you as your own hand, but while you are training you may need to refer back to them sometimes.

'Providing reflexology' (pages 38–65) takes you step by step through the procedures that should be followed from the moment a patient arrives in your practice room. This chapter covers the different methods of assessing the patient's needs, explains how to keep records of your sessions and covers the essential techniques used in reflexology. It also answers some of the frequently asked questions about reflexology.

'Body systems' (pages 66–155) is the largest chapter in the book and will take you system by system right through the workings of the entire body, explaining how you can use reflexology to treat the problems that might affect each different organ or system. While the trainee should study this chapter from start to finish, qualified practitioners may want to use it whenever they have a patient with relevant problems, to refresh their memory

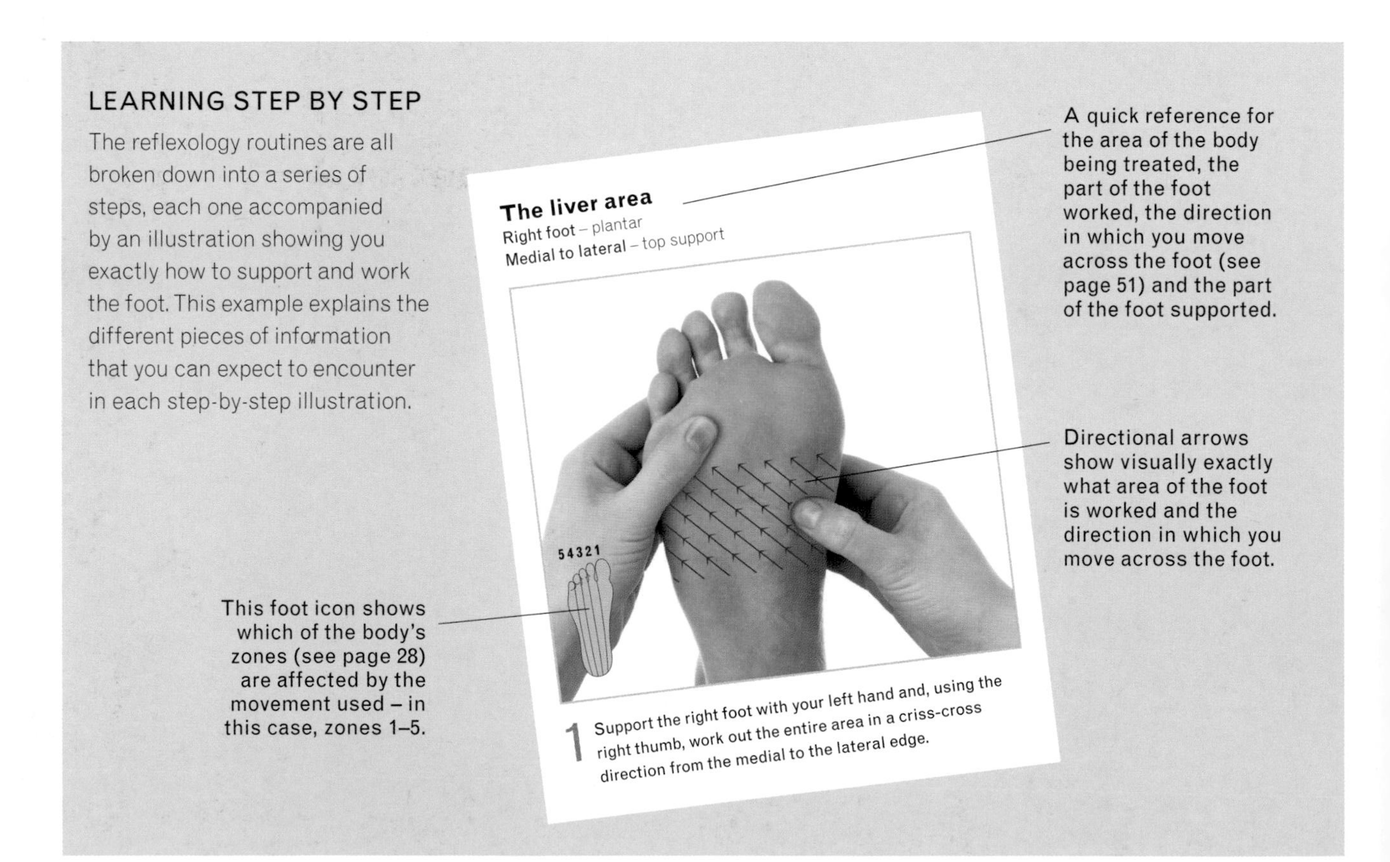

of how to treat the reflexes of specific systems. Detailed step-by-step photographs are a visual explanation of how each reflexology movement works, making the instructions very easy to follow.

'The whole routine' (pages 156–161) combines all the movements described in 'Body systems' to provide a comprehensive treatment routine. 'Hand reflexology' (pages 162–187) explains how to use hand reflexology, when the feet can't be worked on for some reason. You can also teach patients hand reflexology as a self-help technique that they can do by themselves at home.

The following chapters, 'Reflexology for better health' (pages 188–205) and 'Specialized reflexology' (pages 206–233) both look at specific illnesses and special health conditions, giving advice on treating pregnant women, babies, sufferers from cancer and heart disease and the terminally ill. There is also a directory of many common ailments that can be helped by reflexology.

Finally, 'A reflexology practice' (pages 234–247) explains how you can set up your own reflexology practice and attract patients.

Good luck with your studies!

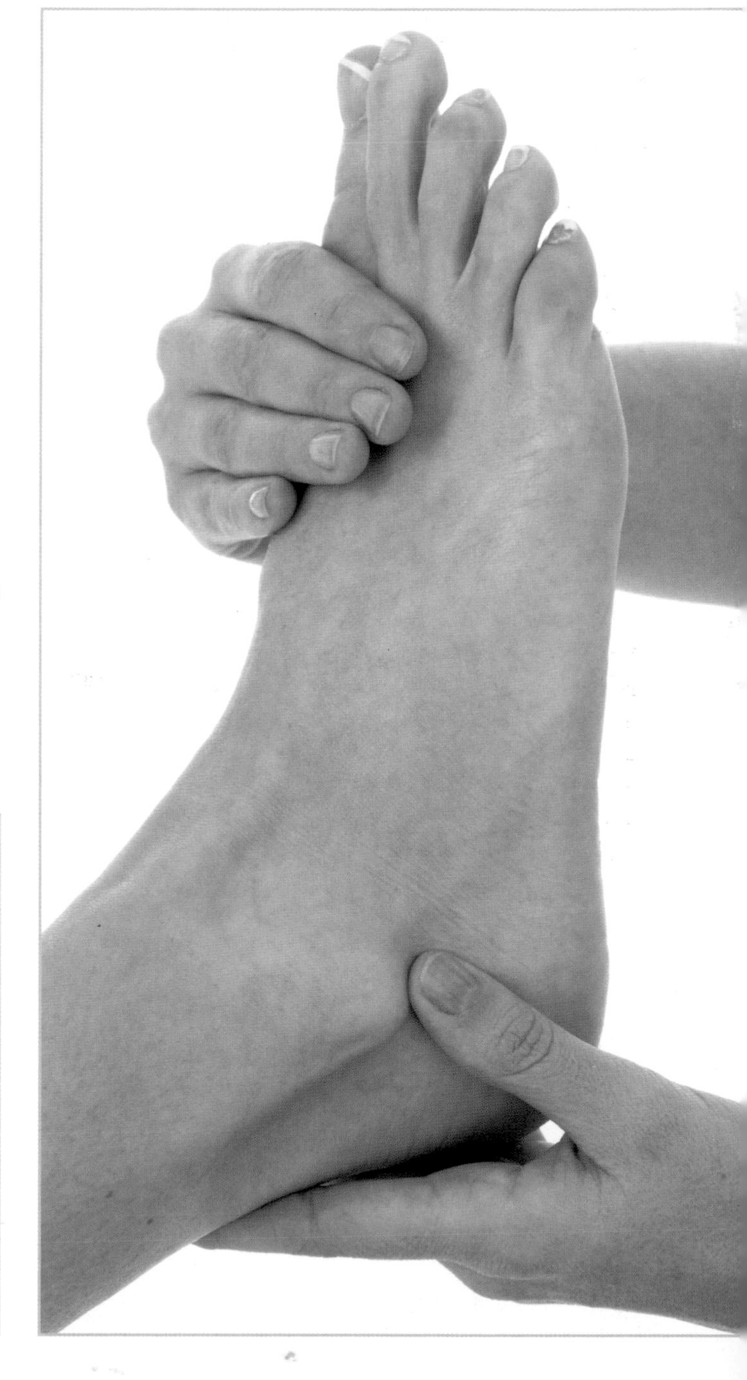

SAFETY NOTES

- Seek professional advice from a doctor or qualified reflexologist before treating someone with diabetes, thrombosis or phlebitis, or cancer patients who are undergoing conventional treatments.
- Do not treat women in the first 14 weeks of pregnancy, particularly if they have a history of miscarriage.
- Do not treat people who are in the acute stage of an infectious illness.
- Do not attempt to diagnose problems according to reflex sensitivities.

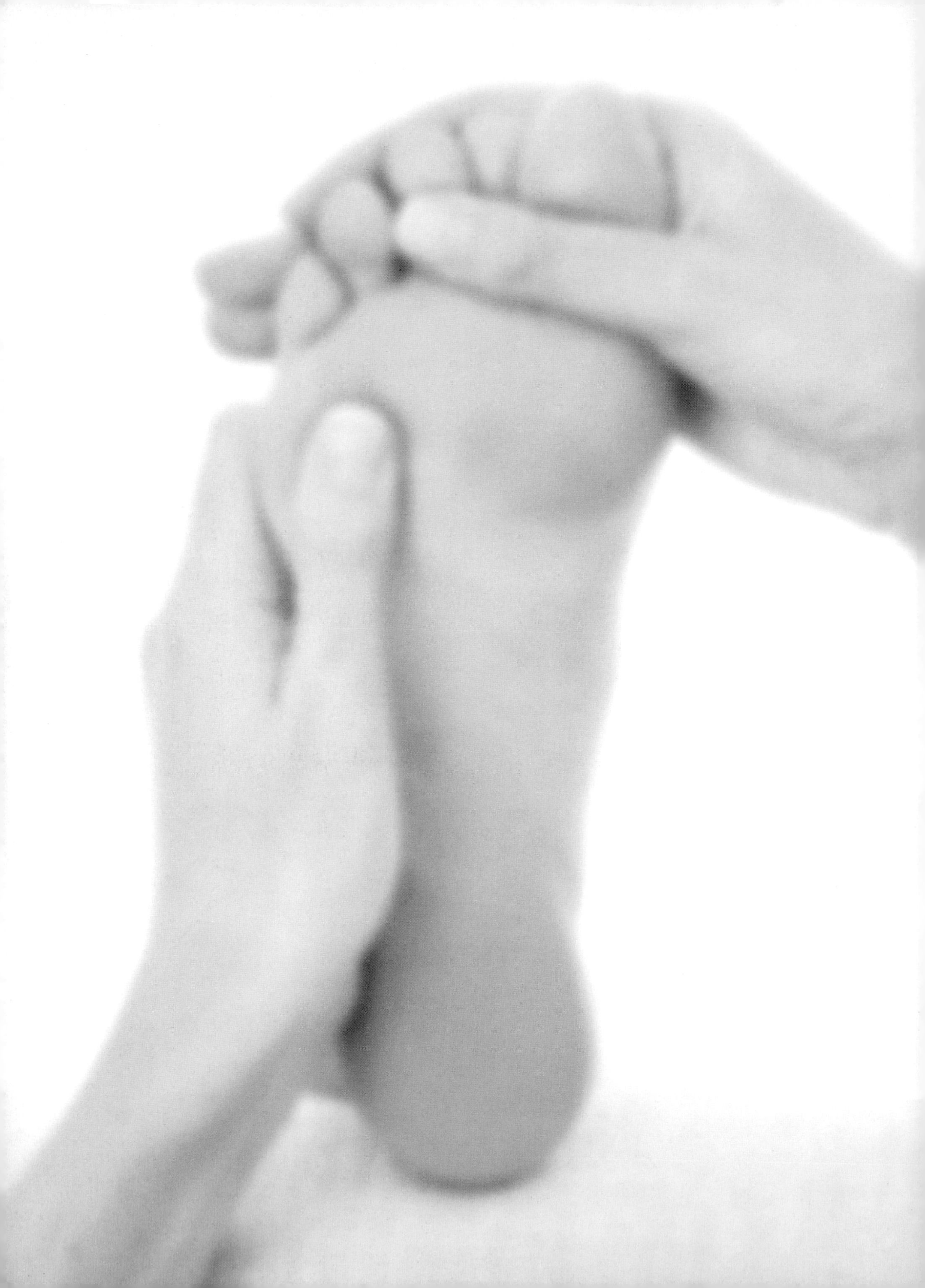

The origins of reflexology

Modern reflexology is less than 100 years old, but promoting healing through the feet and hands has been practised by many cultures for centuries, even as far back as the ancient Egyptians. Since its development during the course of the 20th century from 'zone therapy theory' in the USA, reflexology has always been holistic in nature, treating an individual as more than just a set of symptoms, and wellbeing as much more than a mere absence of illness.

A history of reflexology

There is evidence that reflexology was practised way back in time, by many different cultures throughout the world. Although we cannot actually determine the true relationship between reflexology as understood by the Egyptians 4,000 years ago and the practice as we know it today, it is established that the ancient Egyptians used many different healing skills.

Archeologists have even uncovered various surgical implements and skulls that show evidence of 'cranial surgery'. In this early technique, bore holes in the skull were often used to let out the evil spells that had penetrated an unfortunate sufferer's brain. Dr Shelby Riley, a pioneer of reflexology during the 1930s (see page 14), maintained that it was from Egypt that the practice of reflexology spread throughout the Roman Empire.

Some theorists also believe that a certain form of reflexology was passed down to the native Americans by the Incas of South America. The Cherokee people are certainly known to apply a type of pressure therapy to the feet, often using wooden probes to work on the reflex points in order to unblock energy pathways and restore balance in the body.

The Physician's Tomb

In a tomb at the huge burial ground at Saqqara, Egypt, there is a famous wall painting dating back to 2330 BCE. The tomb is often referred to as the 'Physician's Tomb', because the painting within depicts two figures giving what is clearly a form of reflexology to two patients. One practitioner is treating his patient's feet, while the other works on his patient's hands. According to the translation of the ancient hieroglyphs, a patient is saying: 'Don't hurt me', while a practitioner replies: 'I shall act so that you praise me.'

The painting shows the practitioner who is working on the feet as sitting with his back to the patient. This position would have been used to avoid the insult of one person raising his feet to the face of another. The picture also shows both patients holding one hand under the armpit. It was thought that energy was released from the body during the session, and that placing one hand under the armpit would ensure that energy would go back into the body instead of being lost. Loss of vital energy was considered to cause a weakening of the system.

THE PYRAMIDAL SYMBOL OF ENERGY

The representation of the pyramid as a channel of energy appears in many cultures. The ancient Egyptians always placed their dead within the structure of a pyramid in order of importance, with a king or queen at the top of the pyramid, other relatives further down and the slaves and lowly workers at the very base. The classic church spire of Christianity is also essentially a pyramid, its shape encouraging an atmosphere of peace, calm and spirituality. Even witches are traditionally depicted in tall pyramidal hats, the better to 'catch' energy for their craft and spells, and the shape is echoed exactly by the classroom dunce's cap, put on in an attempt to bring energy to a dull brain.

The pictograms used in the wall painting also put an emphasis on the concept of energy: the blue zig-zag line is symbolic of the great waters of the Nile and, by extension, the vital life force of the universe. The pyramid drawn above the heads of each couple is a further symbol of energy (see box).

Acupuncture

In the 4th century, a Chinese acupuncturist called Dr Ko Hung discovered that using his thumbs to apply a deep pressure to the soles of the feet while acupuncture needles were in place was a means of enhancing healing and encouraging energy to be released. Sometimes reflexology is still referred to as 'acupuncture without the use of needles'.

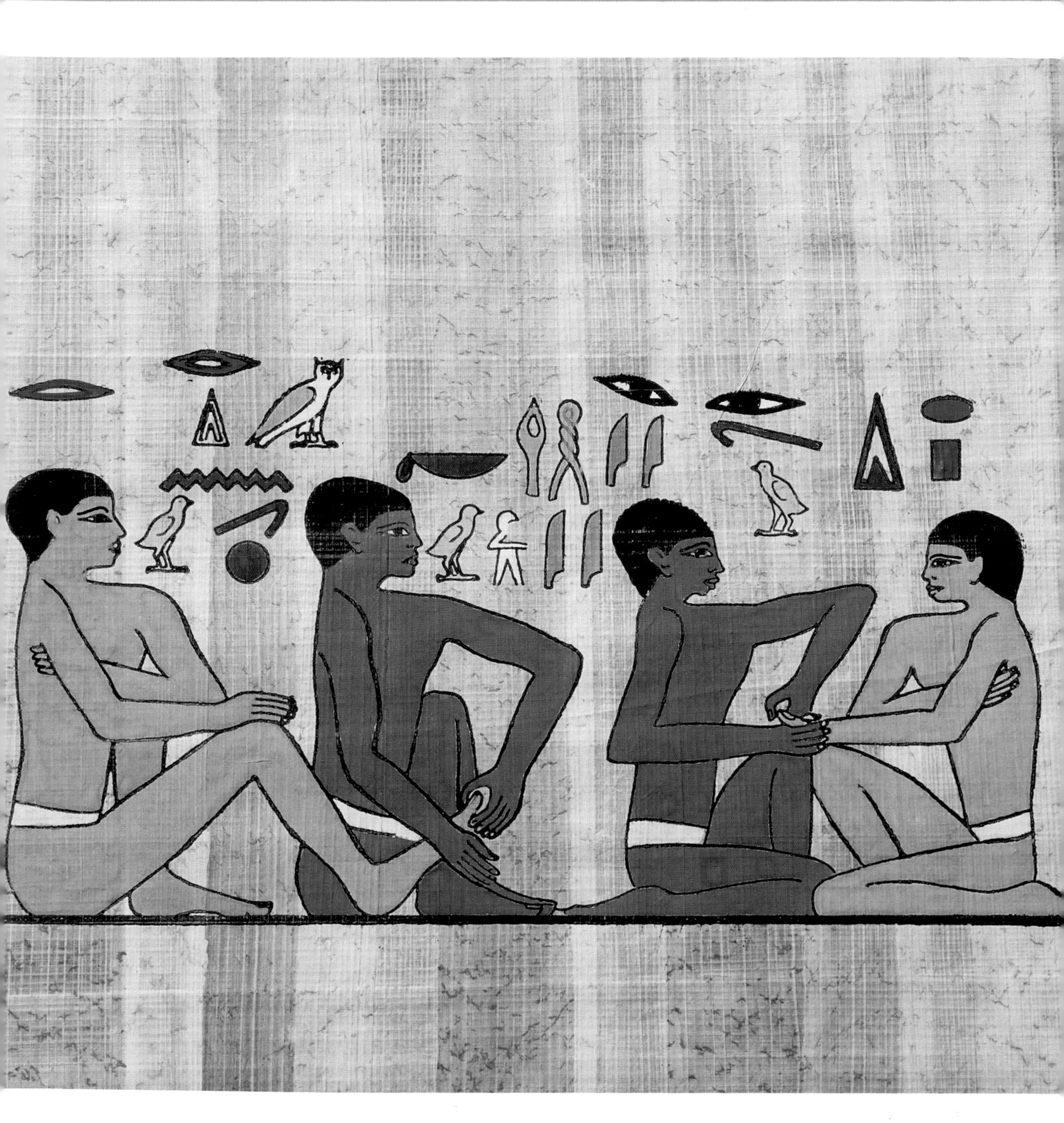

Treating feet and hands in the Physician's Tomb Images above the figures include symbols of energy and 'the white bird of peace and paradise', which is a sign of peace, prosperity and goodwill.

The birth of zone therapy

Zone therapy was the precursor to modern reflexology, which was reborn through the work of William H. Fitzgerald MD in the early 20th century. Dr Fitzgerald was an ear, nose and throat specialist at the Boston City Hospital and St Francis Hospital in Connecticut, USA. He discovered that by applying pressure to the tops of the fingers with metal clamps, and winding tight elastic bands around the middle section of each finger, he created an anaesthetic effect on the facial area. By this intervention he was able to do simple ear, nose and throat surgery without any form of anaesthesia.

Dr Fitzgerald would also encourage patients who were suffering from painful conditions to hold a comb in each hand and allow the teeth of the comb to press firmly into the palm of the hand. Practising this procedure several times a day, he found, reduced the pain experienced. Pressure was also applied to the thumbs of each hand to bring relief. Given our present level of knowledge we can see now how this might be so, since the thumb relates to areas of the brain and to the release of endorphins. Endorphins create a feeling of relaxation and freedom from tension and consequently reduce pain levels in the body. Fitzgerald also used pressure points on the tongue, the palate and the back of the pharynx in order to achieve pain relief or analgesia.

Zonal pathways

Fitzgerald called his work 'zone analgesia'. He was responsible for formulating the first chart showing the longitudinal lines of energy radiating through the body, which he called 'zonal pathways'. He wrote many articles on the subject of 'applying pressure to relieve pain' and in 1917 he and Dr Edwin Bowers jointly produced a book entitled *Relieving Pain at Home*. In the foreword they wrote: 'Humanity is awakening to the fact that sickness, in a large percentage of cases, is an error of body and mind.' How true that proved to be.

Dr Fitzgerald went on to discover that the application of pressure on the zonal pathways via the feet, hands or other parts of the body not only relieved pain but in the majority of cases also relieved the underlying cause as well. The same result is experienced through reflexology today, which is based partially on the zone therapy theory.

Dr Shelby Riley, who worked closely with Dr Fitzgerald, developed zone theory further. He added the horizontal zones running across the surfaces of the hands and feet and he also discovered that deep pressure, especially on the feet, stimulated the zonal pathways, improving nerve and blood supply, detoxifying congested areas and reducing pain.

From zone therapy to reflexology

Eunice D. Ingham was a physical therapist who worked with Dr Riley. She was fascinated by the concept of zone therapy and in the early 1930s started developing her foot reflex theory. She had the opportunity to treat hundreds of patients, carefully and thoughtfully checking and re-checking each reflex point until she was able to determine with confidence that 'the reflexes on the feet are an exact mirror image of the organs, functions, and structures of the human body'. Whereas zone therapy relied solely on the zones to identify the area to be worked, reflexology isolated specific areas within the zones that would stimulate particular parts of the body.

Dr Riley encouraged Eunice Ingham to write her first book, *Stories the Feet Can Tell*, in which she documented her cases and mapped out the reflexes on the feet as we know them today. Her book was published in 1938 and was later translated into several languages, spreading the benefits of reflexology way beyond the United States.

Eunice Ingham was called upon to talk at many health workshops and travelled around the USA giving lectures and book reviews. Many people enjoyed the benefits of reflexology, which helped to improve all manner of health conditions, from back pain to migraine headaches. The word spread rapidly and reflexology became better known among the medical fraternity as well as among lay people. Eunice Ingham's second book, *Stories the Feet Have Told*, published a few years after her first, was a compilation of her most interesting case histories.

Reflexology and the world

In the late 1950s Eunice Ingham's nephew, Dwight Byers, started helping his aunt at her workshops and in 1961 Dwight and his sister, Eusebia Messenger RN (Registered Nurse), studied reflexology under the direction of Eunice and began teaching at workshops on a full-time basis. Seven years later they became responsible for the continued teaching of reflexology under the banner of the International Institute of Reflexology. The Institute is still very active today.

Early in the 1960s the practice of reflexology spread further when Ed Johnstone, Ena Campbell and Laura Kennedy, who attended Eunice Ingham's seminars, took foot reflexology to Vancouver in Canada.

Eunice Ingham was still treating patients at the very end of her life. She passed away quietly in her sleep in 1974 at the age of 85. Her undisputable contributions to the world of reflexology are well documented, and she was convinced right to the end of her life that reflexology could aid in easing the suffering of humanity. Her beliefs can be simply explained:

- The reflexes on the feet are a mirror image of all the organs, glands and parts belonging to the body. The right foot contains all the reflexes to the organs on the right side of the body and the left foot represents the body's left side.
- When there is a problem with a body part the corresponding reflexes in the feet will reveal a sensitivity when pressure is applied. Working through these reflexes brings about changes in the body and consequently a reduction of symptoms, as well as a reduction in the sensitivity of the reflexes.
- By applying a deep alternating pressure, a stimulating effect occurs, which is distributed through the zones of the body. This is in contrast to the local anaesthetic effect demonstrated by Dr Fitzgerald when he applied constant direct pressure by the use of clamps or bands.
- Reflexology can be of great benefit in relieving all the stress-related disorders in the modern world, and can be used for all age groups.

Today, reflexology is one of the most popular forms of complementary medicine. One of its attractions is its simplicity; all that is needed are two healing hands, and the knowledge that can be obtained from this book. Reflexology is being embraced in many countries of the world for its provision of enhanced health and mental and physical relaxation coupled with its inherent simplicity and harmlessness.

Reflexology therapists in Taiwan A totally safe, simple and effective therapy, reflexology is now very popular in many countries of the world.

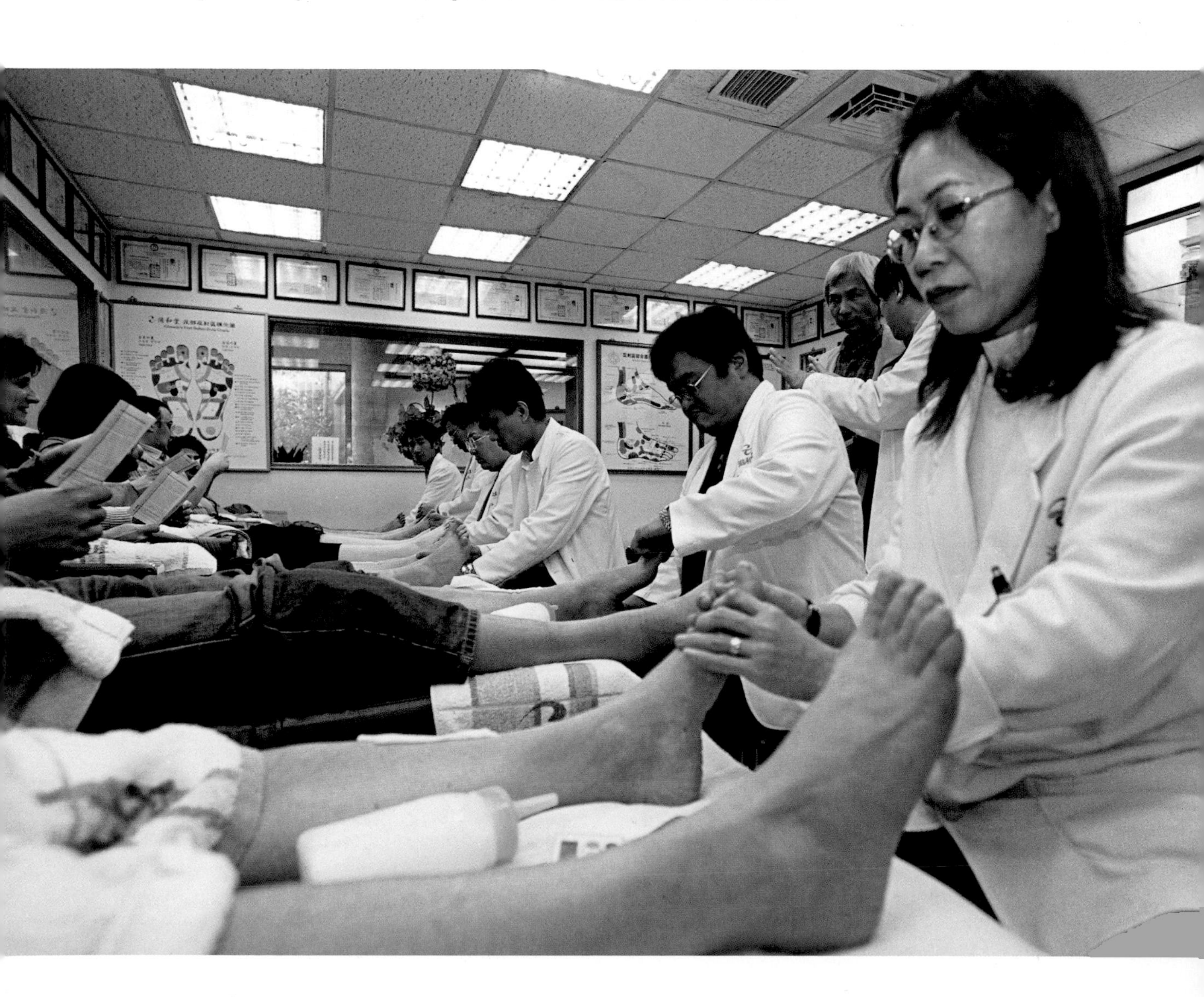

Holistic healing and universal energy

Healing is not easy to define, although most people have an innate sense of what they mean by it. For the majority of us, notions of healing are likely to be based on our own experiences of disease and illness.

In some cultures illness is believed to be caused by bad spirits, perhaps brought about by the sufferer's own wrong actions, by the wrath of a god or imposed by another malicious person. A shaman/medicine woman/witch-doctor will often heal the afflicted person by counteracting these malignant human and spiritual influences with his or her own powers. While some people may regard this as superstitious nonsense, for those living within such a culture, the experiences are real enough and are at the least evidence of the power of belief and suggestion.

In conventional Western culture, illness has been generally viewed as something purely physical, as an invasion of a 'germ' or as the malfunction of a particular body part, just as might occur in an engine. The emphasis is therefore on suppressing the symptoms and making the life of the patient more comfortable by removing offending parts and administering drugs. Each part of the body is dealt with by a different specialist; there are gastrointestinal consultants, respiratory and circulatory consultants, renal consultants and so on.

Between these two extreme views about the nature of health lie the therapies that are often called alternative or complementary, which see ill-health as an outcome of imbalances in the body, mind and spirit. For the complementary therapists, health and wellbeing require a holistic approach.

The holistic approach

Holistic healing means 'treating the whole person' – the body, the mind and the spirit. This entails looking at both the physical and emotional state of the person and their lifestyle. The body is treated as an integrated whole in the understanding that when one system is out of order, every other system is affected.

This is a very different approach from treating symptoms and parts of the body in isolation, which often results in the root cause of the problem remaining untreated. In these cases the patient never really becomes well, and often progresses to suffer yet more disorders, maybe as the result of medication taken for a long period of time. No drug is really safe and all have a negative effect on another body function; they also weaken the immune system, the body's natural defence.

Even 50 years ago most family doctors had little to offer to relieve sickness and suffering, and a bottle of cough mixture, some pain-reducing medication and a good bedside manner were their main tools. Most people with minor illnesses eventually got better even if it did take a little longer than the rapid effect of medications such as the antibiotics that are available today.

Many honest doctors will tell you that their patients would probably recover from most complaints in seven days if they did nothing. Our bodies have remarkable abilities to heal themselves. In fact the body likes to be well and does everything possible to reduce inflammation, rid itself of disease and restore balance. Included in the healing process is the effect of thought patterns, which affect physical illness, as well as psychological factors that may be contributing to the expression or exacerbation of disease.

There is a huge difference between being just free of symptoms and achieving maximum health. True good health means functioning at an optimal level in body, mind and spirit. The well individual is one who is happy, healthy and whole, and who perceives his or her life as one with meaning and purpose.

Energy fields

Everything that is alive pulsates with energy, and all this energy contains information. While it is not surprising that practitioners of complementary medicine accept this concept quite readily, those outside the field may find it harder to come to terms with. Nevertheless, it is worth

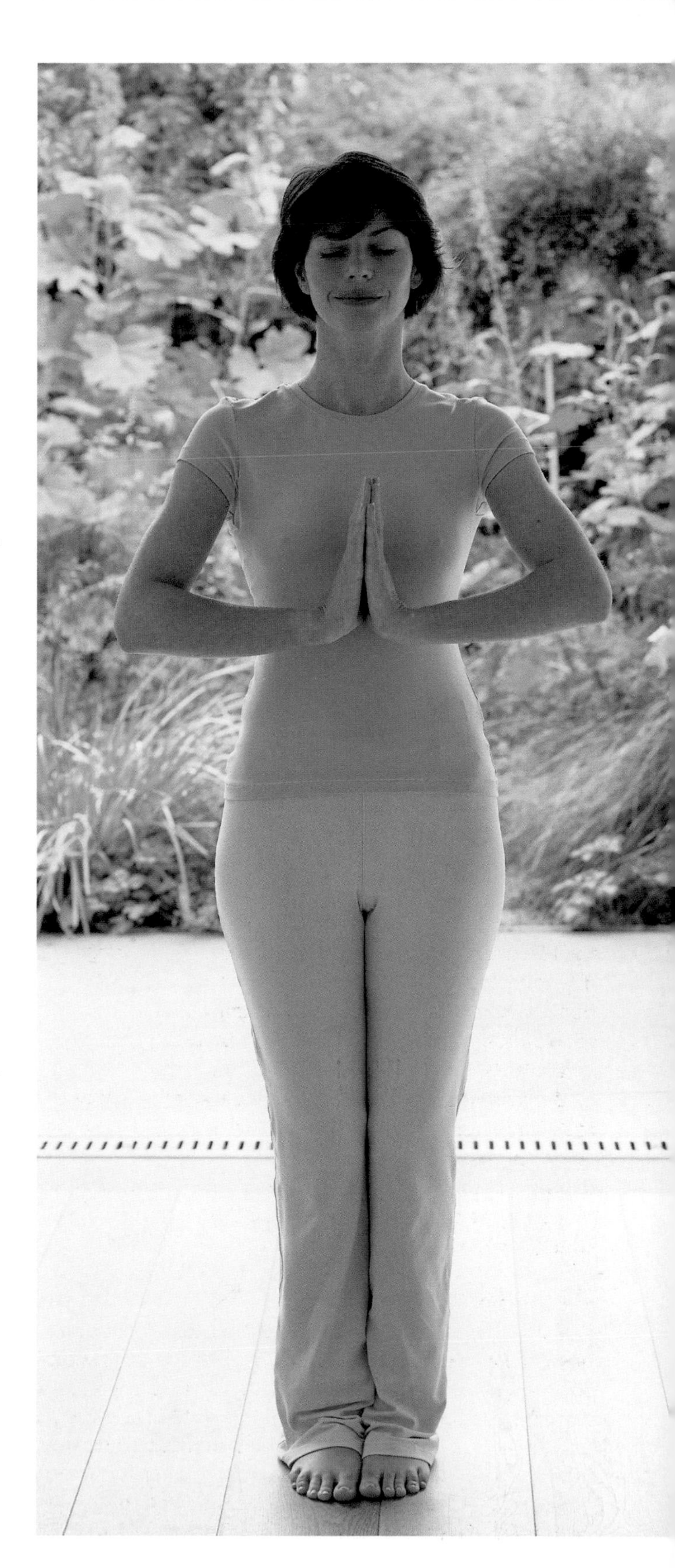

noting that some physicists acknowledge the existence of an electromagnetic field generated by the biological process of the body. Some spiritual teachings also refer to the 'etheric body', which is the term for the emotional or spiritual body that is represented by a balance in the 'energy fields'.

The human body is surrounded by an energy field extending as far as our outstretched arms and along the full length of our body. This energy field acts not only as a communication centre but also as a highly sensitive perceptual system. We are constantly receiving and sending information with every life experience that takes place. The mind is therefore not only in close communication with the body, it is actually present within every cell of the body. Consequently, what we think and believe has a dramatic effect on our wellbeing. In other words, the body and mind act as one. We are aware of our heart beating frantically when we are frightened, we know that it is possible to faint at the sight of a unpleasant situation, so it cannot be too difficult to understand how mental abstractions such as loneliness or sadness can also have a real and disturbing effect on the body.

When depression, fear, anxiety, emotional pain, anger or jealousy form a major part of our emotions, they adversely affect our immune system, which becomes weakened and then disease finds it easy to take hold. The holistic practitioner recognizes that negative emotions are stored as 'negative energy', which causes the body to become out of balance, leading to a state of chronic disease. Complementary treatments, reflexology in particular, restore this imbalance and encourage the healing power of the body.

A holistic approach to health Relaxation techniques such as meditation and yoga help restore wellbeing to the mind and spirit as well as the body.

Kirlian photography

In 1939, Russian inventor Semyon Kirlian discovered by accident that if an object is placed on a photographic plate and the plate is subjected to a high-voltage electrical field, an image is created on the plate. The image looks like a coloured halo or coronal discharge.

Some experimenters think Kirlian photographs reveal a physical form of psychic energy and that this method is a gateway to the paranormal. Another theory is that it reveals the etheric body, one of the layers of the aura thought to permeate all animate objects, or the 'life force' that allegedly surrounds each living thing. This gives rise to the prospect of gaining significant beneficial insights into medicine, psychology, psychic healing and dowsing.

In fact, the Kirlian photographs record the results of quite natural phenomena, such as pressure, electrical grounding, humidity and temperature. Living things are moist. When the electrical charge enters the object on the photographic plate, it produces an area of gas ionization around the object if moisture is present. This moisture is transferred from the subject to the emulsion surface of the photographic film and causes an alteration of the electrical charge pattern on the film. Changes in moisture (which may reflect changes in barometric pressure and emotions, among other things) produce different 'auras'.

Although there seems to be no evidence that Kirlian photographs record a paranormal phenomenon, there is evidence that they change according to the health and emotional state in living things, showing variations in the brightness, colour and patterns of light. At the University of California Center for Health Sciences researchers showed that the aura of a leaf appeared to change when approached by a human hand and picked. Even when part of the leaf was cut off, the flowing portion of the amputated portion still appeared on the film.

Other researchers have found that changes in a person's emotional state can be detected by variations in the brightness, colour and formation patterns visible the photographs. Kirlian photographs of psychic healers and the psychokinetic metal-bender Uri Geller show flares of light streaming from their fingers as they use their powers.

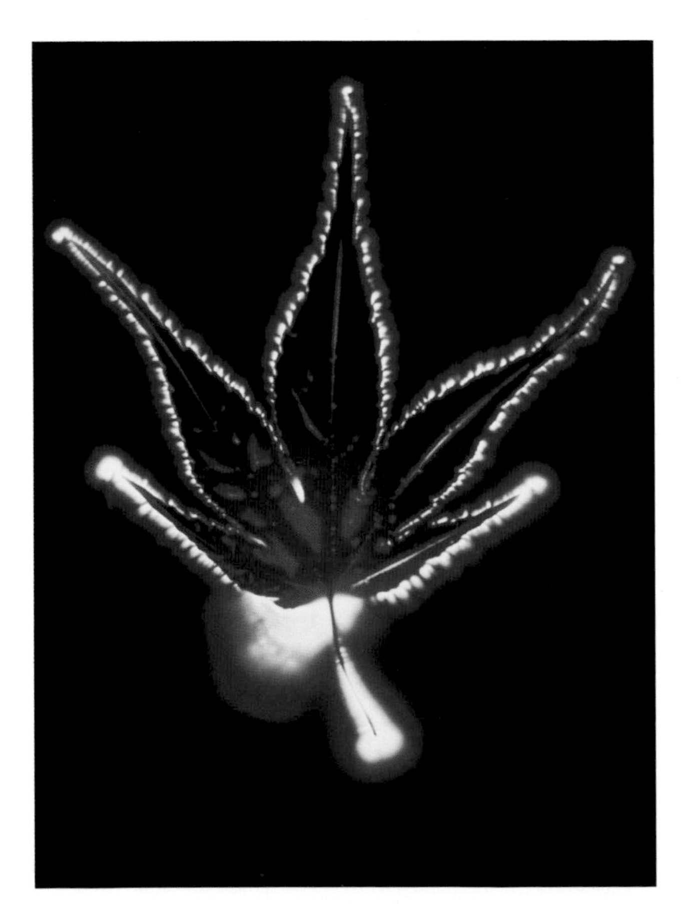

Kirlian photograph of a maple leaf Living things captured in Kirlian photography have been found to vary in brightness and colour according to their state of health.

Chakras

Some religions teach that the human body contains seven energy centres, known as chakras, each of which contains a universal spiritual energy. The chakras keep the body in a balanced state, emotionally and physically. They are vertically aligned from the base of the spine to the crown of the head. The seventh chakra, which relates to the top of the head, draws in our spiritual and creative nature from the universe.

When we hear of a young child who from the age of three is drawn to learn to play the piano and by the age of eight or nine is playing concertos, it is clear that this child has been 'chosen' to receive from the universe a very special creative musical ability and draws in this power to his or her seventh chakra. The same creative energy is given to great artists, musicians, writers and inventors. We say that these people are 'gifted' and indeed they are, because they receive these gifts from the universal energy. Every thought anybody ever had came through the seventh chakra.

Where there is an imbalance in any chakra, diseases can then manifest in the body, as their protective shield or support has been broken. A couple of specific examples may help to clarify this. A person with a long repressed anger over childhood experiences is thought

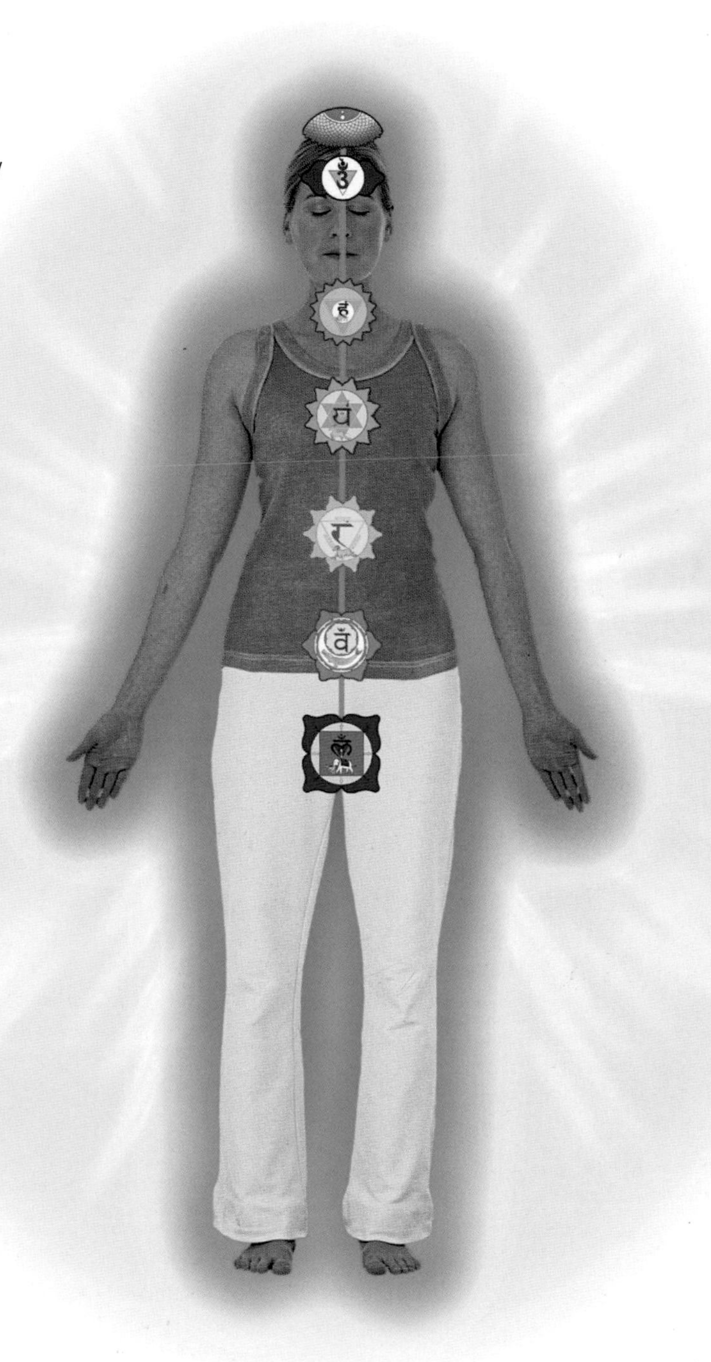

Chakras and the energy field
The seven chakras are whirling vortices of subtle energies. They exist within the subtle body, but each major chakra is anatomically associated with a major nerve plexus and endocrine gland.

to store this anger in that area of the etheric body that controls the functioning of the stomach and duodenum. If harboured in the long term, the effect will be to produce ulcers. If anger is released, it is thought, the ulcer will heal itself. Similarly sadness, especially over someone much loved, can be stored in that part of the etheric body that manages the heart. And we have all heard of the expression 'dying from a broken heart'.

Complementary medicines, in particular reflexology, heal the body's protective shield by restoring its balanced state. As the seventh chakra is directly linked with the central nervous system and endocrine system, it is easy to understand how reflexology, by working through the spinal and nervous system pathways of the body, can stimulate the powerful force of the healing energy to become activated.

Who does reflexology help?

Just about everyone, from tiny babies to the very elderly, can benefit from reflexology. It is important to understand that reflexology is not just for helping sick people become well; it is all about maintaining health and keeping the body in the best possible condition.

Reflexology aids in detoxifying the body and therefore supports the protection of the immune system; indeed if people used reflexology when minor symptoms presented themselves then many serious conditions would never develop.

The feet are contact areas to the entire body and can bring about great changes in relieving pain, improving nerve and blood supply and restoring the body's equilibrium. The greatest results are in alleviating the general, uncomfortable but often minor problems that doctors and clinics spend so much time treating.

Children and teenagers

Young children with colic, digestive upsets or ear, nose and throat infections respond well. (As is described on page 76, many respiratory tract infections have their origins in digestive problems. The respiratory system and the digestive system fall in exactly the same body zones, and by improving and strengthening the function of the digestive system, reflexology can get to the root cause of the problem.) Treatment is extremely effective, although of course very young children find it hard to sit still long enough to be treated!

During puberty, when menstrual and skin disorders may become a problem, regular reflexology treatments can bring relief from period pains, regulate the menstrual cycle and help balance the hormonal overload that plays havoc with hair and skin. It is also highly recommended for bringing mental relaxation during the stress of examination time.

Back pain

Back pain causes more people to take time off work than any other medical condition, and unfortunately conventional medical treatments for it are very limited, other than painkillers and anti-inflammatory drugs. Usually, sufferers will be advised by their physician simply to rest. Physiotherapy is sometimes recommended and, on rare occasions, spinal surgery, although that is not advisable unless all other forms of complementary medicine have been tried. Reflexology practitioners treat more skeletal conditions than any other, including lumbar and cervical pain, whiplash injuries, sciatica, frozen shoulders, arthritic conditions of the spine, hips and knees and sports injuries. The results achieved through reflexology are quite amazing.

Women's health

During pregnancy and childbirth, a reflexologist can relieve morning sickness and, if the weight of the baby she is carrying causes back pain, reflexology can again come to the rescue. Many mothers-to-be also involve their reflexology practitioner during their labour.

In later life, reflexology can help women with uncomfortable symptoms associated with the menopause, such as hot flushes, depression, mood swings and menopausal migraine.

Later life

As they get older, both men and women can be troubled by high blood pressure, angina and heart conditions, as well as all forms of rheumatic aches and pains. Many elderly people have regular reflexology treatments not just to treat specific medical conditions but to maintain their health and vitality for as long as possible.

If surgery becomes necessary, particularly hip or knee replacement, reflexology can assist the body to heal itself as rapidly as possible. Any surgical intervention creates a shock reaction in the body, and anaesthetics lower the protection of the immune system, so regular reflexology treatments post-operatively can be of great benefit.

Children and reflexology Most children enjoy having reflexology, particularly if they can become involved in applying the powder or cream to their own feet!

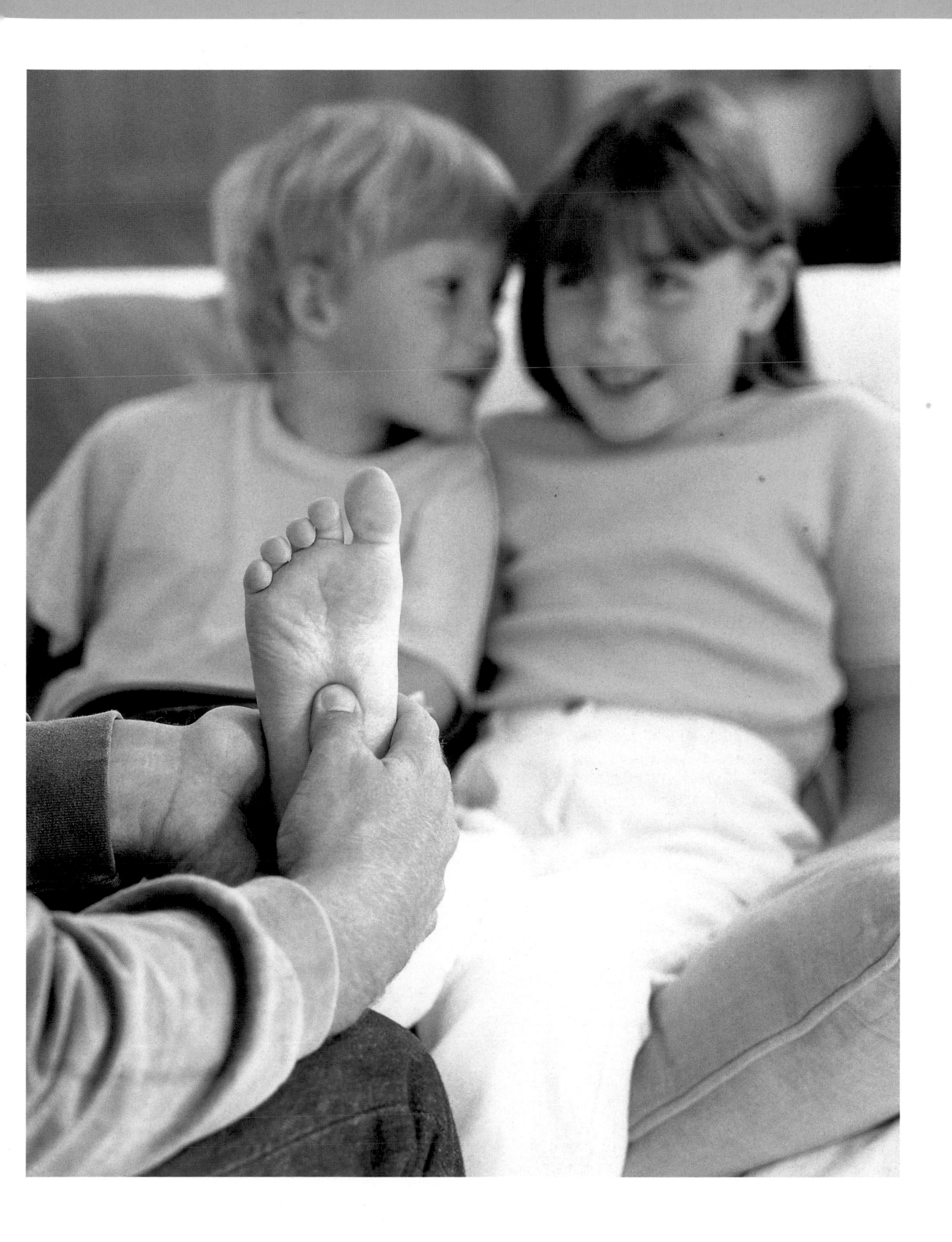

Clinical evidence

Although only a few clinical trials have been carried out to gauge the benefits of reflexology, those that have been published have proved most encouraging. I have also received many accounts over the years from reflexology practitioners about the results they have seen in their particular areas of specialization. Some of these are described below.

Control of blood pressure and reducing pain levels in the elderly

A study of 48 individuals indicated that older adults experienced significant improvements in their mental and physical wellbeing, including reduction in blood pressure and pain levels. Elderly participants experienced considerable improvements in their ability to perform their usual activities of daily living and an increased psychosocial wellbeing. Their resting diastolic blood pressure reduced.

Cancer (pain and nausea)

Reflexology has been shown to modify the distressing symptoms of pain and nausea in patients hospitalized with cancer. In one study, 87 participating patients each received a 10-minute reflexology foot treatment. The results of the study revealed that the treatments produced a significant and immediate effect on the patients' perception of pain and nausea and promoted relaxation. The results were so positive that the researchers recommended that further research be undertaken, using larger numbers of patients in controlled clinical trials into the effectiveness of reflexology in alleviating pain, nausea and anxiety and the management of these symptoms by the family at home.

Cancer (quality of life)

A study that was carried out on patients in the palliative stage of cancer (H. Hodgson, 'Does reflexology impact on cancer patients' quality of life?', *Nursing Standard* 2000; 14: 33–38) indicates the many ways in which reflexology can help cancer patients. The results found that all the participants who received reflexology benefited in terms of improvement in quality of life, appearance, appetite, breathing, communication, concentration, constipation, diarrhoea, fear of the future, isolation, urination, mobility, mood, nausea, pain, sleep and tiredness.

Participants in the reflexology group reported an improvement in all components of the quality of life scale compared with 67.5 per cent in the placebo group. This study suggests that the provision of reflexology for patients in palliative care could be beneficial. Not only did the patients in this study enjoy the intervention, but they were also 'relaxed', 'comforted' and achieved relief from some of their symptoms.

Dyspepsia

In a clinical analysis of the use of foot reflexology in the treatment of dyspepsia (reported at the Beijing International Reflexology Conference by Gong Zhi-wen and Xin Wei-song of the China Preventive Medical Association and the Chinese Society of Reflexology, Beijing, 1996), two groups of patients with upper abdominal discomfort, bloating, belching, nausea and acid reflux (heartburn) with peptic ulcer were studied. One group of 132 individuals received foot reflexology for 30 minutes once or twice a day for two weeks and the other group of 98 received drug therapy for two weeks. The foot reflexology was found to be very effective in 74.2 per cent of patients, effective in 22.7 per cent and failed in 0.3 per cent. The drug therapy group was found to be very effective in 60.4 per cent, effective in 14.5 per cent and failed in 25 per cent.

General fatigue

In a study of the effects of reflexology treatment on general fatigue, 12 athletes were divided into two groups: a foot reflexology group and a control group. The test group received daily reflexology sessions. Both groups underwent the same athletic training and were observed for sleeping, appetite and reactions to training. The group that had received reflexology showed better qualities of sleep, better appetite and quicker recovery from fatigue and muscle soreness.

Headaches

Headaches are one of the most common health problems experienced by adults and it has been estimated that they are responsible for the loss of three million working days in the UK every year. Reflexology is renowned for its ability to help relax and calm patients and for this reason it was considered an interesting therapy to study for the treatment of tension headaches and migraine.

A nationwide research study undertaken in Denmark has shown reflexology treatment to have a beneficial effect on patients who are suffering from migraine and tension headaches. The study was conducted by the Royal Danish School of Pharmacy's Department of Social Pharmacy in cooperation with five reflexology associations, and assessed results from 78 fully trained reflexologists across the country.

Of the 220 patients who took part in the Danish study, 90 per cent said that they had taken prescribed medication for their headaches within the previous month. Of the group who had taken medication, 36 per cent had experienced side-effects. The medicines were predominantly in the paracetamol and acetylsalicylic acid group (81 per cent) and were taken at least twice a week; 72 per cent of the stronger migraine medicines were taken at least once a fortnight, which indicates that the majority of the patients were suffering from moderate to severe symptoms.

Three months after a completed series of reflexology treatments, 81 per cent of patients reported that reflexology had either cured (16 per cent) or helped (65 per cent) their symptoms.

Finding the root cause Persistent headaches, for example, may be caused by digestive problems, an inflammatory condition in the neck or tension around the eye muscles.

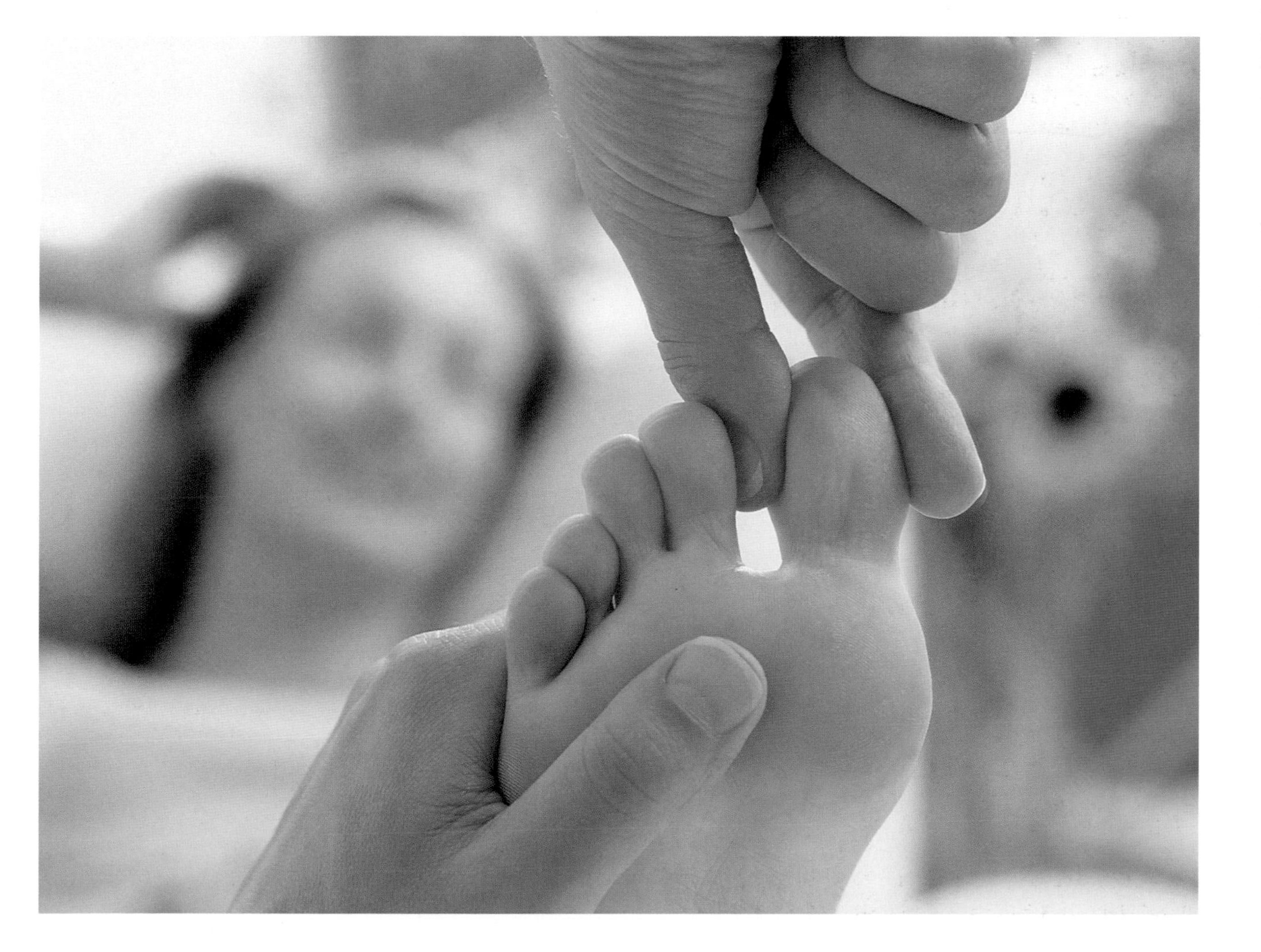

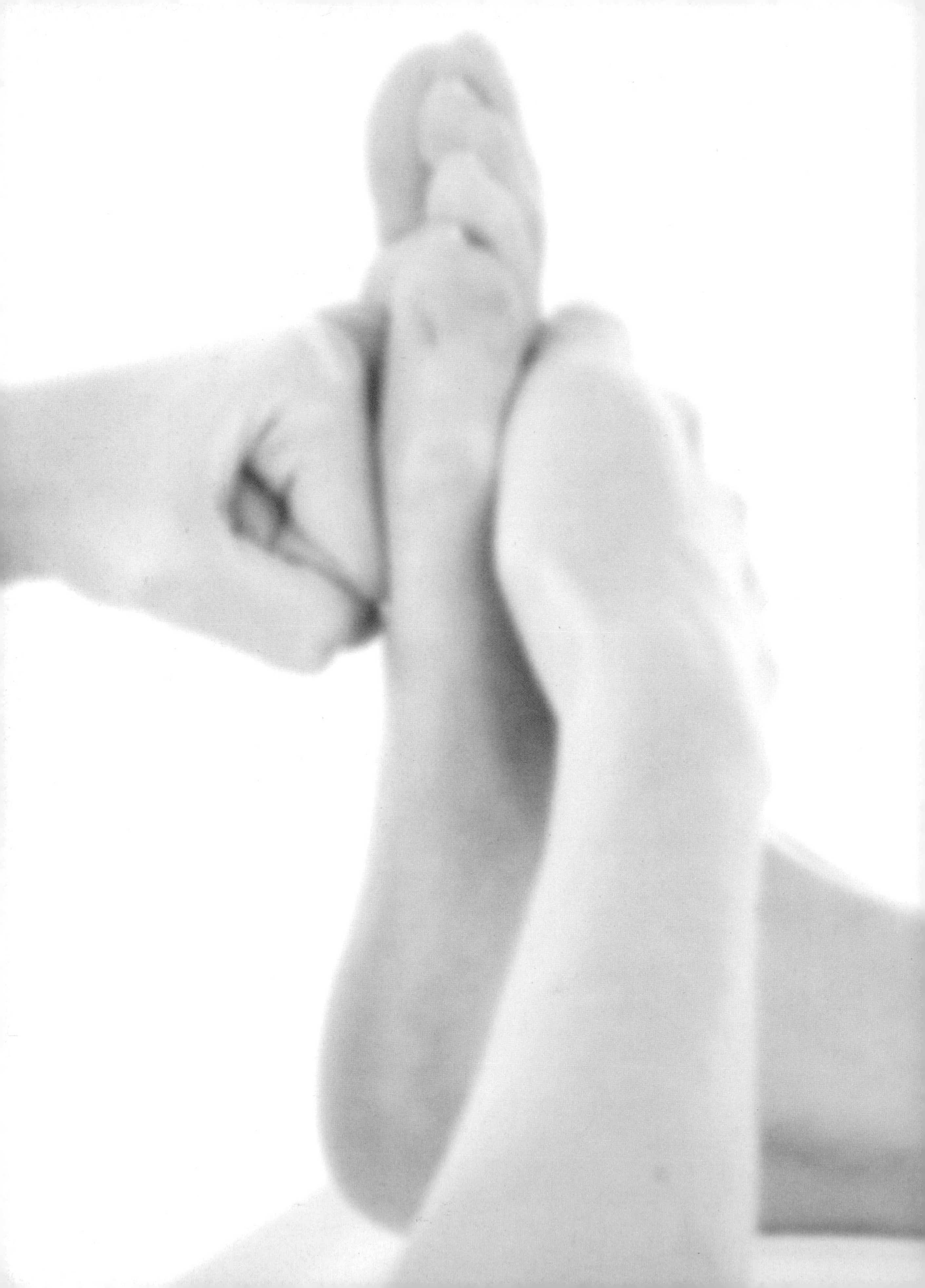

How does reflexology work?

Each part and function of the body is represented by a corresponding reflex point on the body's extremities, most particularly the feet, which contain clusters of ultra-sensitive nerve endings. By stimulating these points, a trained reflexologist can release tensions, clear blockages and help the body to heal many malfunctions. Understanding how the feet are a 'map' of the entire body is key to learning reflexology skills.

How the feet mirror the body

Each part of the body and every bodily function has its own relative reflex point in the foot. This allows an accurate picture of a patient's health to be given by the feet. If an area of the body is suffering from inflammation, tension or congestion, the corresponding reflex points in the feet will be sensitive when pressure is applied.

The feet are miraculous masterpieces of design, exquisitely put together and perfectly coordinating many components. Among the different components of the feet are tissue, 26 bones, 100 ligaments, 20 muscles and an intricate network of nerves and blood vessels.

These marvellous structures reflect comprehensively our state of health. The condition of our feet can give us much information about our physical and mental health. Likewise, how we treat our feet influences not only the performance of the feet themselves but the functioning of our whole body and mind. It's a two-way street – a reciprocal relationship.

Nerve stimulation

By working on the reflex points of the feet, a reflexologist can stimulate, through the nerve pathways, any organ, function or body part that is tense, congested or damaged as a result of accident, injury or illness. Breaking down the tension helps the system to eliminate toxins when necessary, reduces pain quite dramatically and encourages the body to heal itself. Reflexology can also reveal past injuries, as any remaining scar tissue will cause sensitivity in the reflexes.

The principal goal of a reflexologist is to discover and work out the sensitive spots in the feet by an alternating pressure of the thumb and sometimes other fingers on all parts of the foot. The pressure applied to a nerve ending constitutes a stimulus. This is any agent or factor that evokes a functional reaction in tissues, even inducing a physiological change. In reflexology, the stimulus of contact and pressure initiates an electrochemical impulse that changes the nervous processes, transmitting a message through the nerve fibres. Nerve impulses can travel at the rate of about 435 km (270 miles) per hour, while electricity travels at the speed of light. You could say that our bodies are basically electrochemical plants that are in motion throughout the day and night.

Refinement of the pressure and consistent control is of great importance in achieving a result. People treated by inexperienced or unqualified practitioners often complain that it had no effect whatsoever. They are amazed when subsequent treatment by a properly qualified practitioner produces outstanding and rapid improvement.

Reflex points are also found in other body extremities, for example in the hands and ears. However, the feet's sensitivity (they contain over 7,000 nerve endings) and their size make them the ideal area for the reflexologist to work on.

Obstructions in the energy lines

Reflexology teaches that every organ and gland depends for its survival on the ability to contract and relax. When an obstacle is placed in an energy channel, for example when acid crystals, waste products or unused calcium deposits form on the delicate nerve endings of the feet, the energy flow is impeded and the organ it serves is then adversely affected.

Obstructions in the energy lines and fields cause pain to be registered and, in certain conditions, create limitations in motion and functions; for example, a stiff neck or a painful back. Energy blockage also interferes with blood circulation and this is usually first noticed in the extremities. Hands may become stiff, cold and often painful. Waste products accumulate at the lowest point of gravity, and the reflexologist can feel them clearly when working on the feet.

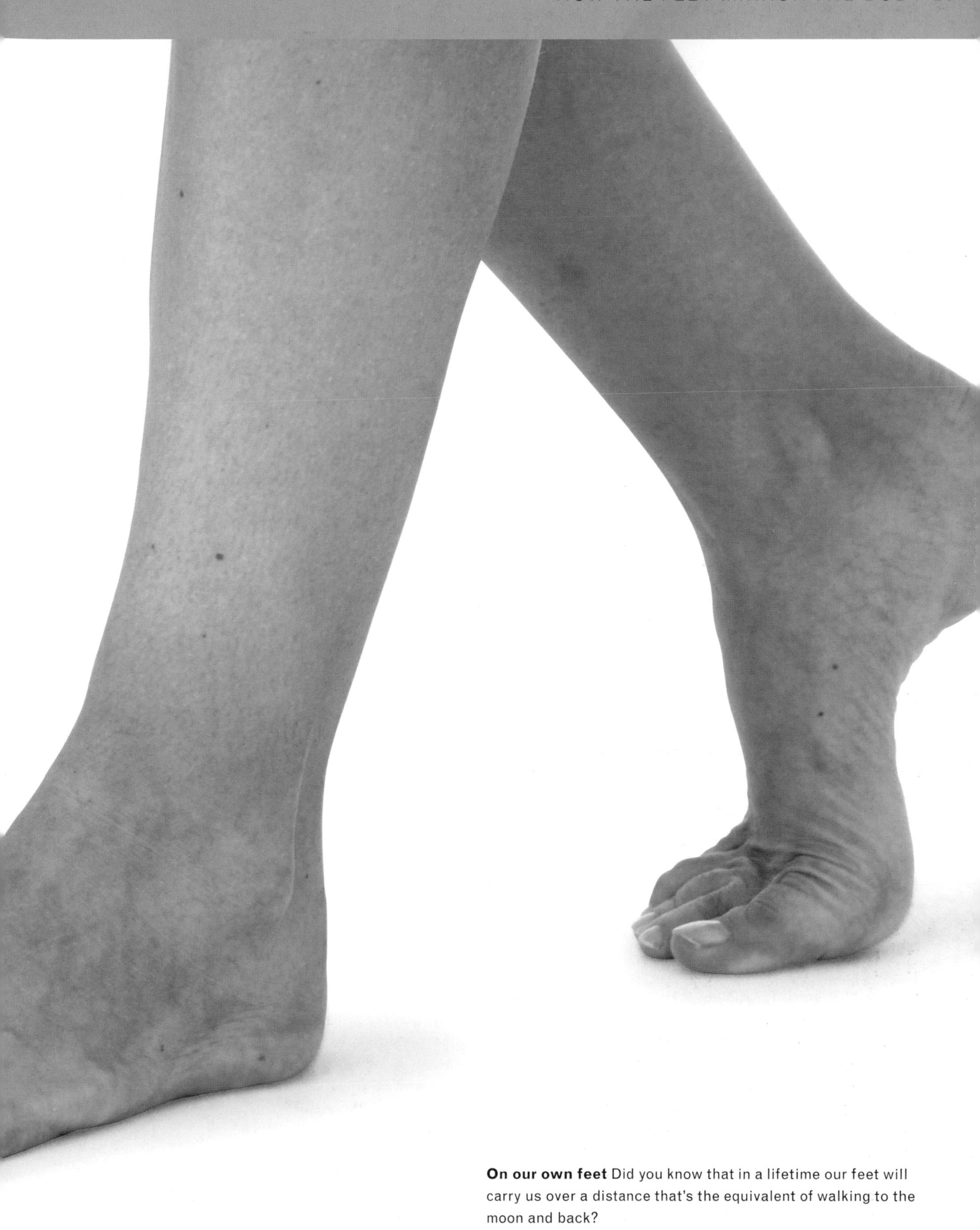

On our own feet Did you know that in a lifetime our feet will carry us over a distance that's the equivalent of walking to the moon and back?

Zones of the feet

Reflexology is based on the theory of zone therapy, which states that there are longitudinal lines of energy, called zones, ascending from the feet to the brain. As we apply pressure to the feet, we stimulate these lines, producing a rejuvenating and healing effect on the entire human body.

There are ten zones in all, five on each foot, and they are represented by a simple numbering system, with each zone beginning at the toes:

- **Zone 1**: big toe
- **Zone 2**: second toe
- **Zone 3**: third toe
- **Zone 4**: fourth toe
- **Zone 5**: fifth toe.

The fingers link up to the zones in the same way, with the thumb being Zone 1 and the little finger Zone 5.

The zones run up the body from the toes to the brain, with the body being divided into five zones on either side of the spine. A sensitivity in any one spot of the foot creates an imbalance throughout the entire length of that zone. For example, a sensitivity in the right kidney could be the cause of an eye condition, because the kidney and eye are in the same zone.

As we work on the feet from one side to the other, we are systematically working through the whole of the human body.

The primary zone

Although all the zones encompass parts of the body that can cause us problems, by far the most powerful zone is Zone 1. When working on people's feet, you will find that this zone is always the most sensitive. This is because Zone 1 includes so many vital organs and parts. Here, for instance, we have:

- The crucial central nervous system, spine and brain, and also the tiny pituitary gland and hypothalamus. Although only the size of a pea, the pituitary is often referred to as 'the conductor of the orchestra' because it regulates all glandular activity and so has an enormous effect on almost every bodily function.
- The nose and mouth: without these important apertures we would unable to breathe or eat.
- The start of the solar plexus. This nerve complex lies just behind the stomach and is responsible for many moods and sensitivities; in fact, it is an emotional barometer.
- The reproductive organs, essential for procreation.
- The navel. This represents the important link between the placenta and the fetus prior to birth. The umbilical cord that connects the mother and child delivers life-giving sustenance to the fetus at the same time as it removes damaging impurities.

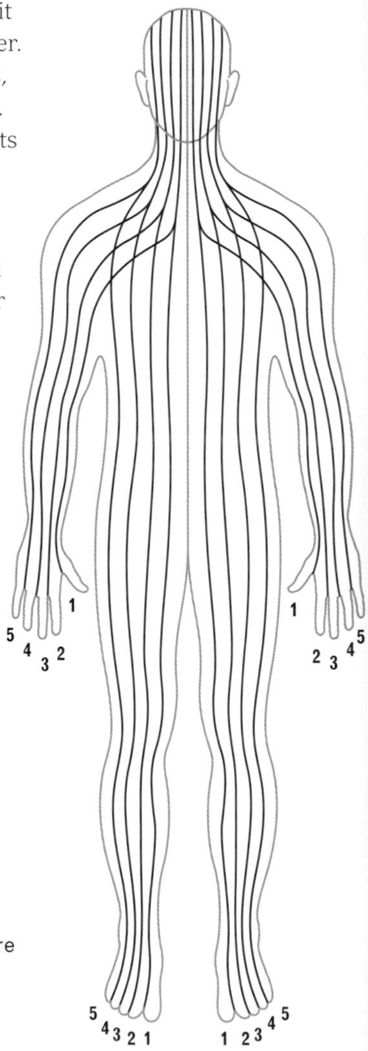

The five zones These longitudinal lines of energy are similar to the meridian lines found in acupuncture.

Guidelines of the feet

In addition to an understanding of zones, the reflexologist also needs to know about the principle of the guidelines of the feet and how they relate to all parts of the body. Like the zones, the guidelines are fundamental to the understanding and practice of reflexology.

The guidelines are quite easily identified by certain outstanding features of the feet. There are five guidelines in all, relating to the diaphragm, waist, pelvis, ligament and shoulder.

The diaphragm line

The diaphragm line is found under the bases of the metatarsals. A distinguishing feature of this guideline is that the colour of the skin on the metatarsal area is remarkably different from the skin of the underside of the instep. The darker skin is above the diaphragm line and the lighter skin below, so it is almost as if nature had provided an identifying line to help us.

The waist line

The waist line is found by running your finger along the outside of the foot until you feel a small bony protrusion about midway. A line drawn across the foot from this point denotes the waist line; it is normally in the narrowest part of the foot.

The pelvic line

The pelvic line (sometimes called the heel line) is found by drawing an imaginary line from the ankle bones on either side of the foot and crossing over the base of the heel.

The ligament line

The ligament line is the ascending line that runs along the plantar ligament, that taut elastic-like structure that you can feel if you retract your big toe.

The shoulder line

The shoulder line is found just below the bases of the toes and we refer to this as a secondary line.

The five guidelines These divisions enable you to find reflexes more easily. In a larger foot, they are relatively spaced out; in a smaller foot, they appear more condensed.

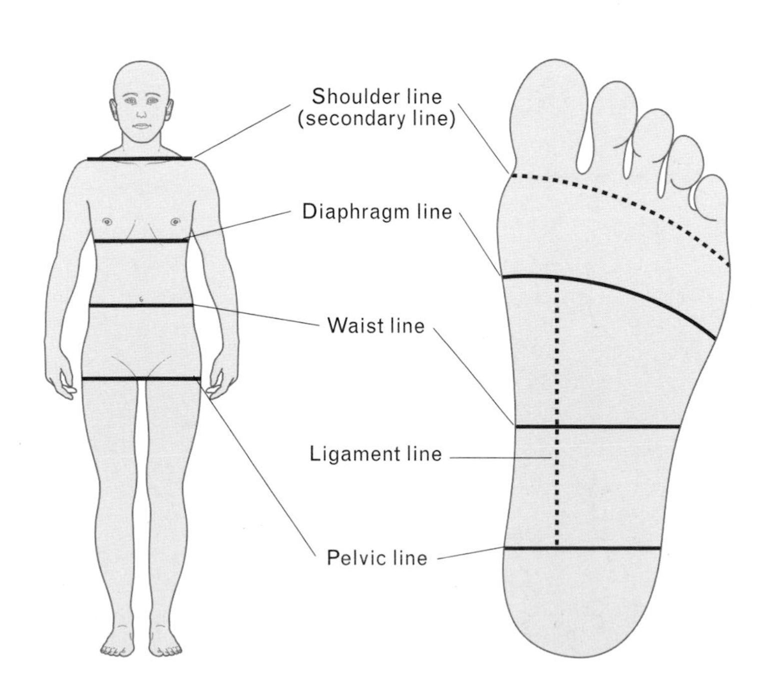

Anatomy of a foot

The arrangement of the bones in the foot allows us to stand steadily and to walk and run while still keeping our balance. To allow our feet their extreme flexibility, there is a complicated structure of ligaments, tendons and muscles supporting and interacting with these bones.

Bones of the foot

The bones of the feet consist of seven tarsals (ankle bones), five metatarsals, which run the length of your foot and 14 phalanges, two in the big toe and three in each of the smaller toes.

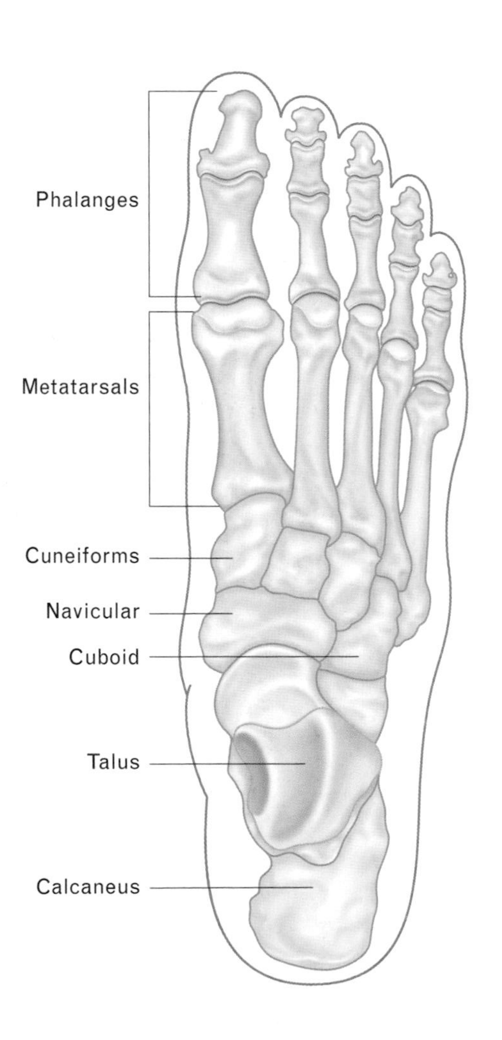

Arches of the foot

The bones of the foot are arranged in flexible arches, supported by ligaments and muscles. These structures support the weight of the body, enable the feet to be flexible and provide leverage while walking. There are three arches in the foot:

- **Medial longitudinal arch**: found on the inner border of the foot
- **Lateral longitudinal arch**: found on the outer border of the foot
- **Transverse arch**: runs from side to side.

Veins and nerves in the foot

The principal veins in the foot are superficial (lying just under the skin). They are known as the saphenous veins. The lesser saphenous vein runs along the lateral side of the foot (outer edge) and behind the ankle joint, then ascends the leg to join the deep popliteal vein around the back of the knee. The greater saphenous vein, which is the longest in the body, begins in the vicinity of the big toe, runs along the medial side of the foot (inner edge) and then rises up the calf, past the knee to the thigh and connects to the femoral vein in the groin.

The tibial nerve serves the muscles and skin of the sole of the foot, and also the nerves of the toes. It descends the lower leg from the knee, where it is linked to the sciatic nerve, which runs the length of the thigh from the buttock. The sciatic nerve is the thickest nerve in the human body, about the thickness of a little finger, whereas most nerves are as thin as a hair.

Bones of the foot We have more bones in our feet than in any other part of the body. It is this complex arrangement of bones that allows us to stand, pivot, dance and run.

Arches of the foot The longitudinal arch runs from the front to the back of the foot and has two parts: the medial and lateral longitudinal arches. The medial arch is the higher arch of the two.

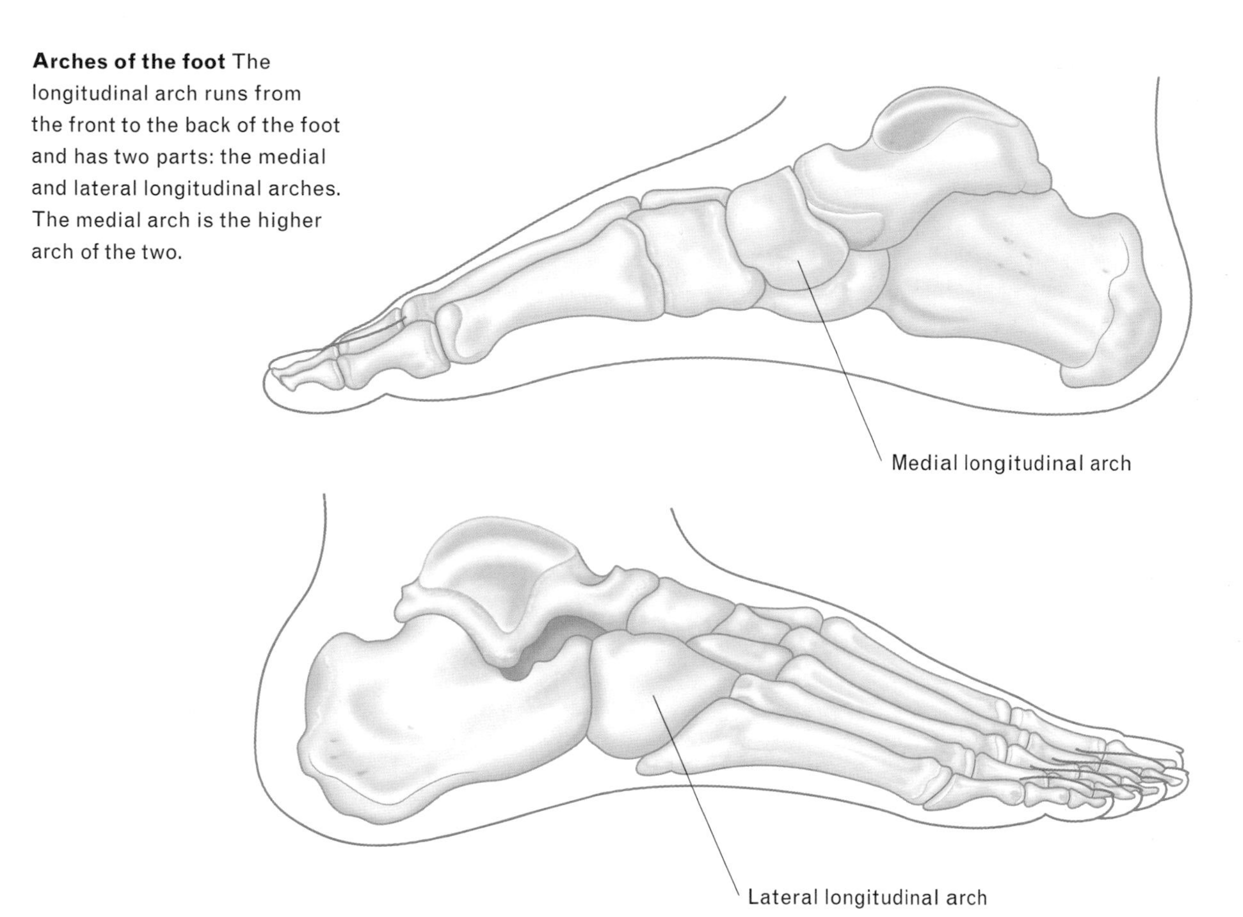

The feet and physical problems

In addition to sensitivities in the reflex area, problems in parts of the body can be manifested in the feet in other ways. In the next chapter (see pages 48–49), the causes and effects of foot problems are looked at in more detail, but here are a few indicators you can easily observe.

- As the reflex area of the cervical spine is found on the medial side of the foot, at the edge of the big toe, a protrusion such as a bunion on the toe joint in this area could indicate a neck condition.
- Someone with flat feet is more likely to be troubled with aches, pains and stiffness in the lumbar spine.
- The area under the fifth toe reflects the shoulder area, and hard skin that builds up on the lateral sides of the feet here can reflect tension and pain in the shoulder joint, often called 'a frozen shoulder'.
- Any deep-seated corns or calluses can interfere with the energy flow and cause inflammation and congestion in the part of the body represented by the reflexes in that area.

A SENSE OF PROPORTION

It is fascinating to see how the feet reflect our overall body shape and size. If you are a tall, slim person you will have long, slim feet with slender toes. If you are slim with narrow shoulders, the width of the foot at the diaphragm line (see page 29) will also be narrow. Your hands, too, resemble the shape of your feet. You will not find a person with long, slim feet but short, fat hands!

Foot maps

The maps on the following pages show the reflex areas for different organs and parts of the body. Each area mapped (for example, the heart, liver or lungs) contains many reflex points, rather like pins on a pincushion. To keep things simple, they are referred to as a single point: the heart reflex, liver reflex and so on. The reflex areas also overlap, so when you work one area you often contact the reflex points of another area.

Plantar right foot

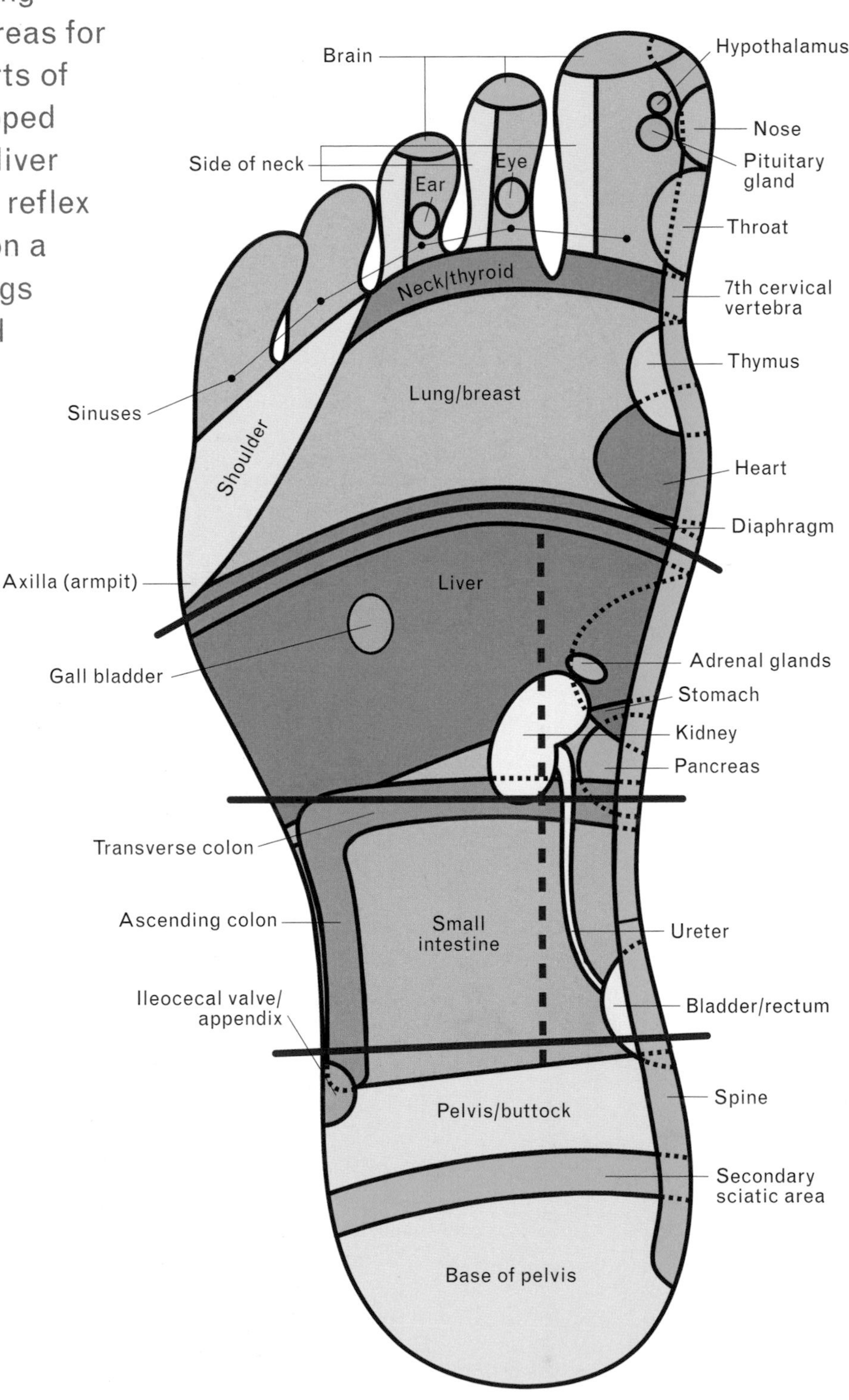

Plantar left foot

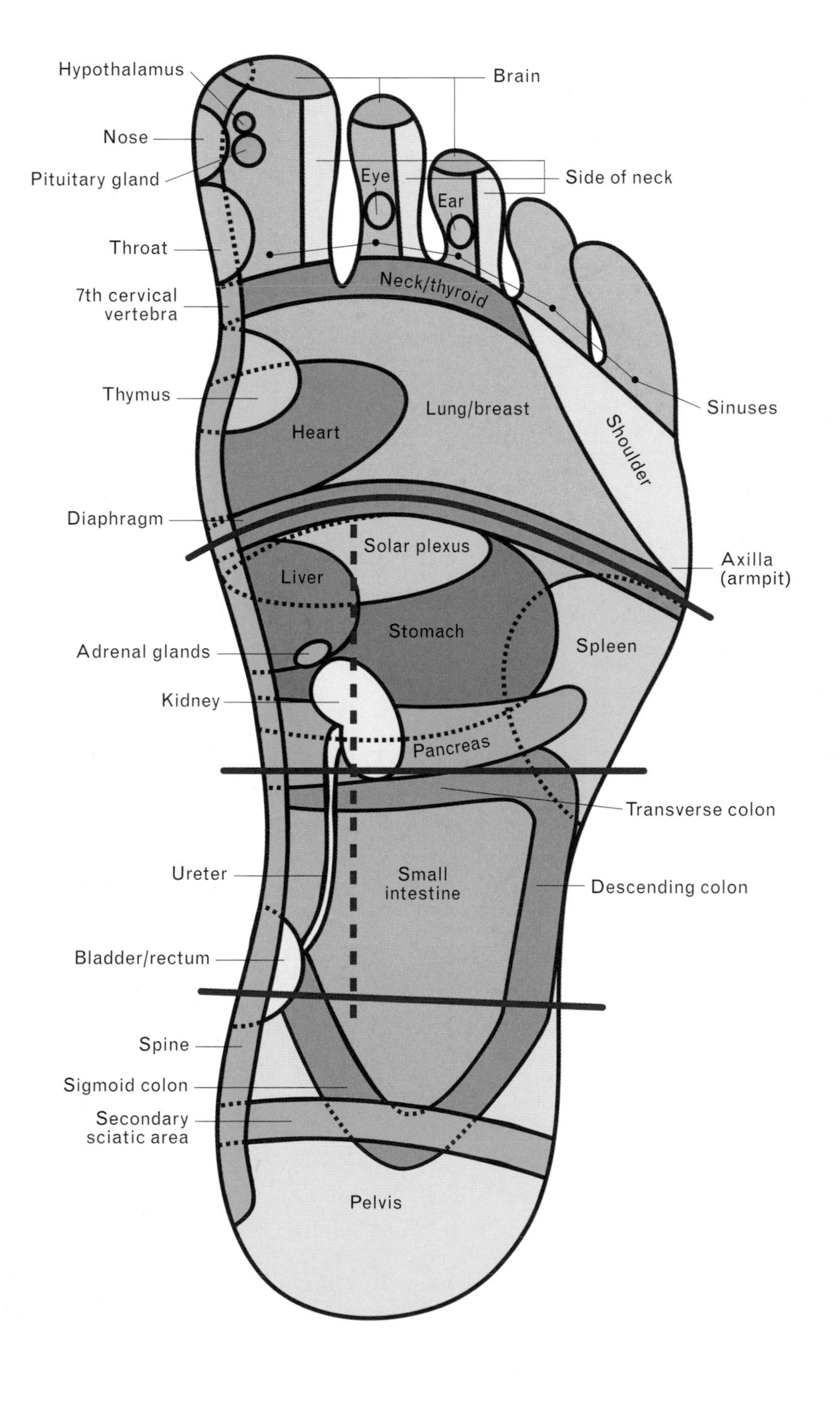

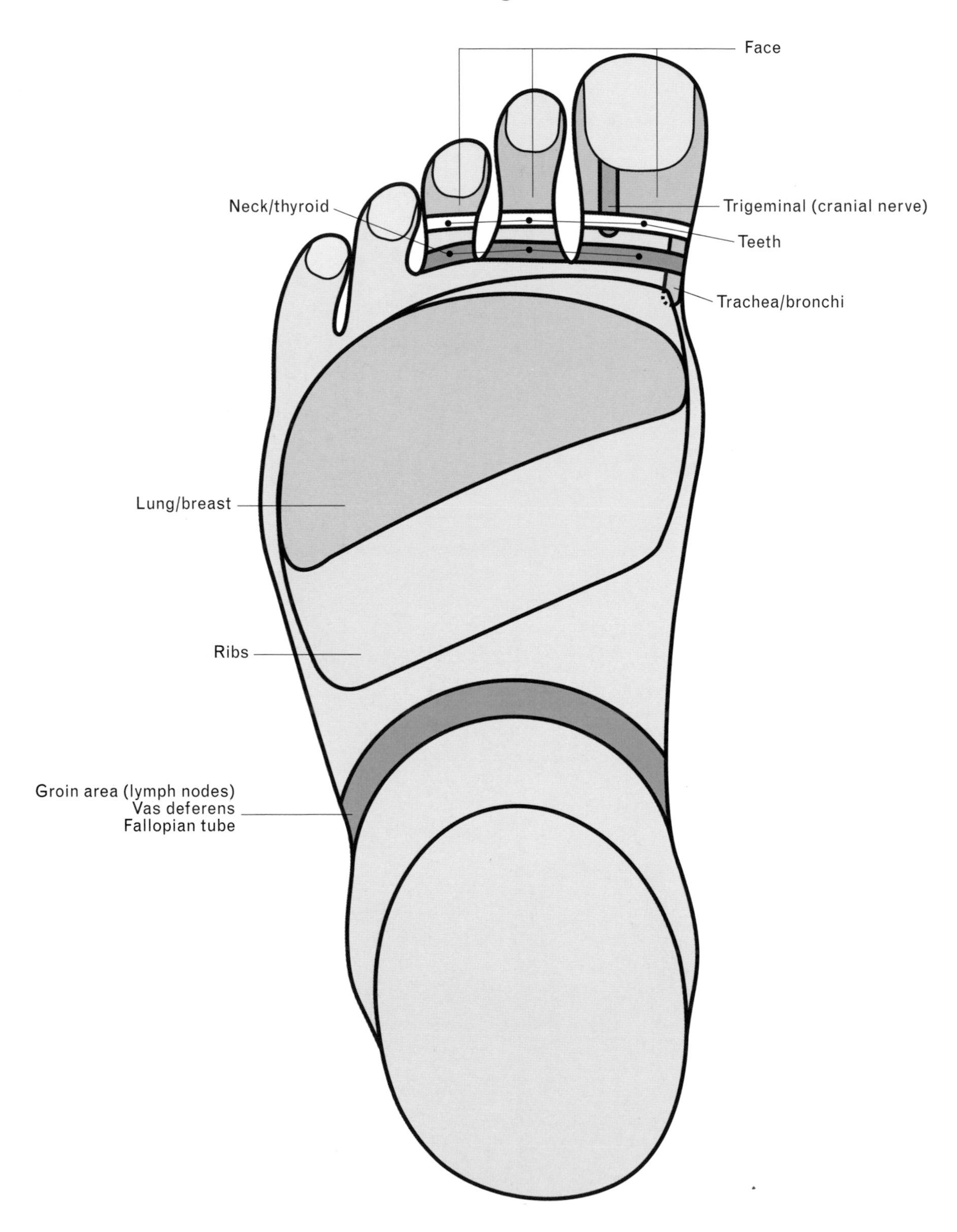
Dorsal right foot
Face
Neck/thyroid
Trigeminal (cranial nerve)
Teeth
Trachea/bronchi
Lung/breast
Ribs
Groin area (lymph nodes)
Vas deferens
Fallopian tube

Dorsal left foot

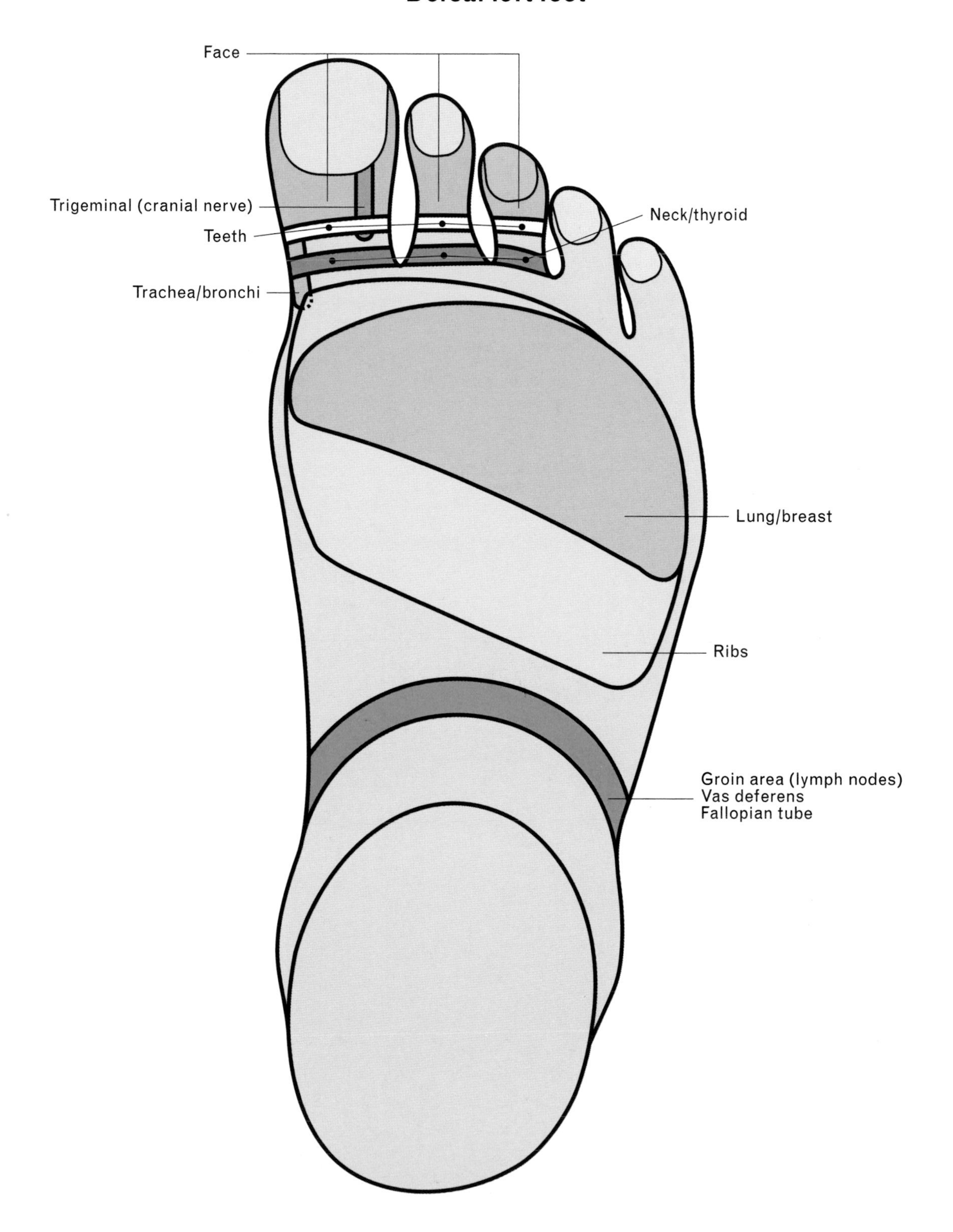

Medial right foot

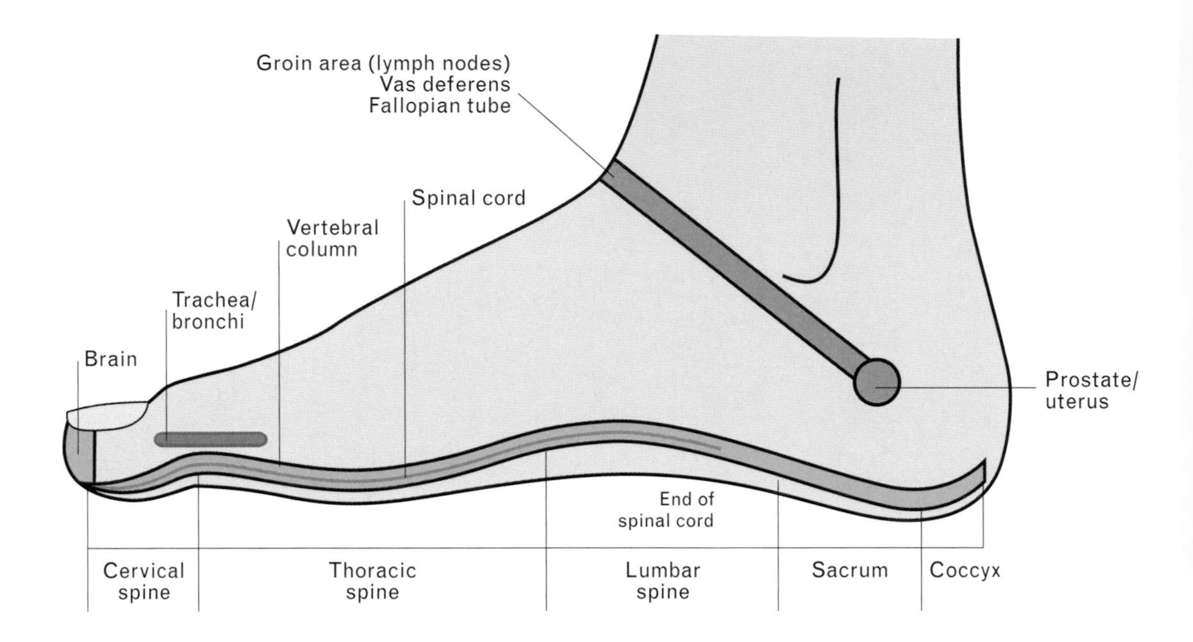

Medial left foot

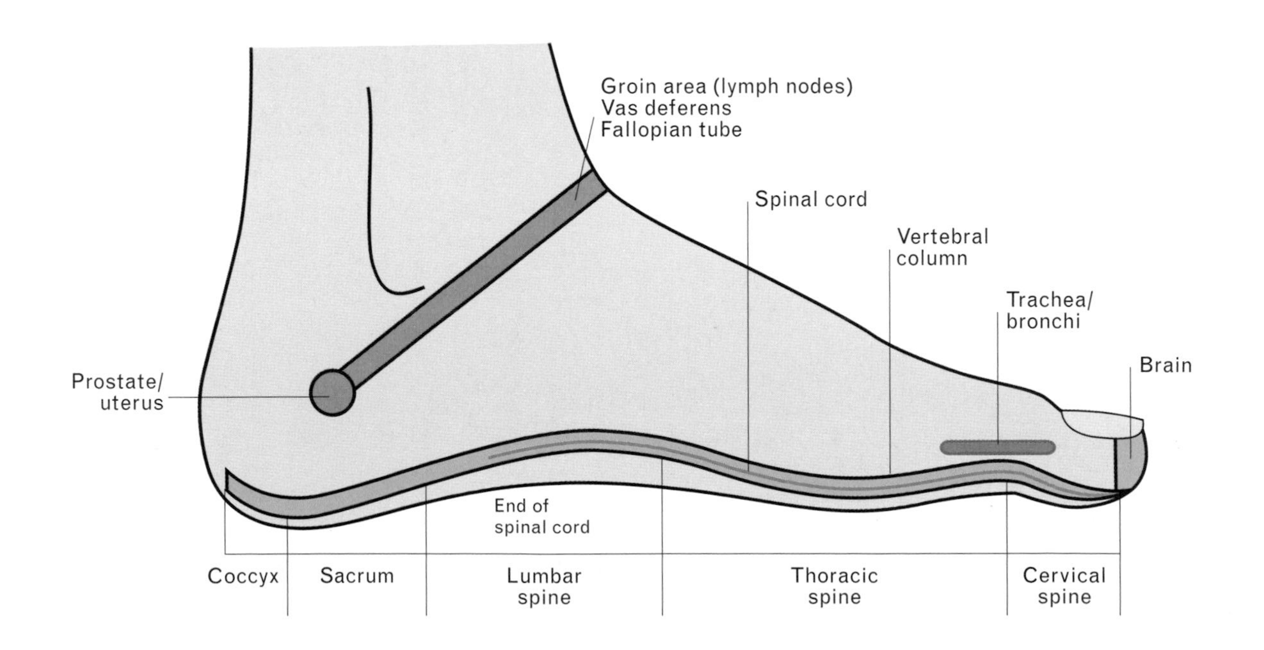

Lateral right foot

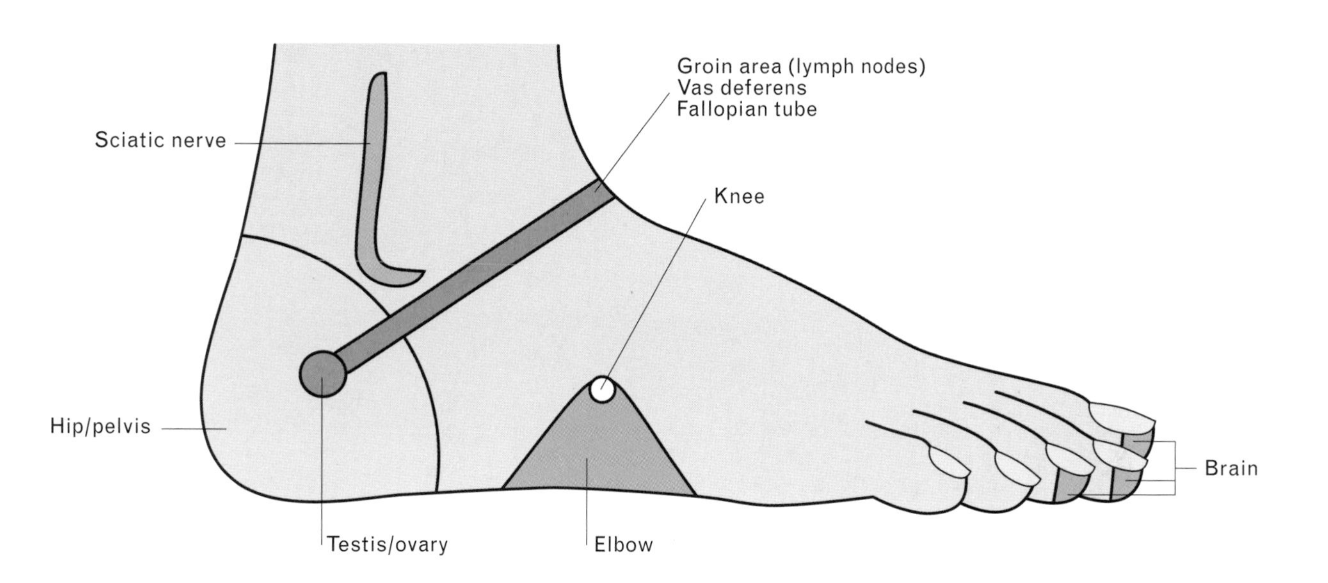

Lateral left foot

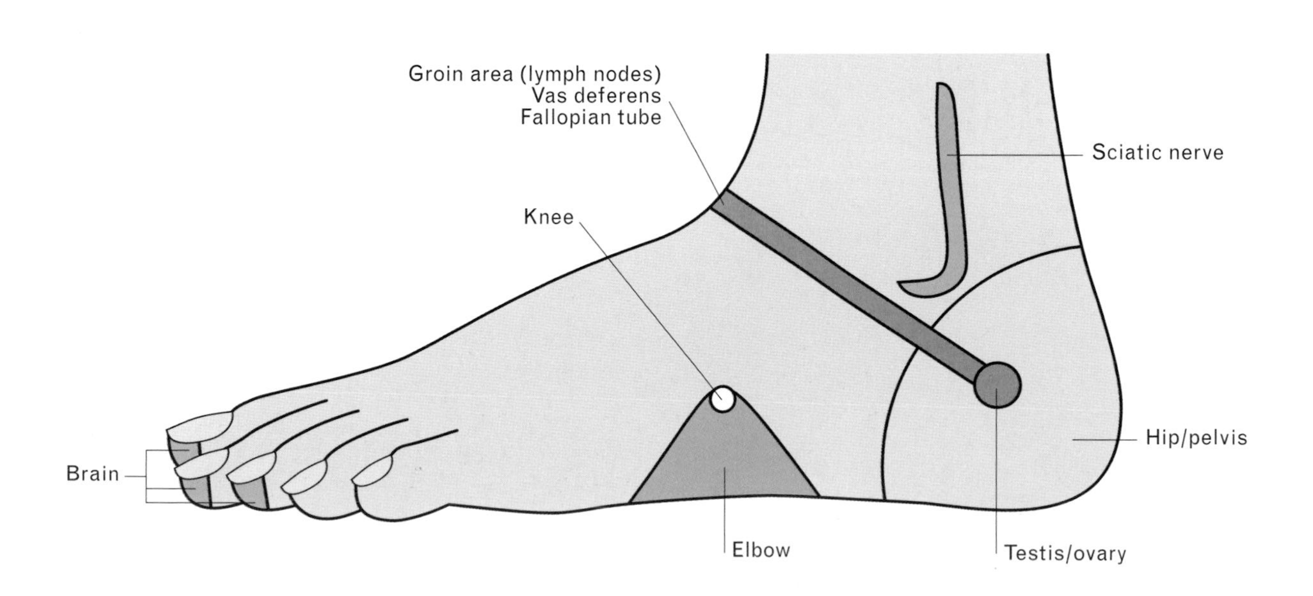

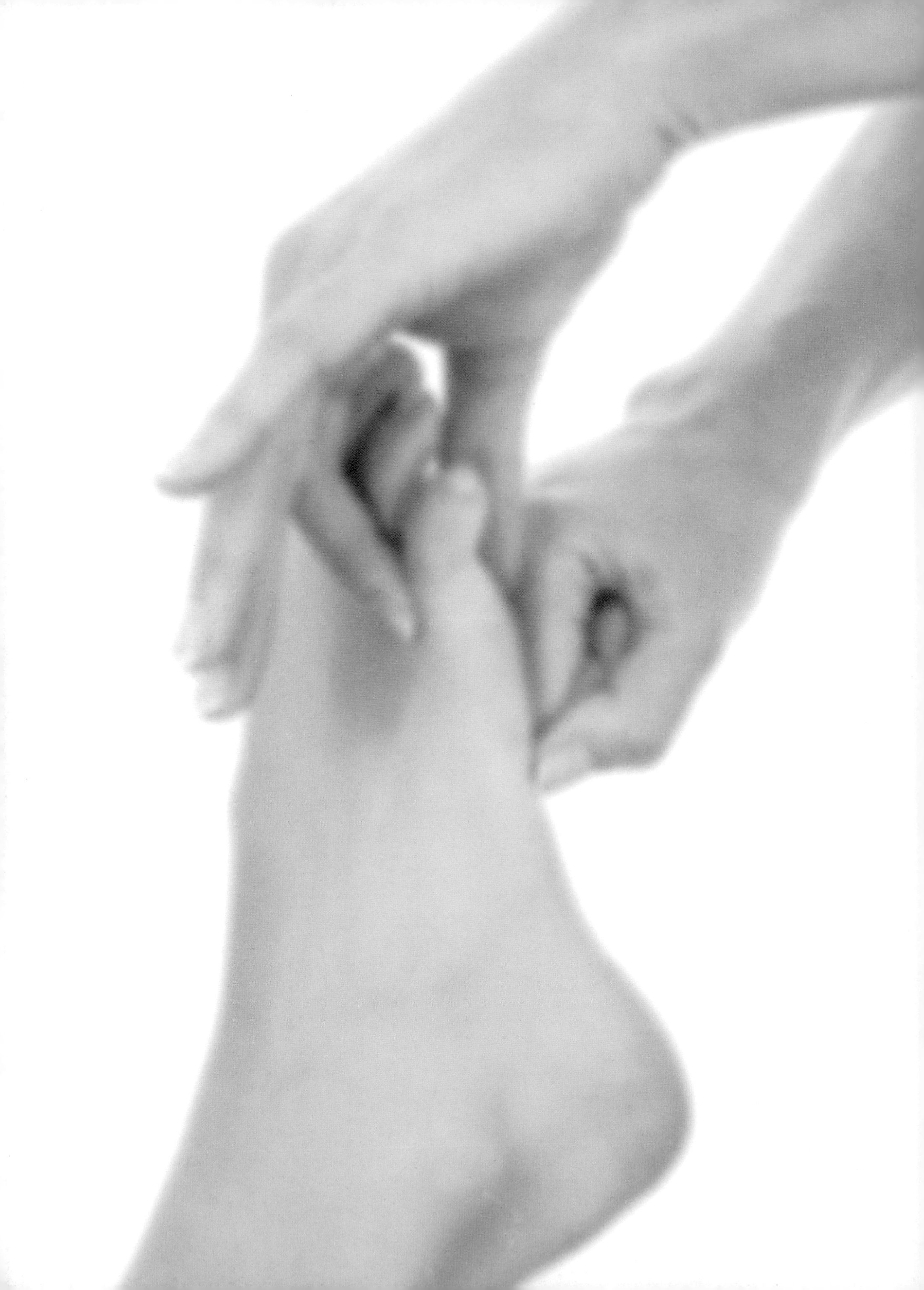

Providing reflexology

Reflexology is about helping the body towards complete wellbeing so it is important, in addition to mastering the techniques used to treat the feet, to put patients at their ease and create a peaceful ambience that will lift their spirits. A reflexologist will need to take and use a patient's case history, to be able to discuss competently the normal reactions to treatment and to know where and when not to treat.

Preparation

A reflexology session should be an hour of blissful relaxation for the patient, so offering a calm, comfortable environment alongside reassuring competence is an important part of the experience. Both you and your patient should always feel relaxed and at ease.

You should make sure that the room you are planning to use for treatments is sufficiently quiet and that you are unlikely to be interrupted during a session. Everyday noises such as passing traffic, a cacophony of ringing telephones or audible conversations in neighbouring rooms may all disturb the treatment and make it difficult for your patient to relax and for you to concentrate on what you are doing.

On the other hand, some pleasant, relaxing music in the background will help to set the mood. You may even like to light an oil burner that will send out a fragrant aroma, to really spoil your patients.

The rhythm of a session

When you are planning your schedule, you need to allow about an hour to spend on each patient with a short break between patients. A break between appointments will give you time to wash your hands, have a refreshing drink and prepare for the next appointment. It also leaves a few minutes spare in case your patient happens to be late. The very worst thing you can do is to rush through a treatment; it undermines the whole principle of reflexology, which is that it is a relaxing therapy.

HOME VISITS

Home visits are becoming popular, particularly for elderly or disabled patients who may be unable to travel to you. Many practitioners are now obtaining work in residential care homes or nursing homes. A weekly visit is very welcome, not only in easing aches and pains, but also in providing an elderly person with someone to chat and listen. Communication itself is a wonderful healer.

When patients arrive I first ask them to take their shoes and socks or tights off, and seat them on the therapy table or in the chair. I start by wiping their feet with medicated wipes, then cover their legs with a large, clean towel and take their case history. This is a chance both to assess the feet and the patient as a whole, to observe and discuss any particular problems and to take relevant notes.

A few relaxation exercises precede and follow the actual reflexology treatment, enhancing the whole experience. The rest of this chapter looks in more details at all the stages of a reflexology session and also covers other considerations, such as how to identify the side-effects of any medicinal drugs that your patient may be taking. Medicinal drugs can often affect the sensitivity of different reflex points.

Seating arrangements

Your patient should be in as comfortable a position as possible. A reclining chair or therapy table is very useful as it allows patients to stretch out and relax with their legs in an elevated position. Make sure you are sitting in a comfortable position as well. I would recommend you invest in a therapist's adjustable stool, which has five wheels and allows you to rotate with ease from the right foot to the left.

Another useful piece of equipment is a portable footstool known as a reflex stool. This is ideal for home visiting. If at any time you want to give a lecture where a demonstration will be needed, the reflex stool is light and easy to carry about.

A professional approach

Dress as professionally as possible: trousers and a plain top or a white tunic look smart, or you may prefer some other form of dress, but it is important to look clean and tidy. Do not wear bracelets, jangling earrings or rings with large stones. In particular, make sure that your

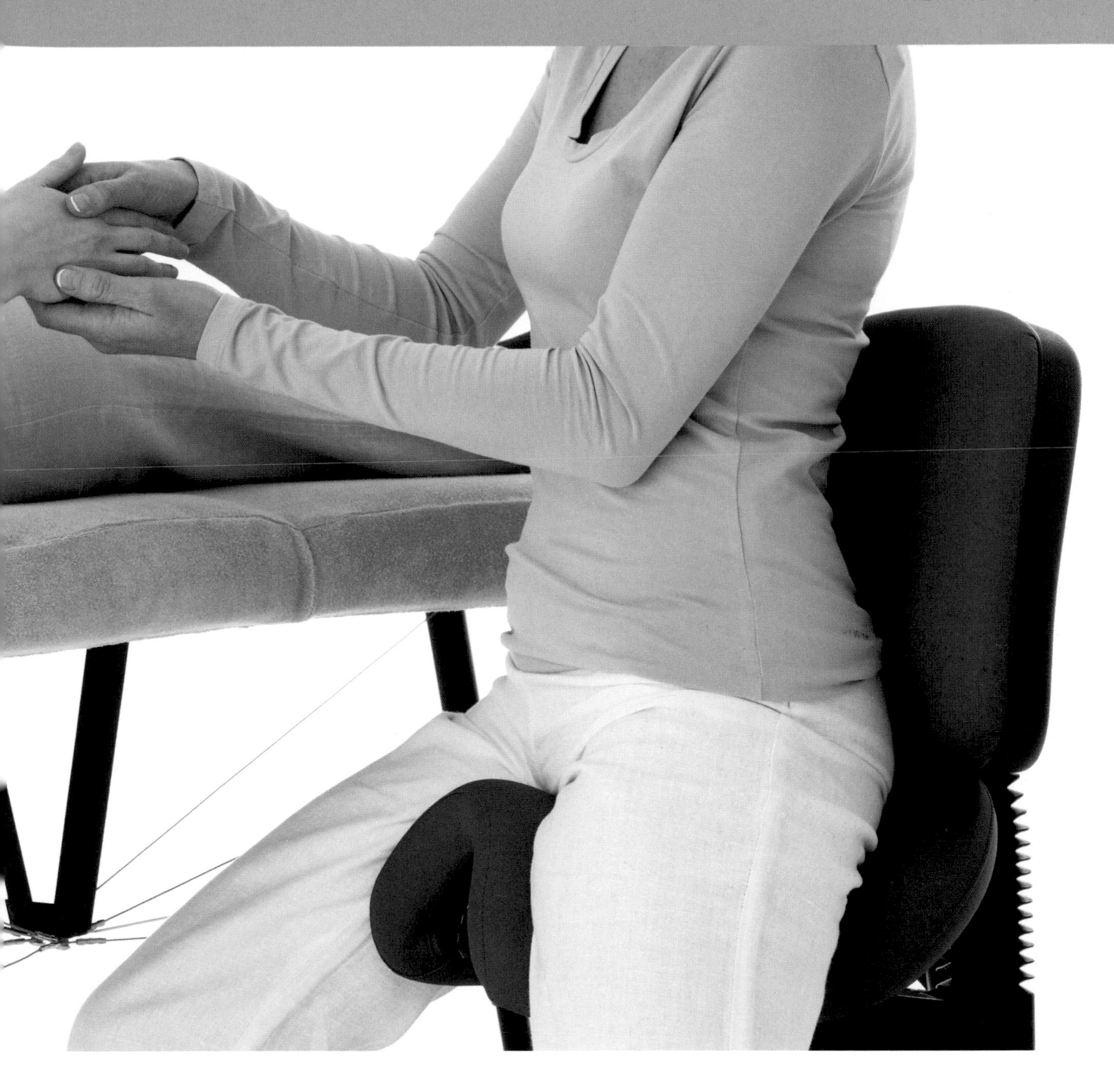

hands are well manicured with short, clean fingernails – your hands are the tools of your trade!

It's a good idea to display your Diploma of Reflexology on the wall of the room in which you are working, together with any certificates you may have showing membership of associations, a first-aid certificate and a certificate of insurance. Patients have the right to see when and where you were qualified and to be able to reassure themselves that you are a member of a recognized association, that you are insured to practise and that you would be able to handle competently and confidently any situation that could occur during treatments.

Seating arrangements You will be spending a lot of time in your chair, so choose a comfortable model that can be adjusted to suit your height and the size of your therapy table.

Taking a case history

In order to obtain good insight into a patient's lifestyle and medical history you need as much information from them as possible. Taking a detailed case history will give you a very clear picture of the person you are about to treat.

A record form or card such as the one shown opposite will cover all the questions you need to ask to obtain a full case history of your patient. You can either ask questions and fill it in yourself or get the patient to complete it. When the form is completed, the patient should sign it, thus giving their permission for you to treat them.

When you start treatment on the patient, you should bear in mind any diseases, operations or injuries that have been mentioned, taking care around corresponding reflex points.

Infectious illness

It is inadvisable to treat a patient during the acute stage of an infectious illness. The stimulating effect of reflexology tends to create a detoxifying effect on all the eliminating functions of the body: the lungs, kidneys, bowels, sinuses and skin. During an acute infection, the body is already desperately trying to rid itself of an accumulation of toxins. Stimulation through reflexology will encourage the body to go into overdrive to eliminate even more toxins, and make the patient feel even more disturbed and unwell than before.

Do by all means work on techniques to create a feeling of relaxation in the patient, but avoid those organs of elimination at an acute stage of illness. In cases of high temperature you may also like to work on the reflexes of the pituitary gland; this is beneficial in lowering temperature. In general, however, it is best to begin treating the patient after they have recovered from their illness, in the 'passive' stage.

WHEN NOT TO TREAT A PATIENT'S FEET

If a patient has a sprained ankle, any broken bones in the feet or legs or ulceration, perhaps associated with diabetes, you should work on the hands rather than the feet (see 'Hand reflexology', pages 162–187). If there is a fungal infection, such as athlete's foot, make sure it is securely covered with a large piece of sticking plaster before you start work.

Intensity of treatment and its effects

Although reflexology is a gentle treatment it is also very powerful and there is the possibility that it can cause someone, particularly an elderly person or someone in poor health, to have an extreme reaction. Under these circumstances, a patient may not feel confident in returning for a further appointment.

When patients who have had a long history of frequent medication and who are perhaps not in good health are being treated, I always suggest that the reflexologist under-treats on the first occasion, to minimize the chances of a violent reaction. Use a very light pressure on such patients, do not exceed half an hour of working over the feet and wait for a report from them as to how they felt the day after.

On following up the first session, you might ask your patients whether they feel that their condition has worsened; if they had any bowel or bladder problems; whether they suffered from a severe headache, and so on. Be guided by these reactions.

If all is well after the initial treatment and the patient reports a general feeling of improvement and wellbeing, then it is quite in order to increase the duration of the treatment session and perhaps use a slightly more intense pressure. Remember, the patient is your guide.

See pages 44–45 for evidence of drug reactions that you might find when working on the feet, and for more on foot problems, see pages 48–49.

Sample client record card This card covers the basic information you need to record about your patients' medical history and current state of health.

Client record card

Name ___ Age ___ Date of birth ___

Sex M/F ___ Marital status ___ Occupation ___

Address ___

Home tel. ___ Work tel. ___ E-mail ___

Children (no./ages) ___

Referred by (doctor's name) ___

Doctor's address ___ Tel. ___

Emergency contact details (name, relationship, tel. no.) ___

Patient's medical history

Medication/Pill/HRT ___ Vitamins/minerals/self-prescribed supplements? ___

☐ Anaemia ☐ German measles ☐ Chickenpox ☐ Diphtheria ☐ Measles ☐ Mumps ☐ Pneumonia ☐ Whooping cough

☐ Rheumatic fever ☐ Sinuses ☐ Glandular fever ☐ Scarlet fever ☐ Shingles ☐ Polio ☐ Other

Operations (appendix, tonsils etc.) incl. dates ___

Accidents/injuries/falls incl. dates ___

☐ Insertions (coil/pacemaker) ___ ☐ Back problems ___

General state of health ___

Patient and family-related conditions

☐ Diabetes ☐ Epilepsy ☐ High blood pressure ☐ Thrombosis ☐ Heart ☐ Chest ☐ Migraine ☐ Kidney ☐ Bladder ☐ Digestion

☐ Constipation ☐ Varicose veins ☐ Allergies ☐ Hepatitis ☐ Hay fever ☐ Asthma ☐ MS ☐ Cancer ☐ Arthritis ☐ Colitis

☐ Lupus ☐ Other ___

☐ Pregnant ☐ Regular periods ☐ Date of last period ___ ☐ PMT ☐ Symptoms of PMT ☐ Breast feeding

☐ Hysterectomy ☐ Menopause ☐ Skin problems ☐ Infectious diseases/HIV

Lifestyle

☐ Smoke/no. daily ☐ Drink (alcohol) ☐ Balanced diet ☐ Eat regular meals

☐ Take exercise/what? ___

☐ Sleep/insomnia? ☐ Stress ☐ Depression

Any other observations (e.g. disabilities) ___

The information I have given about my health in this case history is true to the best of my knowledge and belief, and I hereby give my consent to myself/my child being treated by natural therapy.

Signed ___ Date ___

Observation of feet

RIGHT FOOT ___ LEFT FOOT ___

Skeletal deformities ___

Muscle tone ___

Flat foot or high arch ___

Nail condition ___

Skin condition ___

Area/zone of hard skin build-up ___

Other comments ___

Drug reactions

As we all know, drugs have side-effects, such as inflammation and congestion, which upset the functioning of other parts of the body. It is essential to take into account the side-effects of a variety of medicinal drugs, to understand how they increase the sensitivity of different reflex points.

When I started in my practice some 32 years ago, I often encountered a sensitivity in the foot that did not really seem to relate to the condition that I was treating. For example, in treating a patient with severe hayfever I would pick up a sensitivity in the sinus and lung reflex areas, which I expected, but I would also find that the kidney area was extremely sensitive. This was confusing. What on earth had the kidneys to do with hayfever?

Over the ensuing months I encountered more and more of these oddities. Sensitivities appeared in the feet which just did not link up with the problem the patient had come to me with. Maybe the chart I was using was incorrect, or there was some other hidden mystery concerning reflexology that I knew nothing about? Perhaps I would have to try to work this out for myself.

I then noted that patients showing signs of these various unexplained sensitivities were all on medication of some kind or another. Eventually, after consulting an encyclopedia of drugs, I realized that what I was picking up were the congested areas in the body caused by the medications that the patients were taking.

Effects of drugs

The following list describes some of the effects on the body and foot reflexes of some common groups of drugs.

- **Antihistamines**: Used for allergic reactive illnesses, such as hayfever, skin rashes, troublesome irritant coughs and eczema. Antihistamines create a sensitivity in the kidney reflex area.

- **Steroids** Frequently used to treat inflammation caused by arthritis, heart conditions, cancer and severe allergic reactive illness such as asthma that has got out of control. Steroids can create insensitivity in the foot and you are likely to find no reaction at all, but it is still worth giving treatment as it has a beneficial effect upon the body. Steroids lower a person's vitality.

- **Non-steroidal anti-inflammatory drugs (NSAIDs)**: Used in the control of arthritis, rheumatism, gout and inflammatory conditions of the spine. NSAIDs can be the cause of sensitivities in the liver, kidneys and stomach reflexes.

- **Aspirin**: Commonly used to kill pain. Aspirin causes stomach inflammation and sometimes stomach ulceration. Many people are allergic to aspirin. It produces a sensitivity in the stomach reflexes.

- **Painkillers**: Painkilling drugs have a disastrous effect on the intestine and normally cause chronic constipation. They can lead to a reaction in the intestines, in the ascending, transverse and descending colon reflexes.

- **Antibiotics**: These are commonly used to control infections in the body. Antibiotics destroy the flora content in the intestine, which upsets the balance of the body and can result in either constipation or diarrhoea.

- **Antidepressant drugs/sleeping pills**: These can cause great sensitivity in the brain reflex area.

- **Beta-blockers**: Used in the control of heart conditions and hypertension, beta-blockers dull the sensitivity of the body and thus work as a depressant on the adrenal glands and the heart, causing the heart beat to become slower. They also have an effect on the liver.

- **Statins**: Widely used for lowering cholesterol levels, these cause a reaction in the liver reflexes.

- **Amphetamines**: These drugs are still being used in some private weight-loss clinics but thankfully now only infrequently. Amphetamines are extremely

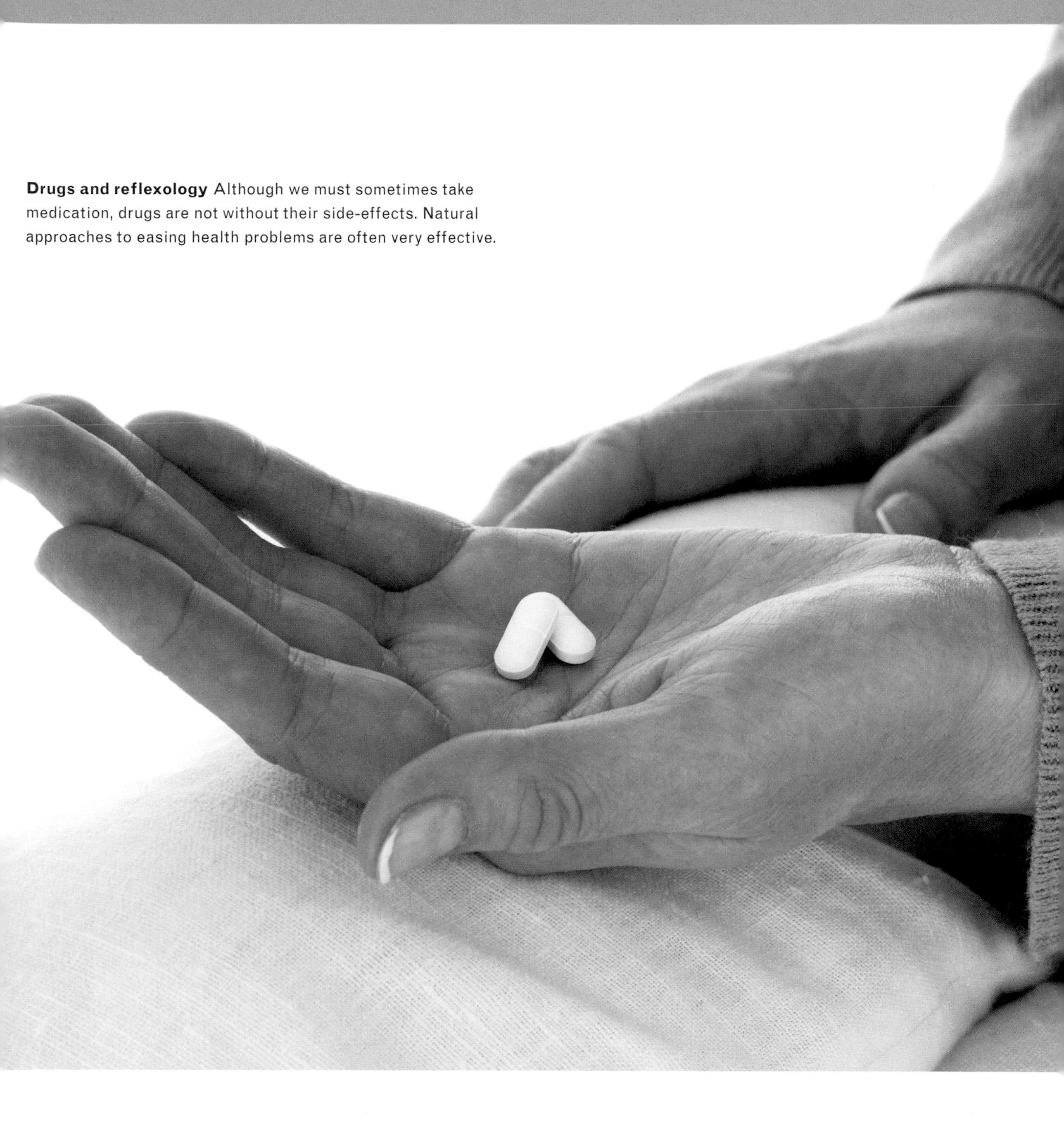

Drugs and reflexology Although we must sometimes take medication, drugs are not without their side-effects. Natural approaches to easing health problems are often very effective.

addictive and stimulate all functioning of the body to work overtime, which creates a drastic effect on the central nervous system. The brain and adrenal gland reflexes are usually acutely sensitive in those taking amphetamine drugs.

- **Antacids**: Peppermint-flavoured and chalk-based medications for digestive disturbances. The chalk content of antacids has an effect on the kidneys and can cause kidney stones if taken in large quantities over a long period of time. You may encounter sensitivities in the kidney reflex.
- **Chemotherapy**: Patients undergoing chemotherapy to combat cancer will usually have sensitivities in most of the foot reflexes.

Assessing the foot

Touch is all-important when it comes to familiarizing yourself with a patient's feet, but you should also keep alert for signs that may be symptomatic of an underlying problem. It helps to keep a record of your observations on a simple foot chart.

As you talk to the patient about their medical history, you can be gently feeling their feet to identify areas with granular build-up, or reflex points that are especially sensitive. Do not use oils or creams. An oily foot makes it very difficult to isolate the reflex points. Non-oily foot balms often work well or, if the feet are very damp, give them a light dusting of talcum powder.

There is no substitute for the human hand. No machine can give you the information that your own sense of touch can, and that is why I am totally against the use of all devices like electrical stimulating machines in reflexology. We have far too many machines in our lives. It is vital that we now reach back to the natural ways of healing, and use our hands. Hands were meant for healing.

During each session, I like to fill out a foot chart, like the example shown opposite. I also update a simplified version of the patient consultation record card (see page 43) after every appointment. It's a good idea to note down any significant personal information the patient has told you, such as a first grandchild due to be born imminently, or exams being taken by children, or concern over sick relatives. When the patient arrives for the next appointment, you can ask about whatever they mentioned last time, helping to create a good rapport.

Client record card

NAME .... DATE ....

ADDRESS ....

....

....

....

TEL. NO. ....

DATE OF BIRTH ....

ANY SURGICAL OPERATIONS ....

....

....

....

MEDICATION ....

....

....

....

HISTORY OF ....

....

....

....

....

COMPLAINS OF ....

....

....

....

....

ANY OTHER OBSERVATIONS ....

....

....

....

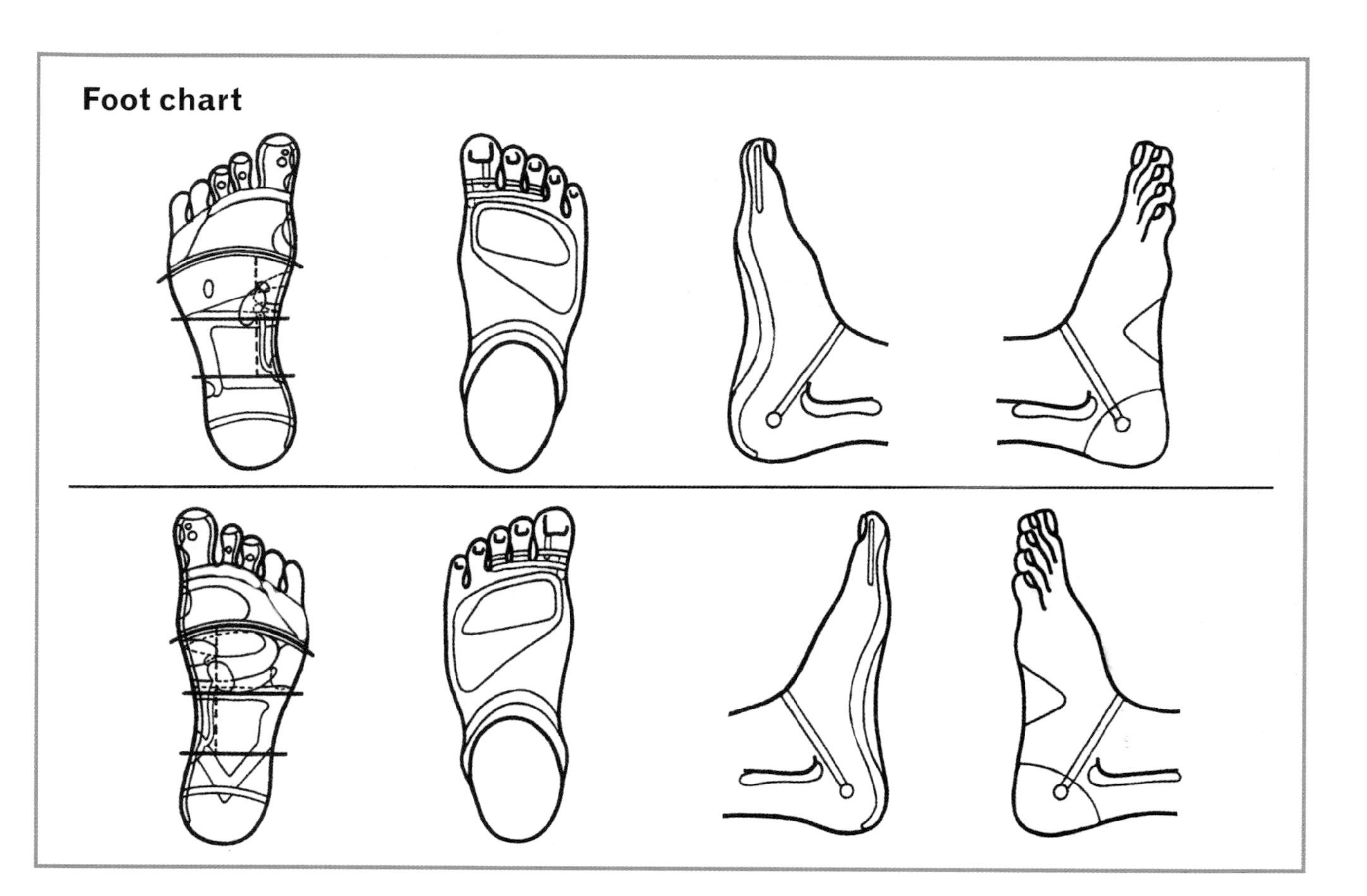

Foot chart You could make a number of photocopies of this blank foot chart and then use it as your 'x-ray' during each reflexology treatment, recording your findings.

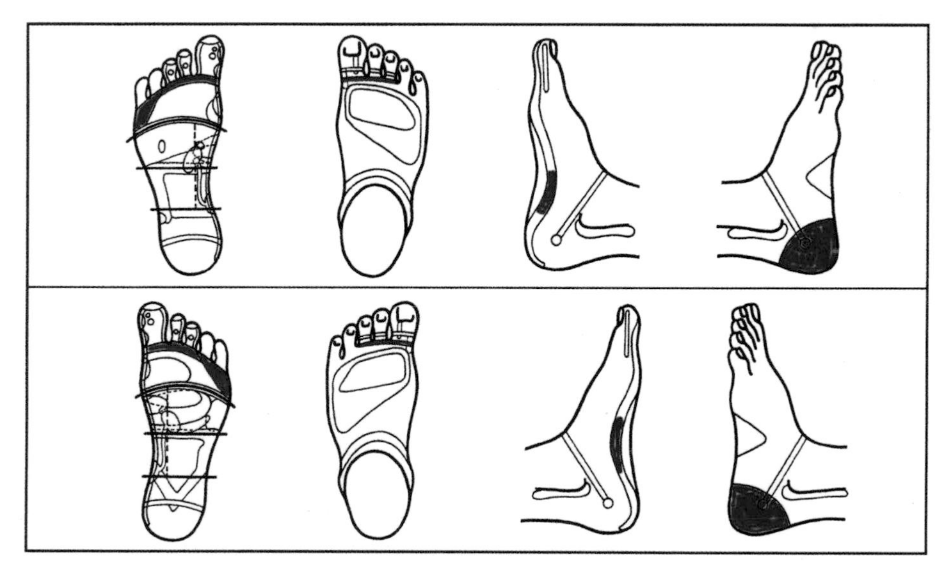

Sensitivities This example of a filled-in foot chart indicates a patient with sensitivities in the shoulder, neck, lumbar spine and hip/pelvis areas.

Simple record card A simplified version of the full record card is useful for updating patients' notes after every consultation. You could photocopy this one or reproduce something similar on your computer.

Foot problems

Medical statistics reveal that two out of three people are plagued with one or more foot problems, and these can often either lead to or stem from more serious disorders.

Abuse of the feet and the consequent foot misalignments cause blisters, bunions, calluses and corns. These in turn often lead to general fatigue and bodily aches. The converse is also true: systemic or general body disorders, such as arthritis, diabetes, multiple sclerosis and some types of heart disease, show up in the feet. Often this is the first place they show, some time before the malfunctioning organs have exhibited other symptoms.

Foot pain can camouflage serious diseases, so foot discomfort of any kind demands immediate attention, not only to the foot but to the rest of the body. What may appear to be merely a foot problem could in fact be a symptom of a systemic disease. Consultation with a chiropodist to remove hard skin and deal with corns and calluses prior to commencing reflexology treatment sessions is highly recommended.

Below, some of the more common problems a reflexologist may encounter are described.

Athlete's foot

Although not a disease in itself, athlete's foot describes an entire set of symptoms commonly including scaling between the toes, an itching sensation and a softening of the flesh. It may initially be the result of a fungus, but if it becomes chronic, roughening of the skin can follow, known technically as hyperkeratomycosis. Athlete's foot occurs more frequently in men than women; it may be a local problem but it can also be the result of an allergy, a drug overdose or sunburn.

Naturopathic doctors believe that athlete's foot is exacerbated by the body's poor elimination of waste; that is, the skin, lungs, bowel and kidney are not performing their elimination duties very efficiently. As a result the feet are used as an area of elimination, through perspiration. Sweat is normally made up of a highly proteinous material, in which the virus that creates athlete's foot thrives in abundance. Often, attention to the body's eliminating processes in the form of extra exercise, hot and cold showers and body scrubs gives the body a chance to eliminate its waste through the proper channels, and allows the condition to disappear.

Bunions

A predisposition to develop bunions might be inherited, but a bunion can also be caused by wearing poorly fitted shoes. In some but not all cases the 'bursa' or sac over the joint of the big toe becomes inflamed and swollen, sometimes twisting the big toe under the two next to it. Pressure must not be applied to painful swollen areas, so when bunions are painful, you must work on the corresponding place on the hand instead.

Corns and calluses

Millions of people suffer from corns and calluses on their feet. They can be the result of friction, abnormal foot structure, systemic problems or can even arise through imbalance of mental or emotional upsets. A chiropodist or podiatrist will usually prescribe salicylic acid plasters to remove them.

Castor oil rubbed twice daily into the affected area softens the corn or callus so that it can eventually be peeled off with the fingers. Other home remedies include the application of a thin slice of lemon or a piece of cotton wool dipped in witch hazel. Either of these should be secured in place overnight with sticking plaster or adhesive tape. After a number of applications over a period of days the skin usually softens enough to remove a corn or callus gradually.

Verrucae

A friend of mine, who is a very good chiropodist, informs me that a good first-aid remedy for the removal of a verruca is to cut a small square from the skin of a banana, place the inside of the skin on to the verruca and cover it with a piece of sticking plaster. Replace with a fresh piece daily and within a week the verruca will fall out. I certainly think this would be worth trying.

Fallen arches

Many people are born with a predisposition to fallen arches. Shoes with arch supports may be helpful in certain circumstances but specifically designed exercises are preferable. It is interesting to note that through the centuries superstitions or myths have developed about the arches of the feet. One such myth is that high arches are a sign of aristocratic descent. Low arches may be an ethnic characteristic and yet cause no pain. It is said that strong arches are important for healthy feet and for good support of the spine.

Rheumatoid arthritis

In its early stages, rheumatoid arthritis may appear as pain, stiffness or swelling in the joints of the feet. The appearance of tiny lumps beneath the skin, known as subcutaneous nodules, is an early warning sign of this serious ailment. You can feel these nodules and they may cause discomfort if pressure is exerted too enthusiastically, particularly during the first reflexology treatment session. When the disease has reached the degenerative, chronic stage, deformities such as hammer toes and bony spurs may appear.

Gout

This painful condition is more common in men than in women. It is possible to be genetically predisposed to gout. Its appearance is often marked by a sudden change in the big toe, which becomes shiny, swollen, inflamed and extremely painful. The initial point of irritation is usually the joint at the base of the big toe (known as the metatarsophalangeal joint), but other joints in the feet may also be affected.

Gout may at first be mistakenly viewed purely as a foot problem, but it is caused by a disturbance in the uric acid metabolism, which results in raised levels of this acid in the blood. Because of the build-up of waste products in the system, insoluble uric acid salts accumulate around the joints and in the tissues in the form of crystalline deposits which can be felt when they are pressed.

Cardiovascular diseases

These affect the heart and circulatory system and may cause pain, swelling and a burning sensation in the feet if the blood circulation is impaired. Swelling and oedema in the feet and legs can be caused by heart inadequacy. Body fluids then accumulate in the extremities since they are restricted in their flow.

Arteriosclerosis

This is the hardening and thickening of the arteries, which seriously reduces blood flow, with the consequent loss of oxygen to the tissues of the feet and removal of deoxygenated blood. This leads to poor gaseous interchange in the tissues. Difficulty in walking, pain when the feet are at rest, ulcers and infections, loss of hair on the legs, and thickening of the nails, particularly on the big toes, are all clues to the presence of this disorder.

Diabetes

An early symptom of diabetes is often a numbness and tingling sensation in the feet. Ulcers may develop on the soles and, if infections occur, they heal very slowly.

Neurological disorders

Symptoms of neurological problems or nerve disorders, even brain lesions, can appear in the feet in the form of lack of coordination and muscle weakness.

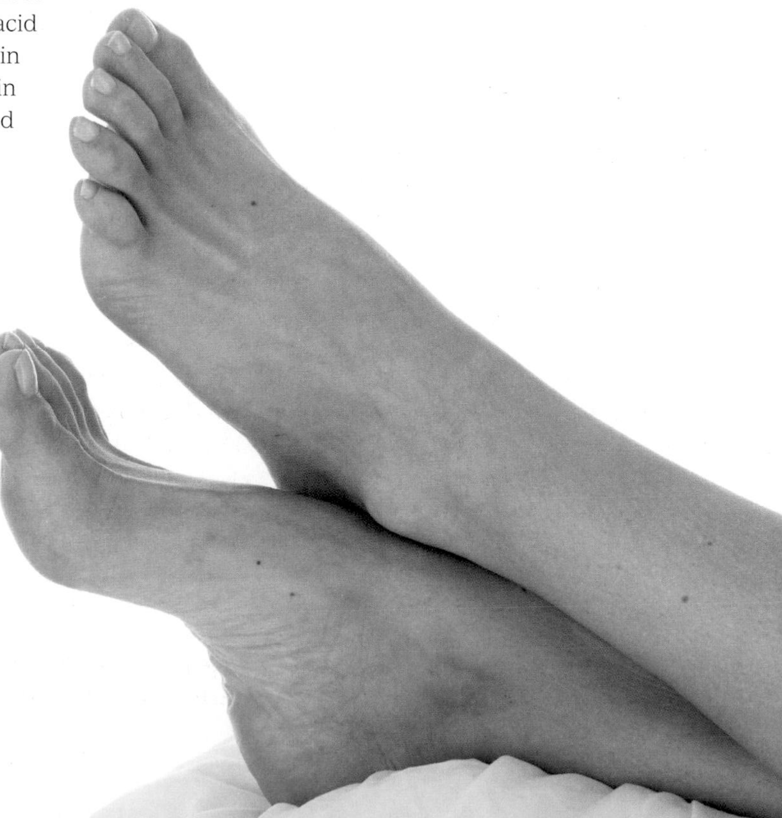

Barometers of our health Many complaints, including some forms of heart disease and diabetes, will be reflected in the feet even before the patient is aware of any problem.

Working on the feet

While the patient's complaints and your own findings will lead to an emphasis on particular reflex areas, it is essential to work all areas of each foot. Follow a routine so that there is no chance of a reflex (the size of a pinhead) being missed out.

To enable practical procedures to be understood and correctly followed, throughout this book certain views of the feet are referred to in a specific way. The views are: plantar (sole of the foot), dorsal (top of the foot), medial (inner edge of foot) and lateral (outer edge of foot).

Working each side of the foot

The following illustrations show the basic procedure for working across each area. 'The whole routine' (pages 156–161) shows how these build into a complete routine, using the techniques described on pages 52–53.

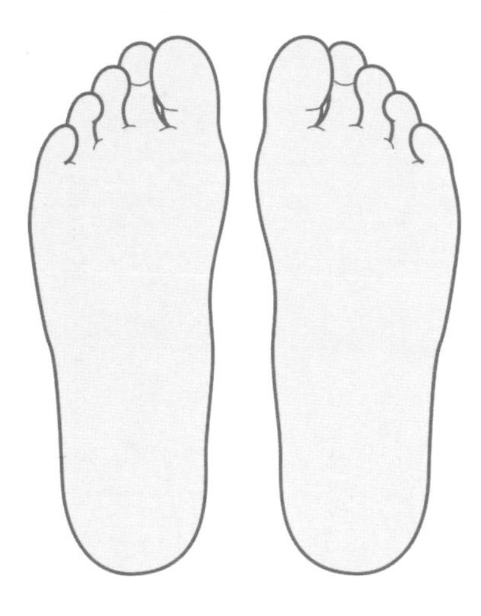

Plantar (The sole of the foot)

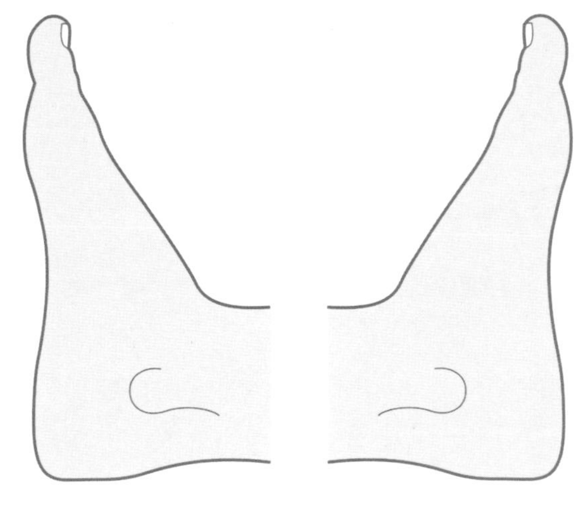

Medial (The inner side of the foot, in line with the big toe)

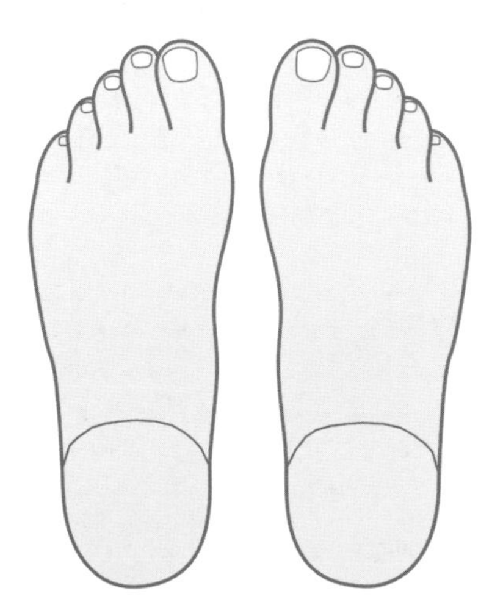

Dorsal (The front, or upper side, of the foot)

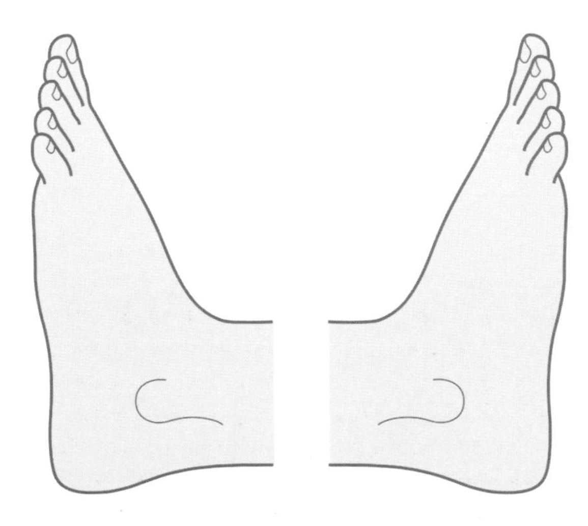

Lateral (The outside edge of the foot, in line with the little toe)

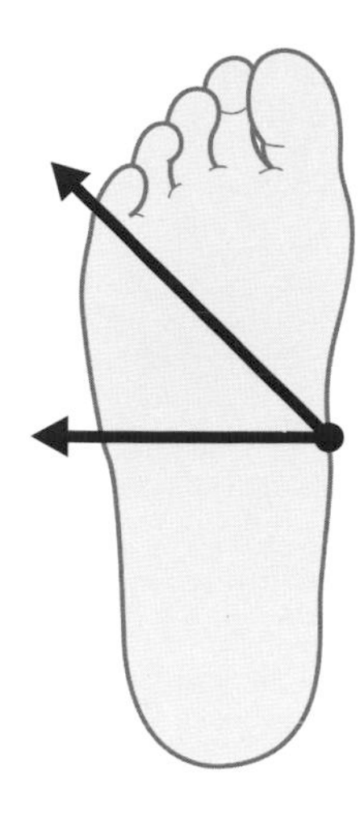

Right foot – medial to lateral When starting to work on the right foot you must support the foot in your left hand and work from the medial side to the lateral side of the foot with the right thumb.

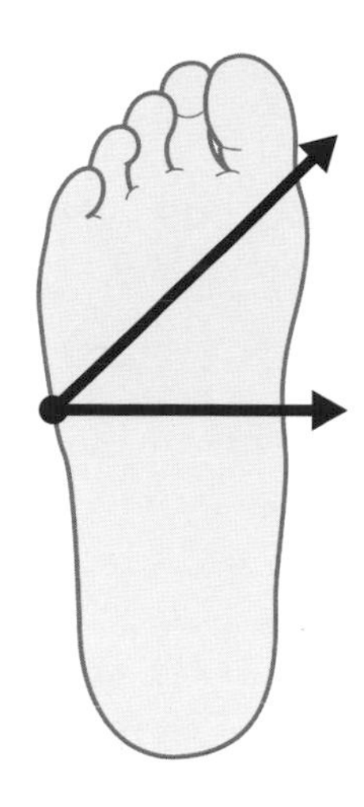

Right foot – lateral to medial As you change direction, you must support the right foot with your right hand and, using the left thumb, work back from lateral to medial.

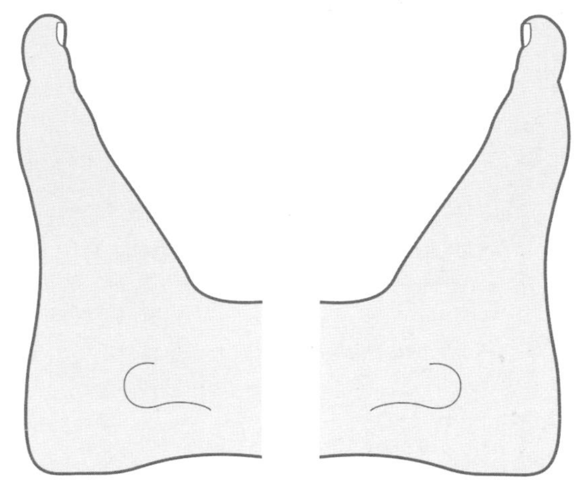

Medial side of the foot To work the medial side of the foot, hold the foot in an upward direction while you support the lateral side.

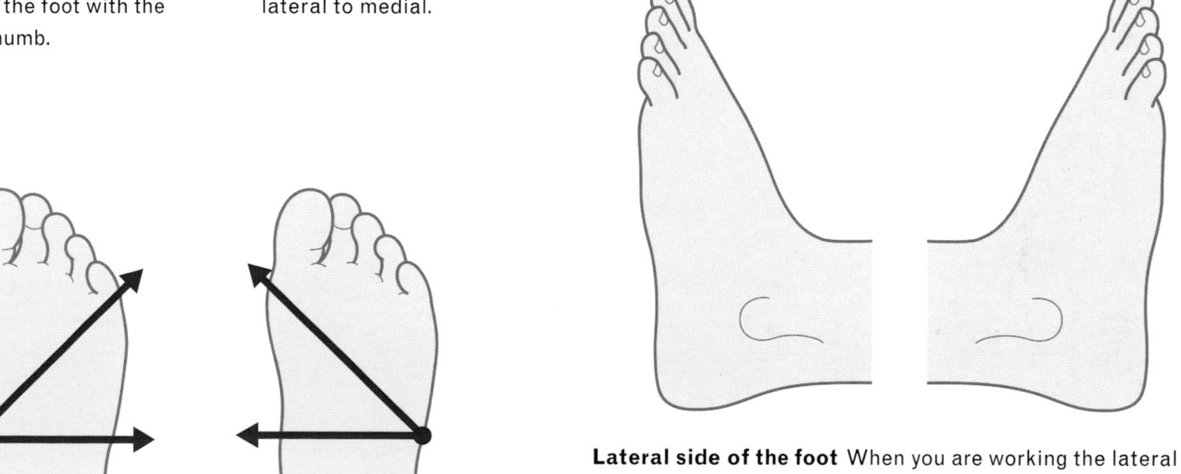

Lateral side of the foot When you are working the lateral side of the foot, hold the foot in an upward direction and support the medial side.

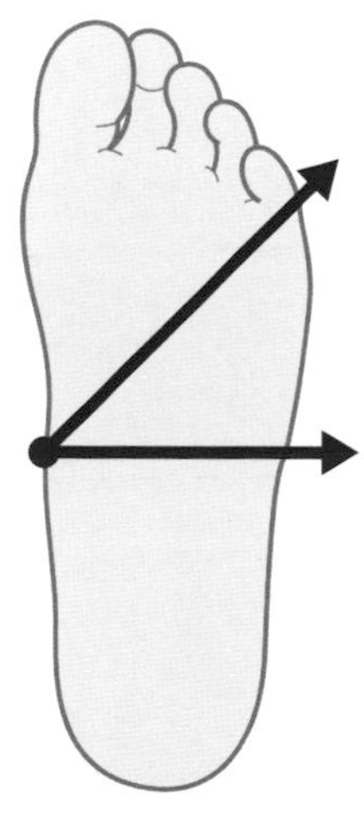

Left foot – medial to lateral When starting to work on the left foot you must support the foot in your right hand and use the left thumb as you work from the medial side to the lateral side of the foot.

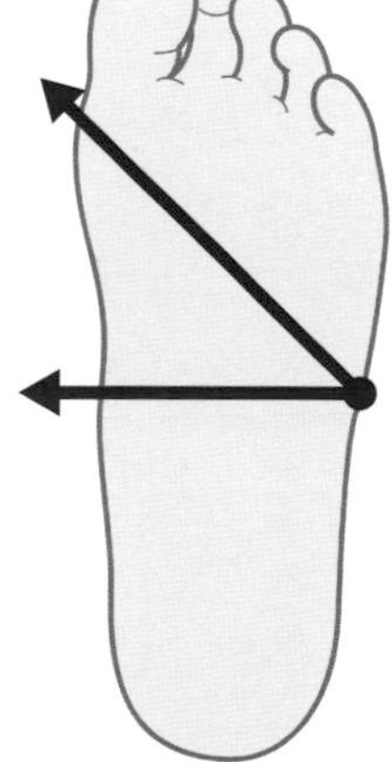

Left foot – lateral to medial As you change direction, you must support the left foot with the right hand and work back from the lateral to the medial side with the right thumb.

SUPPORTING THE FOOT

- Support the top of the foot when working areas above the waist line.
- Support the heel of the foot when working areas below the waist line.

Reflexology techniques

There are four basic techniques used in reflexology: creeping, hooking out, rotating and spinal friction. Practice will build up strength in your hands, especially your thumbs, which are being asked to work in a way that may not be familiar.

Getting the level of pressure just right is simply a matter of experience. The reflexologist should exert enough pressure that the patient feels a reaction in the reflex points, but not so much that the pressure causes pain. As it is necessary to really get into the reflex point, you should aim to exert a firm, consistent pressure with the working thumb and to provide a comfortable support for the foot at all times.

There is no point in working with a 'feather-touch' technique, but you will need to adjust the intensity of pressure according to your patient. A healthy person can generally cope with more pressure than someone who is elderly or unwell. You will also need to use a much firmer pressure when treating, for example, the feet of a tall, strong man than for the delicate feet of a five-year-old child. This is just a question of common sense.

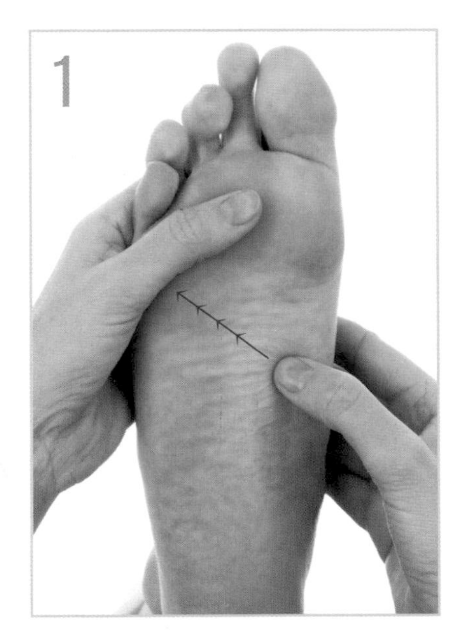

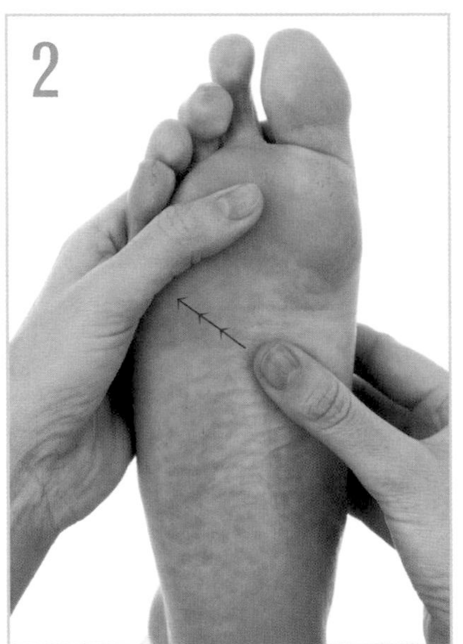

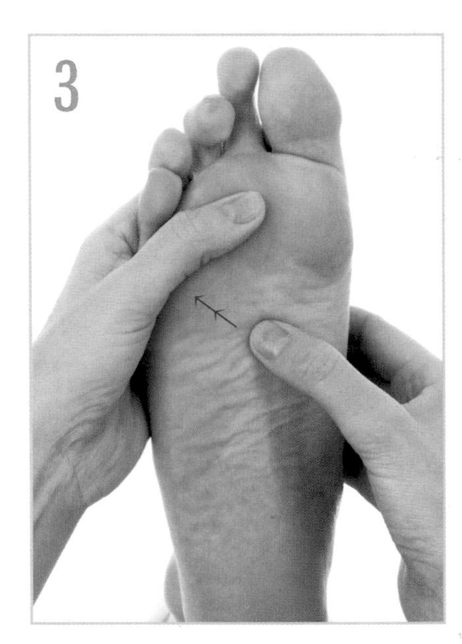

Creeping This is a forward creeping movement of the thumb, bending from the first joint of the thumb. The movement takes time to acquire because it is unusual for the thumb to work in this way. Practice is required to build up sufficient muscle power in your thumb to be able to apply appropriate pressure. After all, your thumbs have never been called on to work in this way before.

The creeping movement is always forwards, never backwards. Work with the flat pad, but keep your thumb flexed and then relaxed as you move across the foot in tiny methodical movements (the action resembles the movement of a caterpillar). Don't rotate in circles or hold a deep pressure for any length of time on any reflex point.

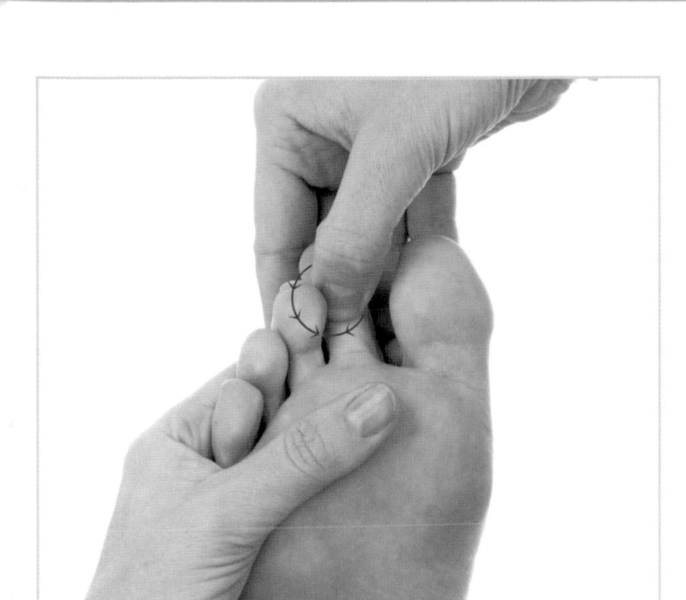

Rotating This is used when certain reflex points need extra stimulation. Place the flat pad of your thumb on the reflex point and rotate it inwards, using small but firm movements. Keep the pressure up for several seconds for the greatest benefit.

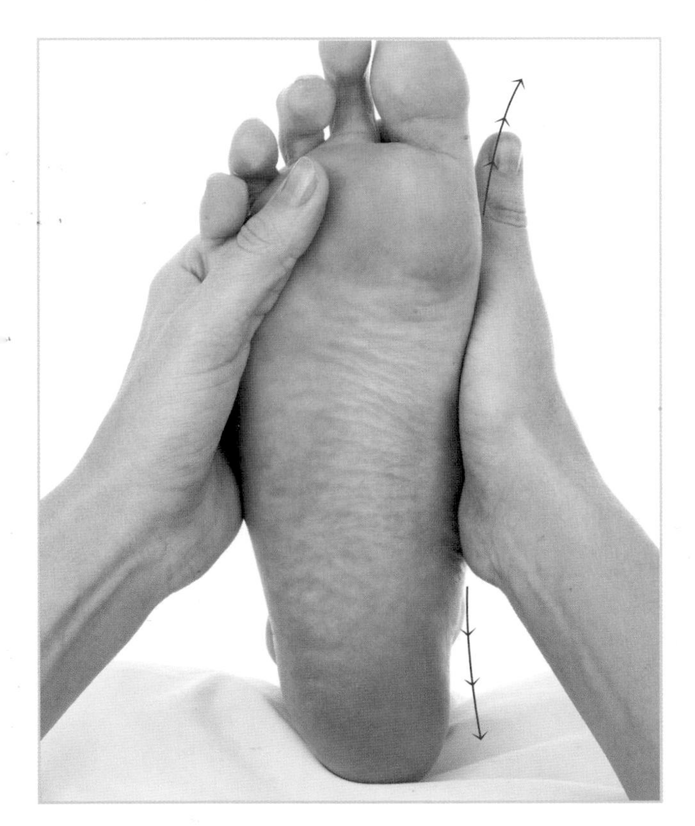

Spinal friction This is a special technique for stimulating and warming the spinal column. Place the palm of your hand on the medial edge of the foot in line with the big toe. Rub your hand vigorously up and down.

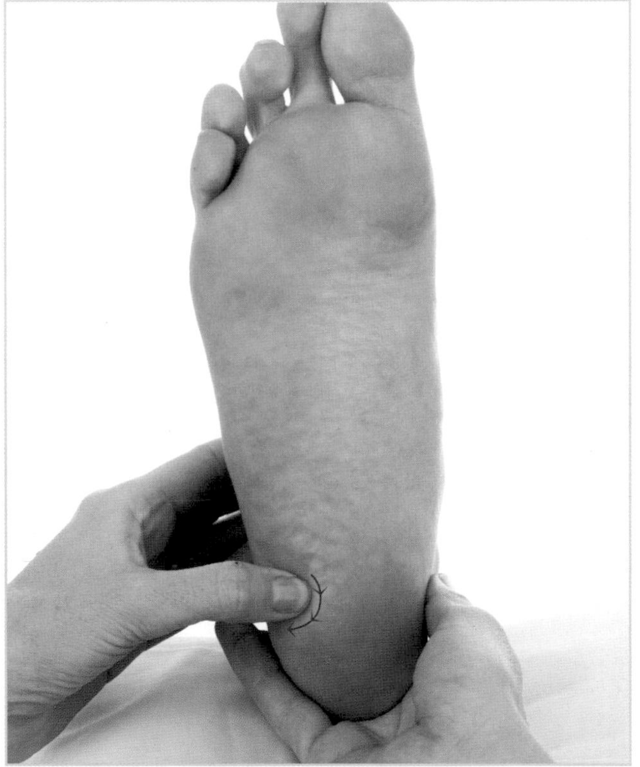

Hooking out Use this technique to stimulate the reflex of the ileo-caecal valve (the valve that joins the large and small intestines). The reflex point is on the lateral edge of the right foot only. Using your left thumb, press firmly on this point, then use the flat of your thumb to make an outward hooking movement in the shape of the letter J.

Relaxing the foot

These exercises are used to enhance relaxation and give the foot maximum movement. They make a good start and end to a treatment session, but are also very soothing mid-session if a specific system in the body creates extra sensitivities in the feet, which may cause a little discomfort to the patient. These exercises are good for students in training too, as they help them to become accustomed to handling feet and to maintaining contact with the patient through the treatment.

Side-to-side relaxation

Right foot

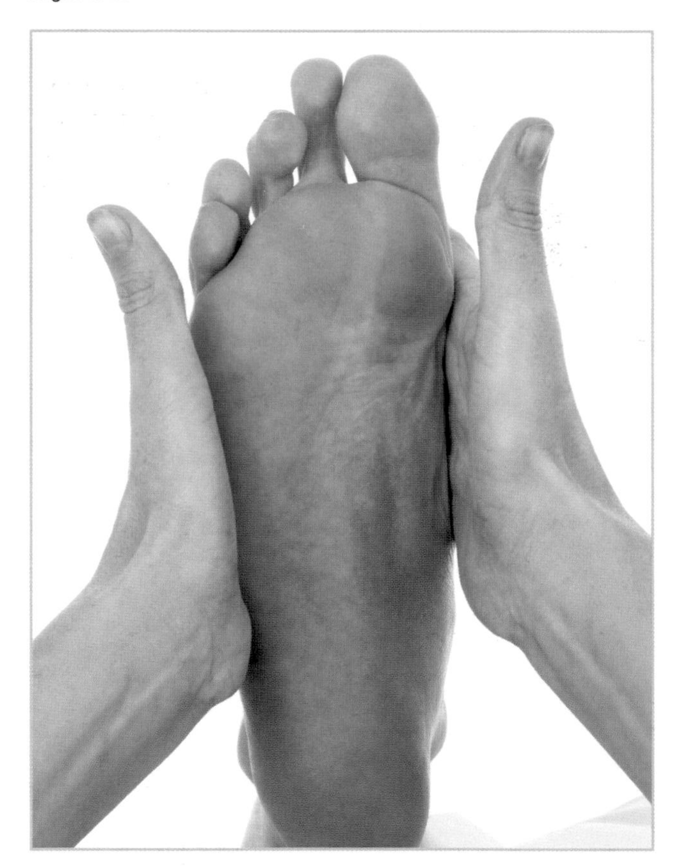

1 Supporting the right foot at the top, use a rocking, side-to-side movement – the foot should move quite swiftly.

Left foot

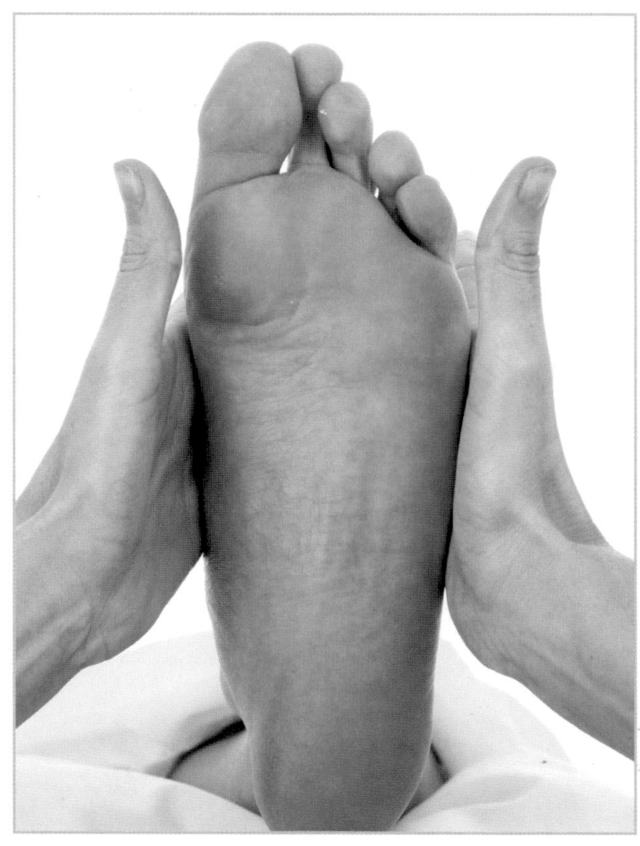

2 Use exactly the same technique when you are working on the left foot, supporting the foot at the top and using a rocking movement.

Diaphragm relaxation

This is a great relaxant of the diaphragm muscle, producing slow, rhythmic breathing. It is recommended to start your treatment session.

Right foot
Medial to lateral

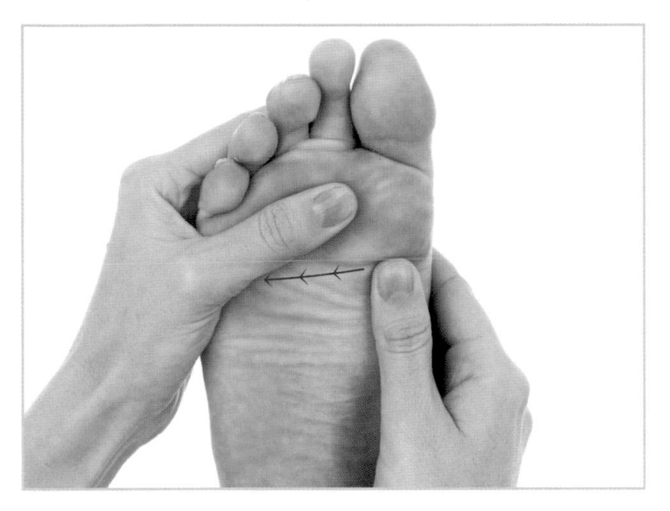

1 Supporting the right foot with your left hand, place your right thumb on the start of the diaphragm line. As you move the thumb from the medial to the lateral side of the foot, bend the toes downwards towards your thumb.

Right foot
Lateral to medial

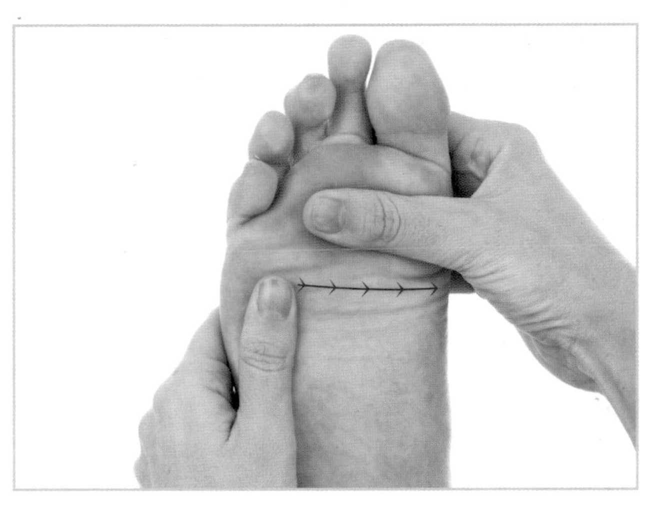

2 Place your left thumb on the diaphragm line as indicated. As you move the thumb from the lateral to the medial side of the foot, bend the toes downwards towards your thumb. At no time should your thumb leave the surface of the foot.

Diaphragm relaxation

Left foot
Medial to lateral

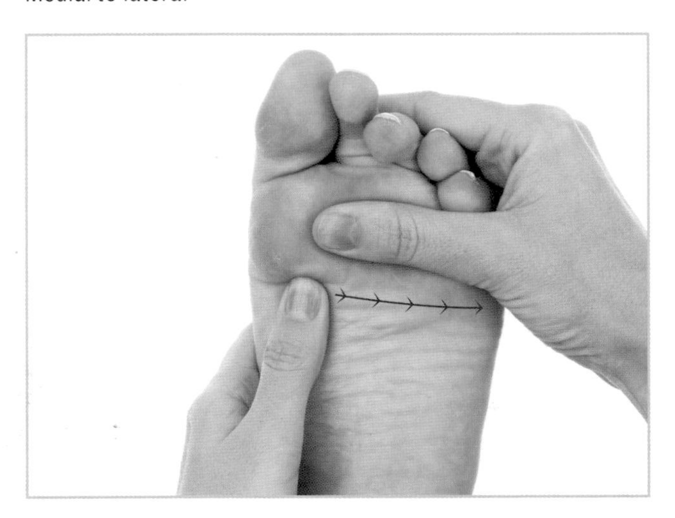

1 Supporting the left foot with your right hand, place your left thumb on the medial edge of the diaphragm line and move it to the lateral edge, bending the toes downwards towards your thumb.

Left foot
Lateral to medial

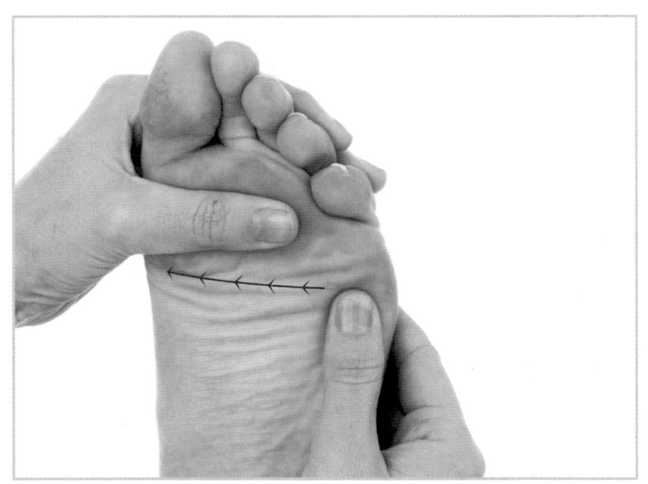

2 Supporting the left foot with your left hand, place your right thumb on the diaphragm line as indicated and move it towards the medial edge, bending the toes downward towards your thumb.

Metatarsal kneading

This is a combined movement using both hands, so your two hands must work in harmony with each other.

Right foot

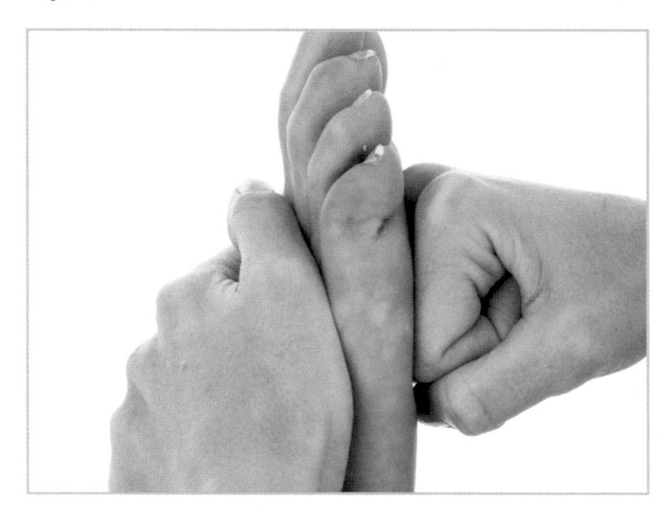

1 Place your right fist on the plantar side of the right foot and place your left hand over the dorsal side of the foot, using a pushing movement from the plantar side.

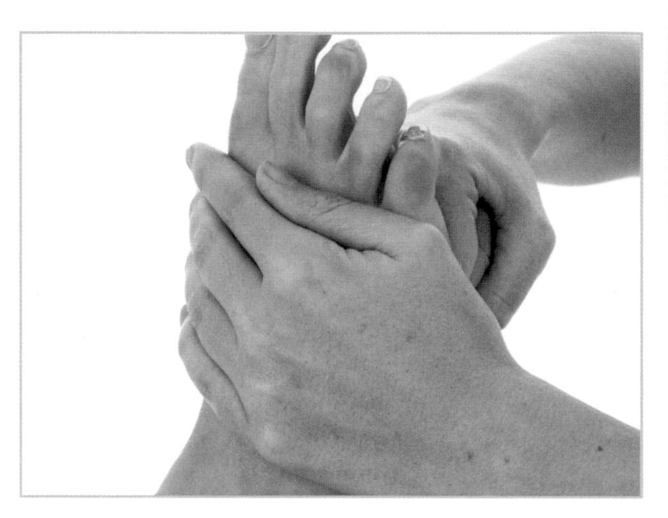

2 As you push the foot from the plantar side, use a gentle squeezing movement from the dorsal side to create a kneading technique.

Metatarsal kneading

Left foot

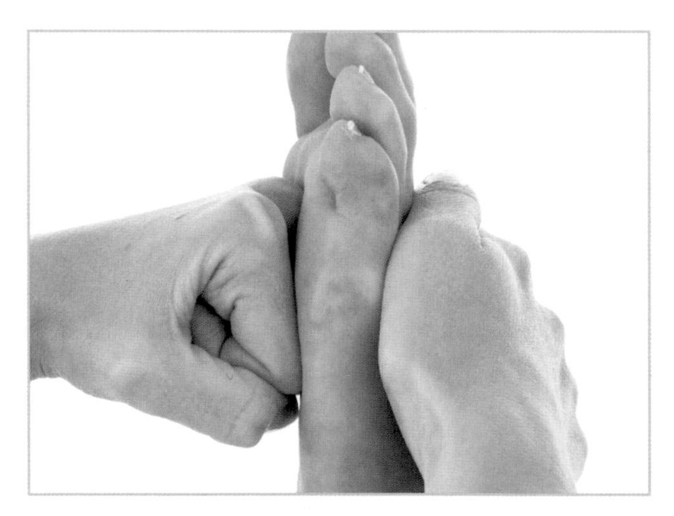

1 Place your left fist on the plantar side of the left foot and place your right hand over the dorsal side of the foot, using a pushing movement from the plantar side.

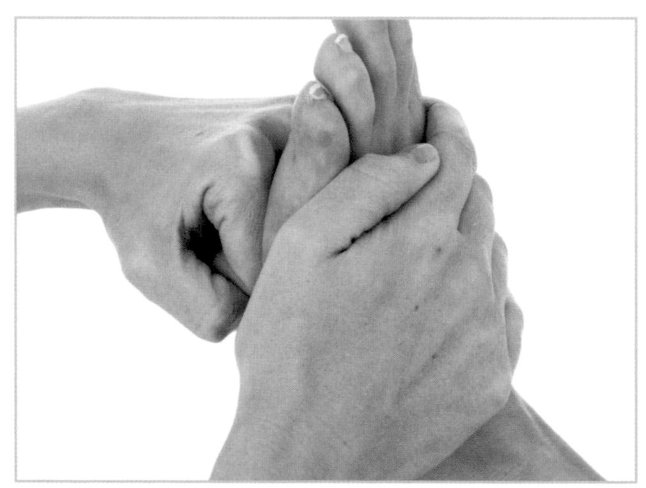

2 As you push the foot from the plantar side, use a gentle squeezing movement from the dorsal side to create a kneading technique.

Ankle freeing

Ankle freeing is an excellent exercise for loosening up your patient's stiff ankles.

Right foot

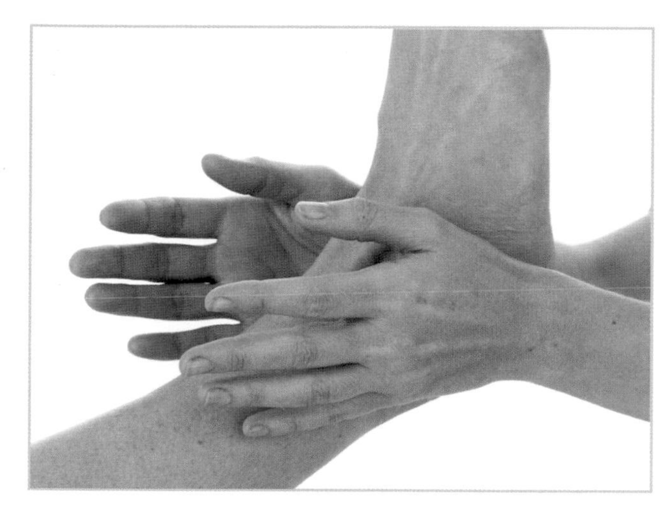

1 Position the pads of your thumb joints in front of the ankle bones of the right foot and rock the foot using a side-to-side motion.

Left foot

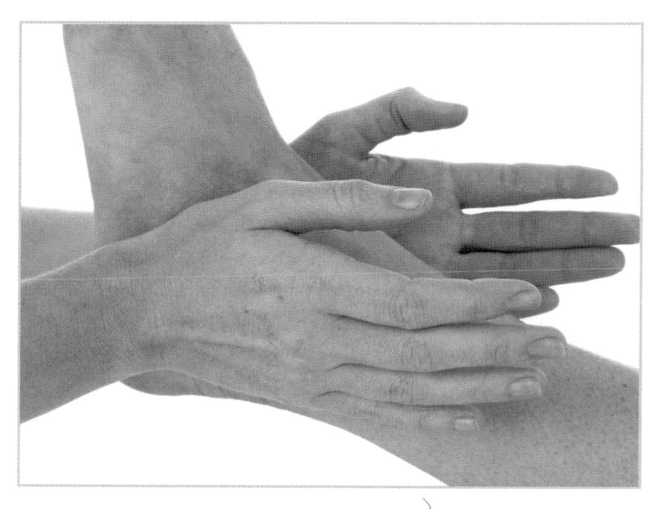

2 Position the pads of your thumb joints in front of the ankle bones of the left foot and rock the foot using a side-to-side motion.

Undergrip

This technique provides great relief when treating someone with swollen legs and ankles.

Right foot

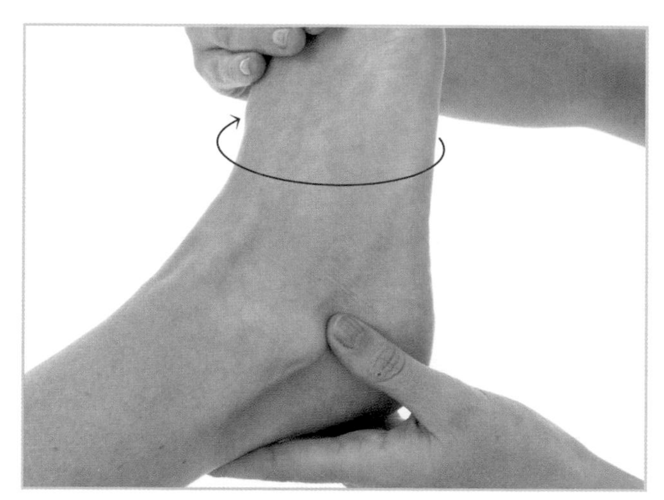

1 Place your left hand under the ankle, with your thumb on the lateral edge of the foot.

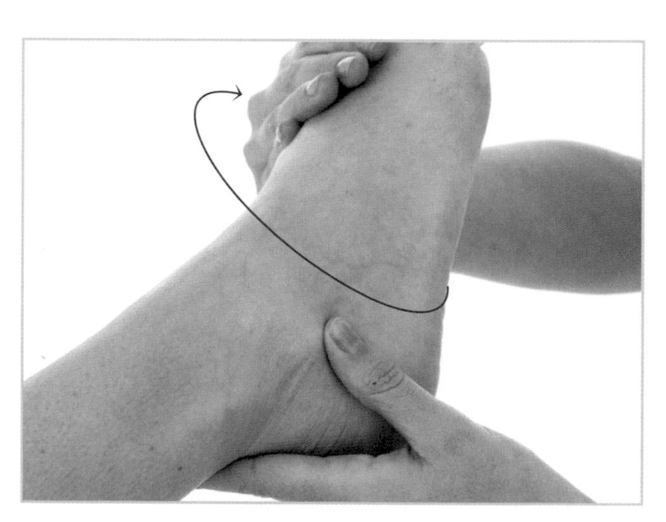

2 Working with your right hand, turn the foot in an inward direction, using a light, circling movement.

Undergrip

Left foot

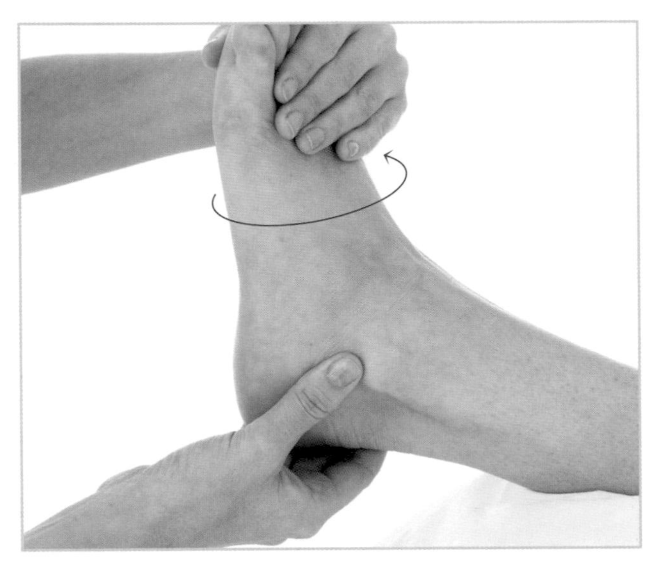

1 Repeat the same exercise, this time placing your right hand under the ankle and working with your left hand.

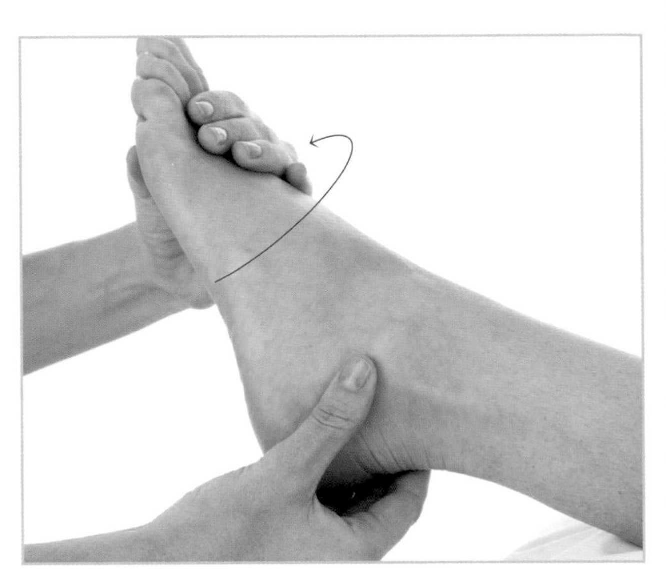

2 Turn the left foot in an inward direction, using a light, circling movement.

Overgrip

This technique is another excellent way of relieving swollen legs and ankles.

Right foot

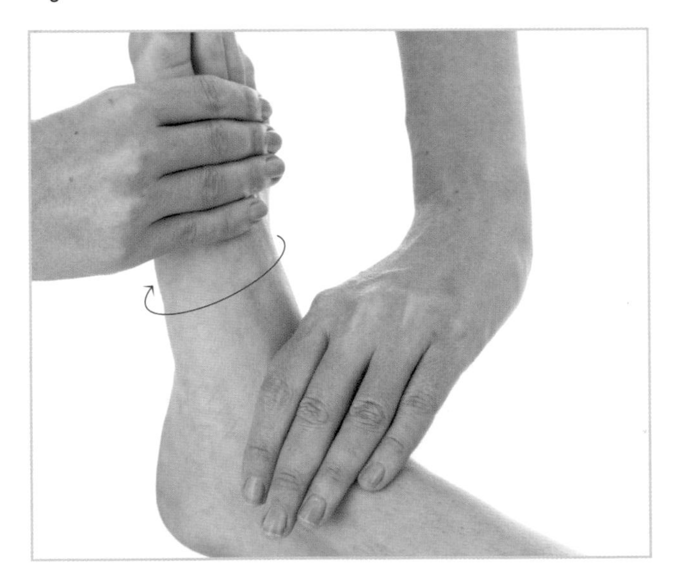

1 Place your left hand over the top of the right ankle, making sure that the thumb of your left hand is on the lateral edge of the foot. Turn the foot in an inward direction, being sure to use a light, circling movement.

Left foot

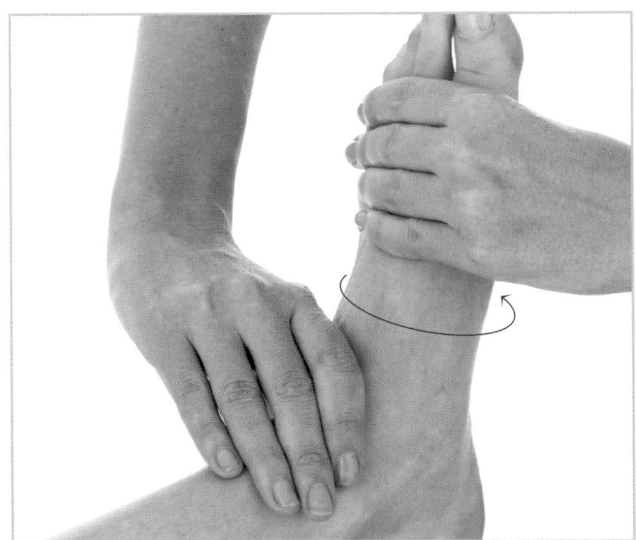

2 Reverse the procedure, placing your right hand over the top of the left ankle and rotating the foot inwards as for the right foot.

Foot moulding

Right foot

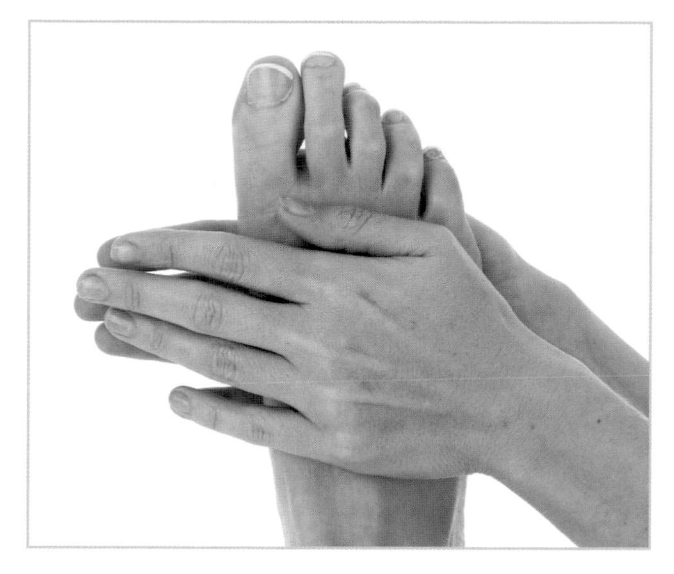

1 Support the right foot from the lateral edge and sandwich the foot between your two hands.

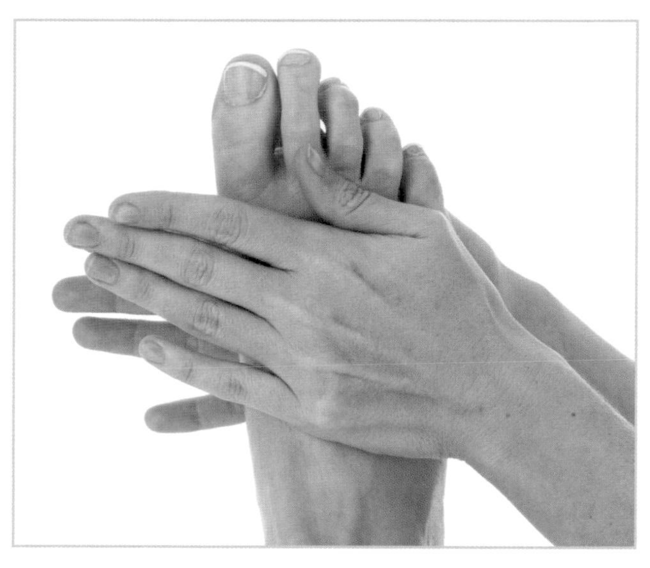

2 Gently rotate both hands. Your hands must be in tune with each other, so the movement resembles the motions of the wheels of a train.

Foot moulding

Left foot

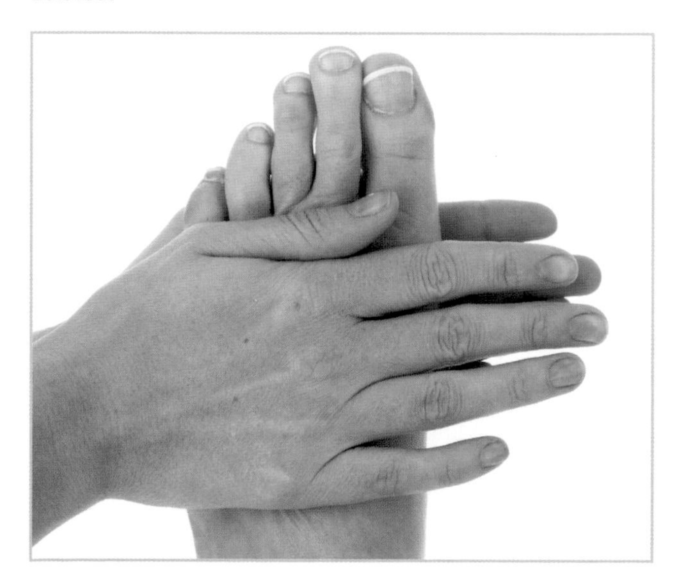

1 Support the left foot from the lateral edge and sandwich the foot between your two hands.

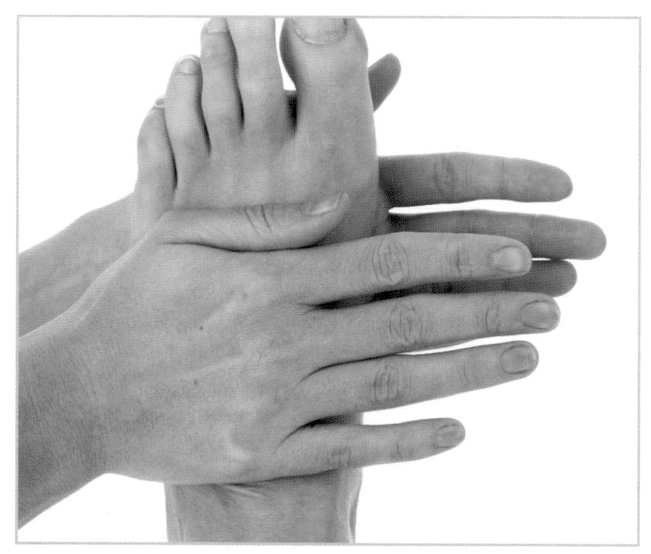

2 Gently rotate both hands. Your hands must be in tune with each other, so the movement resembles the motions of the wheels of a train.

Rib cage relaxation

Right foot

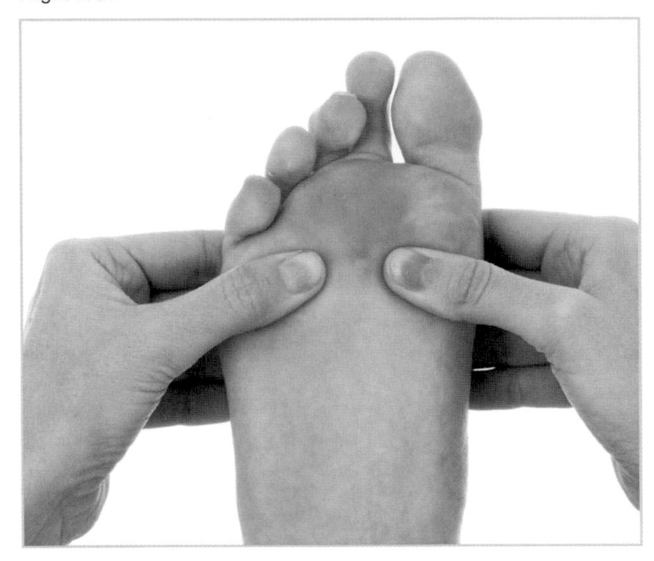

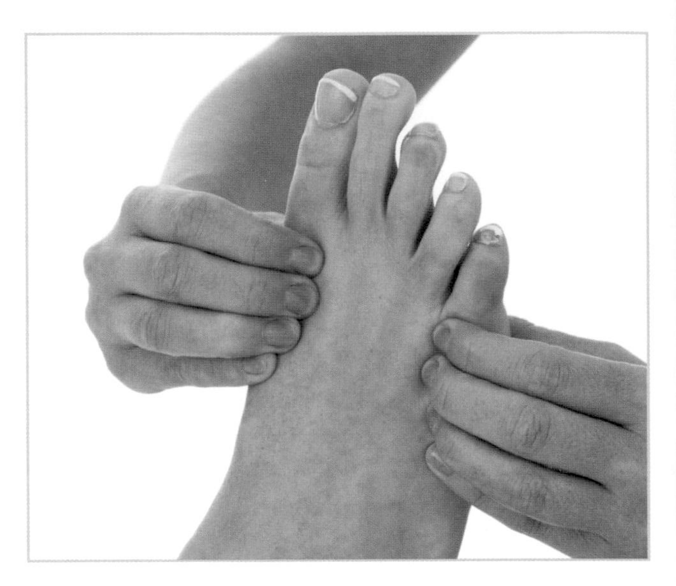

1 Apply pressure to the plantar side of the foot using your two thumbs.

2 At the same time, use all the fingers of both hands to creep around the dorsal side of the foot.

Rib cage relaxation

Left foot

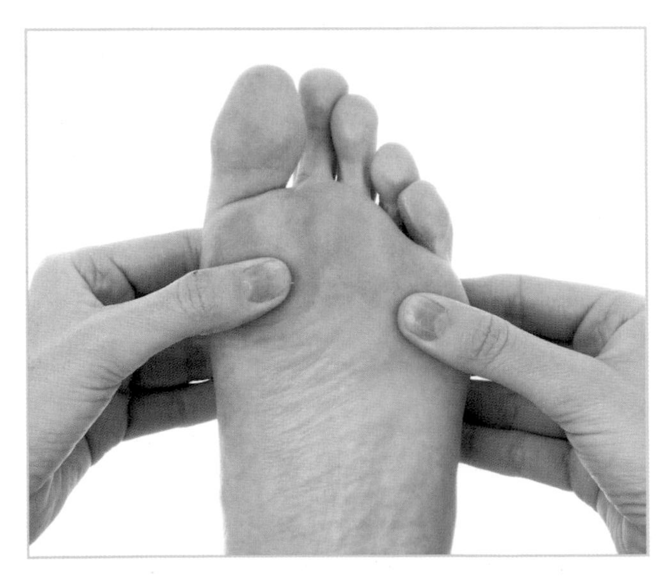

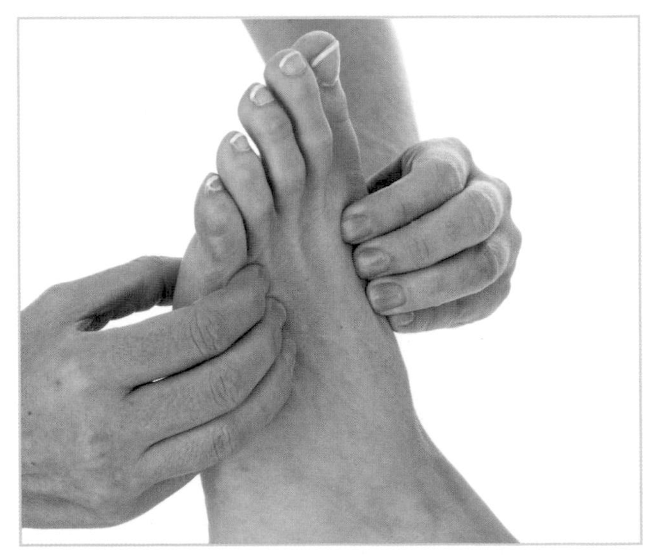

1 Apply pressure to the plantar side of the left foot with your two thumbs.

2 At the same time, use all the fingers of both hands to creep around the dorsal side of the foot.

Reactions to treatment

It is not unusual to get side-effects following, and sometimes during, a reflexology treatment session. It is essential that both you and the patient are well aware of exactly what is going on within the body when these symptoms occur.

Sensations during treatment

As you apply pressure to the reflex points in the feet, the patient may experience a sharp pricking sensation, like a very pointed fingernail 'digging into the foot' (although reflexology practitioners should not have long fingernails, of course). This sharp reaction reveals that all is not well in that part of the body; there is congestion, inflammation or tension, which causes the reflexes to react.

Some sensitive individuals actually feel a 'tingling sensation' in their body as the reflexes are stimulated, while others feel heat or tingling sensations in their hands. Occasionally very stressed patients are overcome by emotions and shed a few tears; others feel a deep sense of relaxation and it is not uncommon for pain levels to be reduced within the very first treatment session.

When treating patients with sinus conditions there is often an immediate release of mucus from the nose as the sinus reflexes are worked upon, bringing instant relief from pain and congestion in the nose.

HELP WITH ALLEVIATING REACTIONS

You may like to advise your patients to drink plenty of pure, bottled spring water and take a large dose of vitamin C (1 g would not be too much on this occasion) following a treatment session, particularly if they suffer from irritable bowel syndrome, arthritis, asthma, migraine or sinusitis. Vitamin C aids detoxification and the extra fluids help flush the toxic waste through the urinary system. This will lessen the possible side-effects of the treatment.

Side-effects following treatment

First, it is worth stressing that there are no dangers in treating with reflexology and it is impossible to make a situation within the body permanently worse.

Symptoms are signals of changes and following a treatment it is not unusual for the patient to discover that symptoms have become exacerbated. Back pain may be worse, for example, or there may be increased frequency of bowel actions. If the patient suffers from a chest infection, quantities of mucus may be coughed up. These are all excellent signs of a healing crisis.

What is a healing crisis? Any build-up or residue of toxins in the body causes a 'stagnation' in one or other vital area and this in turn leads to congestion. In aiming to improve circulation and help the body rid itself of these unwanted substances, reflexologists stimulate the body's systems. This can result in a short-lived worsening of symptoms or manifestation of new symptoms. The same reactions occur with herbal preparations, homeopathic support, fasts and colonic irrigations.

In no way has the patient's condition become worse. A healing crisis has simply been reached as the body, under stimulation, throws off toxins at an accelerated pace. I have known patients come out in a rash following a session, as the skin, a great organ of elimination, provided the means through which the body rid itself of toxins. A healing crisis is proof enough that reflexology works and should not last more than 48 hours.

Some side-effects are very welcome. For example, patients may sleep for many hours following a session, or their general sleep pattern may improve.

When we take medication, we are simply suppressing the problem and eventually it will 'burst through' and express itself in another form. Using complementary medicines and practices, particularly reflexology, means treating the root cause of disease and trying to restore natural balance and harmony, improve nerve and blood supply and help the body to detoxify itself. Once cleansing and relaxation have occurred, the body can heal itself.

It is unusual for side-effects to continue after the first couple of treatments. Thereafter, the patient's condition should improve little by little until, after between six and eight sessions, it has improved significantly.

The aims of reflexology

Reflexology is more than just applying pressure the right way in the right place. A practitioner needs common sense and – something gained through experience – good judgement. It is important to know what cannot be achieved as well as what can be, and to be equipped to answer a patient's questions.

First of all, there are some important do's and don'ts that you should bear in mind. Always be realistic in what you hope to achieve and avoid offering a cure or attempting to diagnose medical conditions.

Be realistic in your aims

If you are a practitioner of reflexology, treating patients regularly, you will need to decide for yourself what your specific aims are and the relief that you expect to be able to achieve for an individual patient. It is obvious that if you are treating a patient who has been confined to a wheelchair for many years suffering from multiple sclerosis, and who perhaps has acute and frequent bladder infections, that the most you would be able to offer would be to improve their general circulation, maybe to reduce the number of bladder infections and generally give them a feeling of wellbeing, improving their quality of life. There is no way a reflexologist, however talented, is going to be able to get that patient to walk again, or make the MS vanish.

Similarly, it would be very unlikely that a middle-aged patient with a long history of asthma, who since childhood has been treated with steroidal inhalers in order to maintain some quality of life, could be restored to full health. Generally speaking, long-term sufferers from asthma have impairment of lung function and often an enlarged heart, which will have been under strain for years in coping with a limited oxygen supply during acute attacks. You could expect to achieve, however, a reduction in the frequency of attacks, and attacks of lesser severity. On the other hand, if you were treating a young man who had strained his back while carrying out some heavy physical work, you could anticipate achieving total relief for him.

Take a realistic approach to the treatment of patients and understand that, although reflexology is a wonderfully beneficial treatment for a host of physical conditions, it is not a panacea.

Don't offer a cure

Professing to be able to 'cure' anything is a bold statement. The aim of the reflexology practitioner is to be able to relieve pain, improve bodily functions and help the body to eliminate its waste more efficiently, particularly through the liver. 'Curing' really means restoring the body to a near perfect state permanently. There is no treatment anywhere, in either the orthodox or the complementary medical fields, that can offer this.

Don't diagnose or prescribe

There is much confusion regarding diagnosis. Reflexology is not able to *diagnose* diseases within the body. However, what the practitioner can do is to find that a certain part of the foot reveals a sensitivity and this in turn indicates that there is congestion, inflammation and tension in the corresponding part of the body. Frequently, by treating the sensitive areas, the inflammation is relieved, tension removed and great improvement is achieved in the functioning of the system that was under duress.

When a sensitivity is found in the foot, it is absolutely wrong to jump to conclusions as to what it indicates. For example, if Mrs Smith's liver reflex points reveal a great sensitivity, do not instantly assume that she must be suffering from a liver disease. This is diagnosing, particularly if you extrapolate to 'I think perhaps this patient is suffering from hepatitis or cirrhosis of the liver'. A sensitivity in the liver reflex can be caused by many factors. It could be due to an over-indulgence of alcohol in the days before a treatment session, or a meal with a heavy fat content (among other things, it is the liver's job to process alcohol and fat). It could also indicate a high cholesterol level, and if you are treating a patient with angina or coronary artery disease, this could well be the cause of the sensitivity.

To give another example, you might pick up a great sensitivity in the heart reflex area. The position of the

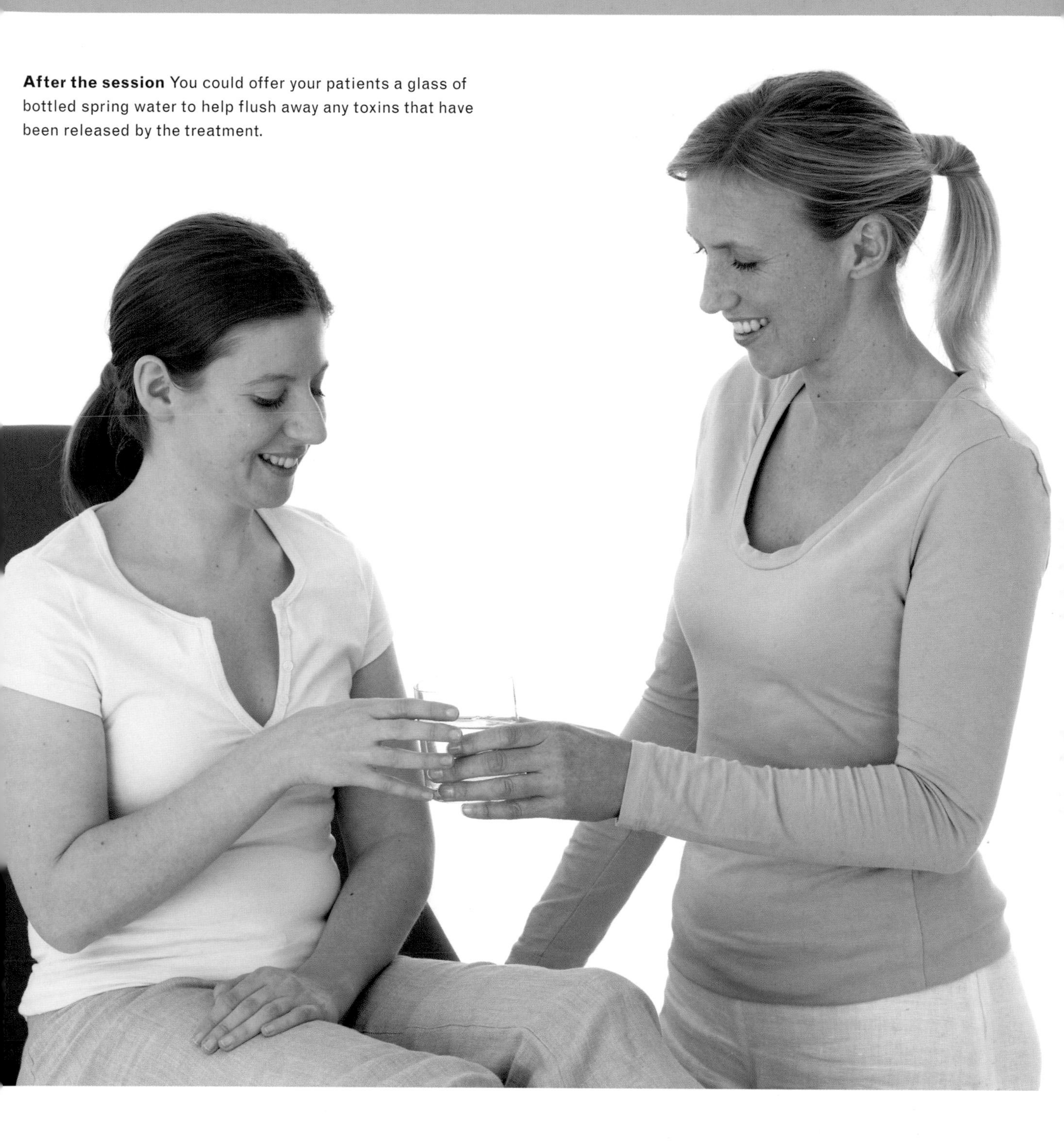

After the session You could offer your patients a glass of bottled spring water to help flush away any toxins that have been released by the treatment.

heart reflex points within the foot also link up to the muscles within the chest (such as the pectoral muscles) as well as the heart muscle itself. Chest muscles can easily become over-strained simply through heavy lifting, gardening or even perhaps carrying a toddler on one side for too long. It would be completely unprofessional to jump to the conclusion that a patient now has a 'heart condition' and it would be totally wrong and unethical to make such suggestions.

Always bear in mind that a reflexology practitioner is in no way able to diagnose these precise problems. Only doctors are able to diagnose, for only they have the access to x-ray machines, equipment for blood tests, scanning devices and so on.

Some common questions answered

Practitioners as well as patients often need reassurance about certain aspects of reflexology. In my many years of experience I have found that the following questions crop up time and again.

How often should patients be treated?

It is totally safe to treat patients daily, although it is unlikely, for practical and financial reasons, that the average person will be able to attend for a daily session. However, a member of your family or a friend may be able to enjoy a daily treatment session and this is particularly beneficial when treating acute back conditions such as sciatica, lumbago, disc lesions and so on. It is also beneficial to treat asthmatic sufferers every day in order to try to relax their lungs and heart function and to benefit their general health.

In general, the average person responds very well in six sessions conducted on a weekly basis. Some people take longer, and chronic states usually take a little longer to improve than acute problems. The best approach is to give treatment sessions weekly until the patient remarks that their pain or symptoms have greatly improved; at that stage lengthen the appointment gap to two weeks. If good results are maintained, it is safe to wait a month before the next treatment. If, after the month's gap, all symptoms and pain have failed to return, it is a very strong indication that a good result has been achieved.

After this, many people like to come back – say, every six weeks – for 'maintenance treatment' and find that this keeps them in tip-top condition for years. Others prefer to have their treatment sessions, gain the maximum possible improvement in their health and then stop treatment altogether and just see how their health continues. Patients may return to their original practitioner after a gap of several years. It is up to the patient to decide.

Can reflexology be dangerous?

No. There are no dangers attached to reflexology, as practitioners are only treating a reflex point in the foot (or hand) that links to a corresponding part of the body. They are not applying any undue pressure on any other part of the body, or manipulating it in any way. They are not giving the patient any medications to ingest or even putting any oils on the feet that could perhaps affect the skin. Effective though reflexology is, there is not even any need to get permission from the patient's doctor or anybody else involved in the medical profession before commencing treatment, the methods are so very safe.

It is totally safe to treat everyone, regardless of age. I have treated infants under a year old and my oldest patient was 99 years old.

Is it safe to treat a pregnant woman?

Yes. Pregnancy is a natural function, not an illness, and most women find that reflexology is of tremendous assistance in helping to prevent fluid retention which causes feet and hands to swell uncomfortably, to keep blood pressure normal and to avoid or ease back pain.

I would refrain from giving treatment to a woman in the early weeks of pregnancy if she has a history of frequent miscarriage. I would be much happier to wait until she was safely past the 14th week. When a miscarriage does occur, patients go through a period of grief and it is quite normal to look for somebody to blame for the miscarriage; it would be very unfortunate if reflexology were to be mistakenly linked to the cause of the miscarriage. See pages 208–213 for more on reflexology during pregnancy.

And what about post-operative patients?

Reflexology is very effective in countering the shock and distress associated with surgery. Surgery also has a very debilitating effect on the immune system, and reflexology can be of benefit in restoring the immune system.

Should you treat patients with cancer?

Many books on reflexology warn against treating patients who have cancer but I have treated cancer patients for years, with only good results. Reflexology can not cure

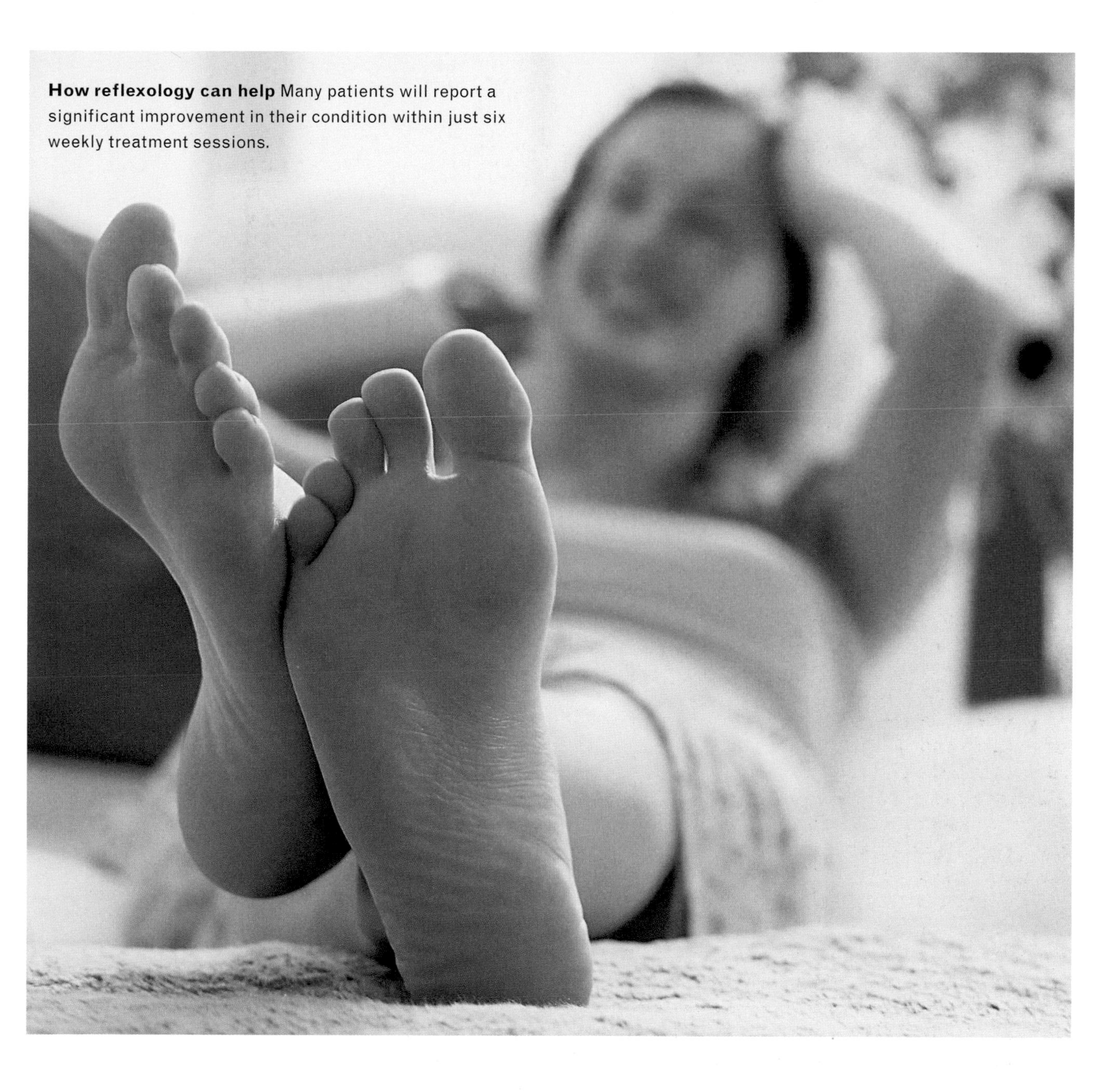

How reflexology can help Many patients will report a significant improvement in their condition within just six weekly treatment sessions.

cancer, but I have found that patients have all expressed how much better they have felt. What they experience is a great sense of relief and, I think, a freedom from anxiety. See pages 220–223 and 228–229 for advice on treating patients with cancer and forms of terminal illness.

Does reflexology always work?

Reflexology can help in nearly all cases. I have found in my years of experience in treating people with all manner of illness that only about 6 per cent of people fail to respond to reflexology treatment.

There is no obvious reason why improvement does not occur in these cases. It may be a simple condition you have treated many times before, but one patient may simply not respond. (Conversely, a complicated, long-term illness can respond dramatically to reflexology after just one or two treatment sessions.) There really seems to be no rhyme or reason why these oddities occur.

In general, people who attend at least six weekly sessions do get good results. There are very few people who can honestly say at the end of the course of treatments that reflexology has done absolutely nothing for them.

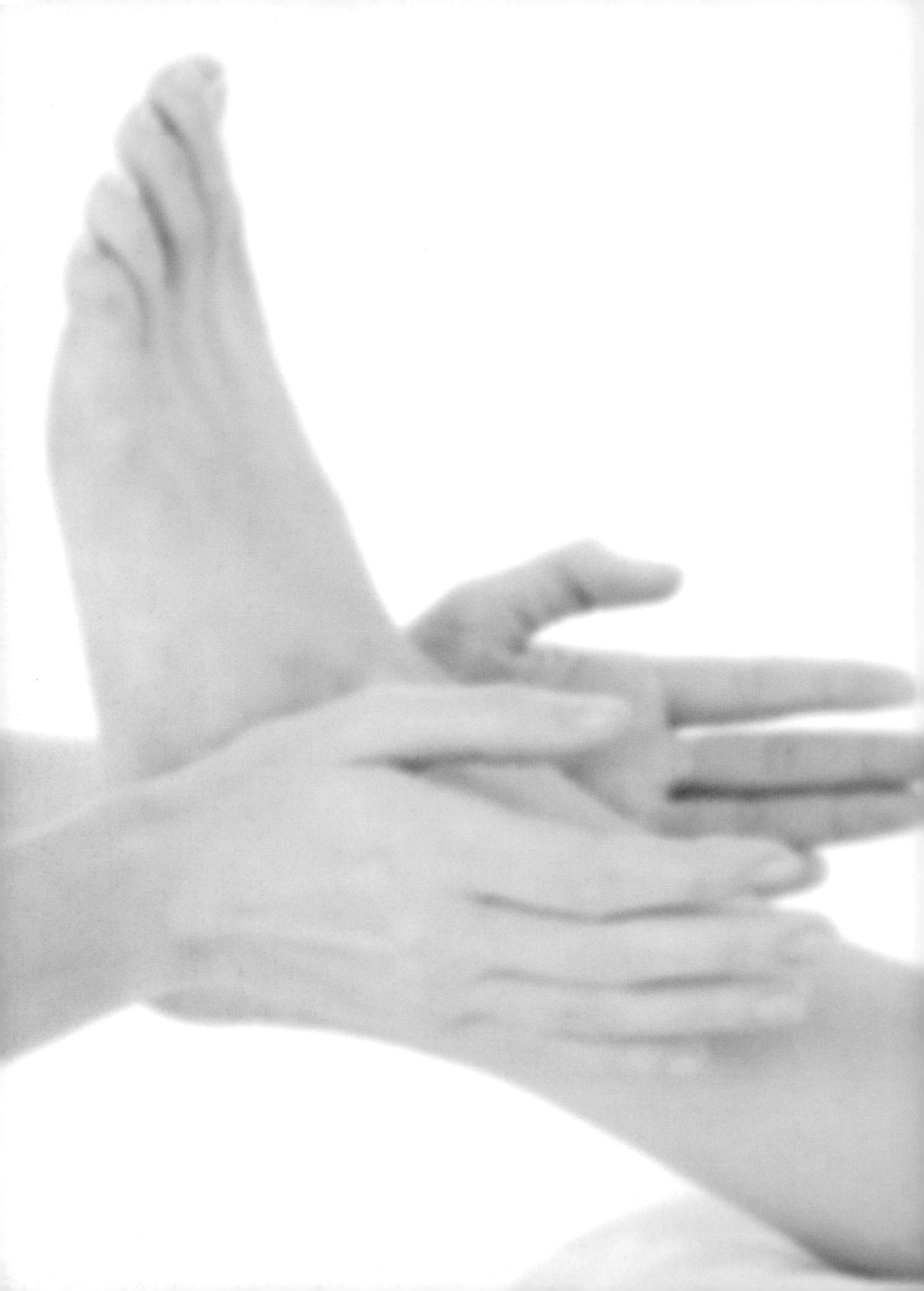

Body systems

It is essential for reflexologists to understand the anatomy and physiology of the human body and to know where the reflexes for every organ, gland, structure and function reside in the feet. They should also have a knowledge of disease and disharmony, plus an understanding of drugs and their effects upon the body. This chapter explains how the various functions of the human body work and how each body system can be treated by reflexology.

Cells, tissues and skin

Cells are the building blocks out of which all life evolves. They divide and gather together to form tissue with specific functions, creating blood, bone, muscle and skin. Tissues group together to form organs, such as the heart, stomach or liver. Each of the organs is an integral component of an overall system. For example, the heart functions as the pump for the body's circulatory system.

Cells

The cell is the smallest structure of the human body but ultimately controls all the processes that define life, including movement, respiration, digestion and reproduction. It is amazing to contemplate that everything about our body, including the colour of our eyes and hair, our approximate height and even our genetic strengths and weaknesses, are influenced by our cellular make-up.

Each of us, a unique individual, begins as a single cell that divides and multiplies, our constituent cells taking on specialist forms and functions. Cells are so minute that most are invisible to the human eye. The female sex cell, the largest cell in the human body, is still only the size of the full stop at the end of this paragraph.

A cell consists of a jelly-like material called cytoplasm contained within a plasma membrane. This membrane protects the cell and regulates the passage of materials in and out of the cell itself.

The nucleus

Within the cytoplasm is the cell's nucleus, which is itself surrounded by a membrane that appears darker than the surrounding cytoplasm. The nucleus is the control centre of the cell and contains chromatin, which forms chromosomes during cell division. A human cell contains 46 chromosomes. Each is a long, coiled molecule of DNA and together they contain about 30,000 genes. Each gene has a minute segment of DNA that controls cellular function by governing the synthesis or manufacture of protein. Proteins have many vital functions in the body; some catalyse biochemical reactions to produce energy or growth, others have structural, signalling or immune functions. Every cell in the body has a nucleus, with the exception of mature red blood cells.

The organelles

The cell also contains a wide variety of smaller units called cytoplasmic structures, or organelles. These play specific roles that ensure the proper functioning of the body. Different types of organelles include:

- **Mitochondria**: These are concerned with releasing energy from food molecules, in a process called cellular respiration.
- **Endoplasmic reticulum**: This is involved in the manufacture and transport of enzymes, chemical activity and protein within the cell.
- **Golgi apparatus**: This organelle produces glycoproteins and secretory enzymes and transports and stores lipids. It also processes proteins and other products of the cell to make them ready either for storage, transporting elsewhere within the cell or secreting out of the cell.
- **Cilia**: These tiny hair-like organelles project from the surfaces of many cells, including the cells lining the respiratory passages, for example, and help move materials outside the cells.

How reflexology can help

Every illness of the body involves some disorder of the associated cells. However, the reflexology routine does not target cells specifically, because contact is made constantly with the cells and tissues whenever any reflex is worked.

Cancer is a condition specific to cell disorders. Britain's Association of Reflexologists has reported very positive findings about how reflexology can improve quality of life and reduce pain and nausea in cancer sufferers (see 'Clinical evidence', page 22). For more information on helping cancer sufferers, see pages 220–223.

Cell The basic unit of all living organisms can reproduce itself exactly. Each cell is bounded by a cell membrane of lipids and proteins that controls the passage of substances in and out of the cell.

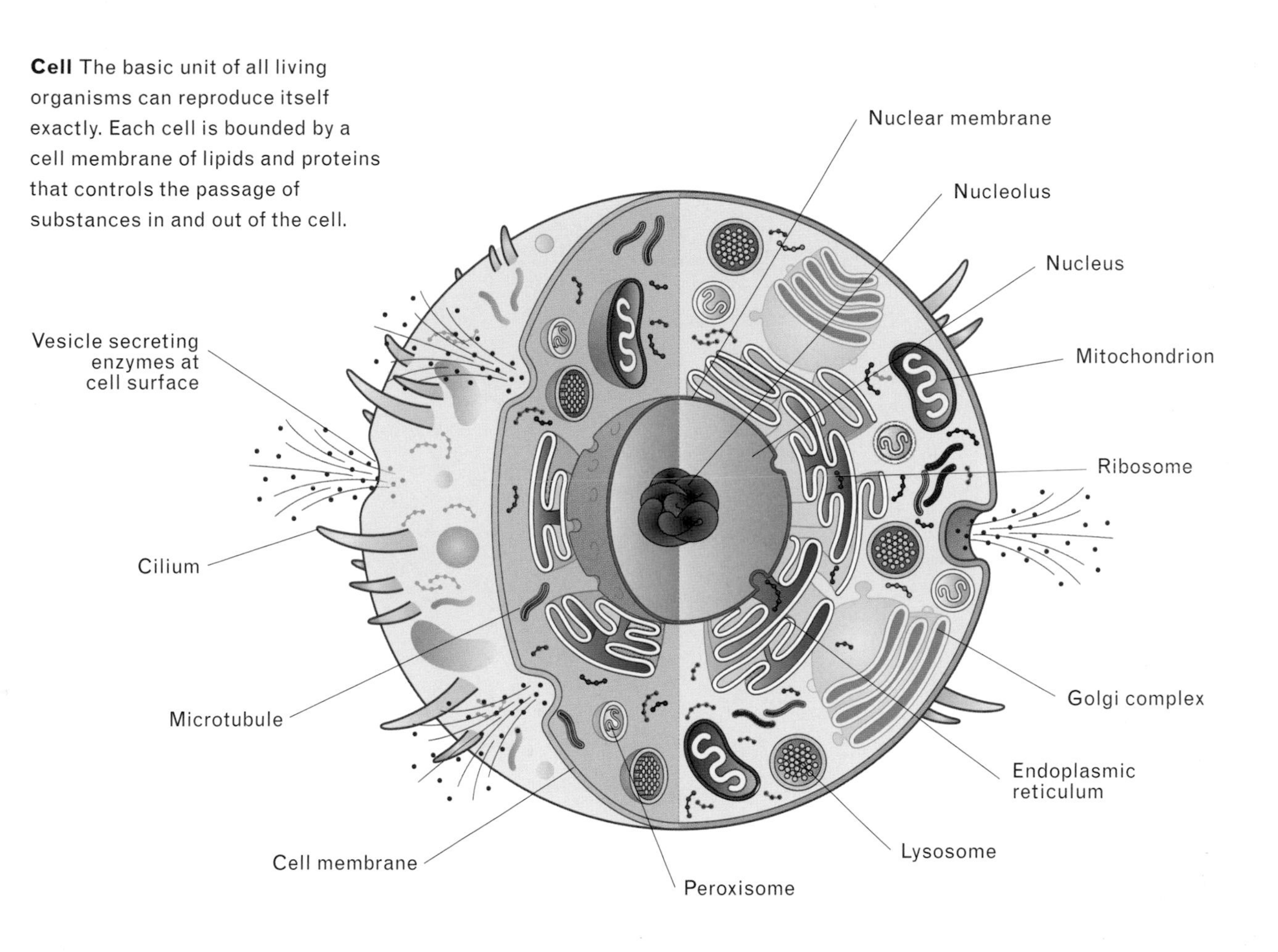

THE BUILDING BLOCKS OF LIFE

Cells group together in a hierarchical structure that, in increasing complexity, makes up the human body:

Structure	Example
Tissue: This is a group of cells with similar structure and function.	Muscle and nerve tissue
Organ: This is the term for a collection of different tissues.	The stomach, which is made up of involuntary muscle, blood, nerves and epithelium that all come together in order to perform a distinct stage of the digestive function.
Body system: This is a group of organs working together and performing a complex set of functions.	The digestive system, in which the mouth, oesophagus, stomach, small intestine, large intestine and associated glands work in concert to process everything we ingest.
Organism: A number of body systems contributes to the life of a single being.	The human body, which is alive and active thanks to the complex interrelated functions of the blood, nervous, musculoskeletal, digestive, respiratory and other systems.

Tissues

The tissues of the body all consist of large numbers of cells, but they vary greatly in form and function. There are four main types of tissue: epithelial tissue, connective tissue, muscle tissue and nervous tissue.

Epithelial tissue

This tissue, also called epithelium, covers surfaces and lines cavities. Its functions are to protect, absorb and secrete. In the respiratory system, for example, epithelial tissue lines our airways. The cells here are equipped with cilia that beat mucus containing trapped dirt and particles away from the lungs. The taste buds in our mouth also consist of epithelium, as do the tubules in our kidneys.

Connective tissue

This forms the packing between organs of the body and, as its name suggests, connects one part of the body to the other. It also supports and protects. The main types of connective tissue are:

- **Connective tissue proper**: This joins body structures, fills spaces between body parts and acts as a reservoir for water and salt.
- **Adipose (fat) tissue**: Consisting of fat cells and acting as an insulator, adipose tissue makes up 20–25 per cent of our body weight. If we are overweight, we tend to carry an excess of it on our buttocks, thighs, abdomen, breasts and upper arms. It is also adipose tissue that cushions our eyeballs and vital organs.
- **Blood and lymph fluid**
- **Lymphoid tissue**: This is found in lymphatic tissues, such as the spleen, lymph nodes, the tonsils and adenoids, the appendix and walls of the intestine.
- **Cartilage**: This is a firm type of connective tissue reinforced by collagen and elastic fibres (see box). There are three types of cartilage. Hyaline cartilage lines the surfaces of the bones at joints, connects the ribs to the sternum (costal cartilage) and forms part of the larynx, bronchi and trachea. Fibrocartilage is found between the vertebrae, in the form of intervertebral discs. Elastic cartilage is rigid but elastic and forms a framework for the pinna or outer part of the ear and the epiglottis, the flap that covers the trachea to prevent food going down the airway.
- **Bone**: Also a form of connective tissue. The skeleton provides support, protection and, together with muscles, moves the body. Bones also produce blood cells (see page 126).

TYPES OF CONNECTIVETISSUE FIBRES

Connective tissue cells are separated by a thick gel, which has microscopic fibres throughout. These fibres can be one of three types:

- **Collagen fibres** are the most abundant. These protein fibres give great strength to structures.
- **Fine reticular fibres** give support to many tissues and organs, such as the kidneys, brain and lymph nodes.
- **Elastic fibres** are an important component of structures that must stretch, for example air sacs and arteries.

Muscle tissue

This sort of tissue is composed of cells that are specialized to contract. We have control over the movement of some, but not all muscle tissue.

- **Skeletal muscle**: This has a striated appearance and comprises the bulk of the body's muscle system. It is attached to the skeleton and is voluntarily controlled. The function of skeletal muscle is covered in 'The musculoskeletal system', pages 128–129.
- **Smooth muscle**: So-called because it is not striated. This is found in internal organs and its movement is involuntary. It occurs in the walls of the digestive tract, blood vessels, lymph vessels, uterus and other internal organs. Its function is covered in more detail in other sections, in particular in 'The digestive system' (pages 72–75), 'The circulatory system' (page 88) and 'The lymphatic system' (page 94).
- **Cardiac muscle**: Found in the wall of the heart, cardiac muscle is striated in appearance but its control is involuntary (see page 88).

Nervous tissue

Made up of two types of cells, nervous tissue comprises neurons, which transmit and receive information, and glial cells, which support and nourish them.

How reflexology can help

As with the body's cells (see page 68), the tissues are not focused on *per se* during a reflexology routine, because they are always being contacted whenever any of the reflexes are worked.

Skin

The skin is the largest organ in the body and has remarkable properties. It provides effective protection for our delicate insides, yet through its sensory receptors we are aware of even the lightest touch.

If we are cold or frightened the erector muscles of hair contract to give us 'goose pimples' and our rapid response if we place our hand or finger on a burning surface is the reflex action triggered by our skin's sensors.

Skin is able to stretch to a quite staggering degree if needed (as in the case of pregnancy), and then return to its normal dimensions very quickly. It is capable of repairing itself rapidly and effectively, and oils secreted by the sebaceous glands keep it soft and pliable.

Layers of the skin

The skin has two main layers. The outer one, the epidermis, is made up of layers of skin cells (epithelial tissue) which, being close to the surface, are involved with protection, absorption and secretion. Below this, the dermis contains fibrous and elastic tissue, blood vessels, sweat glands, nerve fibres, hair follicles and the sensory nerve endings stimulated by touch, pressure, pain and temperature. Beneath the skin is an underlying subcutaneous layer, the hypodermis.

Our skin eliminates large quantities of fluids daily in the form of perspiration, but this porosity is largely one way. Although our skin is absorbent it doesn't let in water when we bathe or swim, for example.

How reflexology can help

The appearance of a person's skin will often give an accurate indicator of their general health. Most skin troubles, other than burns or chemical reactions, have their cause within the body and problems such as eczema, boils, acne and allergic rashes need to be tackled by treating the whole body and looking for the cause within the body, not without.

Most skin disorders have their origin in the digestive system, being caused by allergies to food or sensitivities to external environmental factors, such as dust, animal fur or pollen. Whether these are absorbed into the body through the digestive system or the skin, the results will be the same. Sufferers from eczema usually also have a tendency to asthma.

Regular reflexology benefits skin complaints by strengthening the digestive system, improving bowel elimination and relaxing the body (see pages 76–77). The treatment will lessen internal oversensitivity and improve skin conditions and asthma.

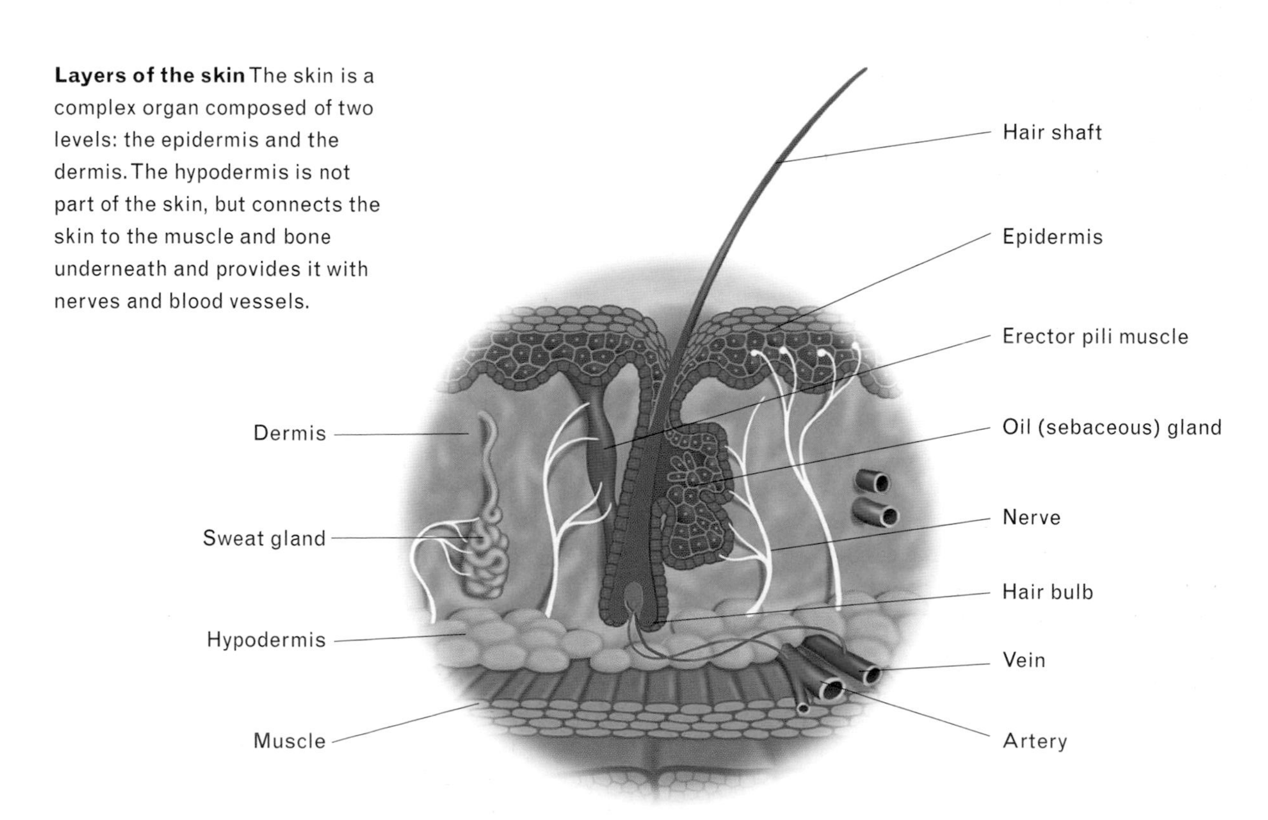

Layers of the skin The skin is a complex organ composed of two levels: the epidermis and the dermis. The hypodermis is not part of the skin, but connects the skin to the muscle and bone underneath and provides it with nerves and blood vessels.

The digestive system

All the energy the body needs comes from ingested food and drink. The complex digestive processes, which begin even before we take a bite of food, gradually break down and simplify the food we eat until it is in a form suitable for absorption and use by the body.

The process of digestion begins at the mouth and terminates at the anus. Between the two, all we eat and drink works its way through the alimentary tract, which although it incorporates various organs with distinctive names, is structurally remarkably similar throughout its length. The main elements are the mouth, pharynx, oesophagus, stomach, liver, small intestine, large intestine, rectum and the anal canal. The salivary glands, the liver and the pancreas are not directly part of the digestive system but secrete digestive juices into it and so are vital to the digestive function.

The mouth, pharynx and oesophagus

As soon as food enters the mouth it is chewed by our strong back teeth, the molars, and mixed with saliva. This helps it become a soft mass, a bolus, that is easy to swallow. There are three pairs of salivary glands: the parotid, submandibular and sublingual.

While food is still in the mouth, you have conscious control of it and can spit it out or swallow it. Once swallowed, it comes under the control of the autonomic nervous system. The entire digestive system relies on a strong muscular function to force the food through the digestive tract. This activity is called peristalsis.

On swallowing, food enters the pharynx and is carried towards the oesophagus. As the pharynx also leads via the larynx to the trachea, or windpipe, there is a potential danger of food or drink 'going down the wrong way'. To prevent this, a flap of cartilage known as the epiglottis folds over the entrance to the larynx as we swallow, blocking the airway. Food is propelled along the oesophagus by muscular force into the stomach.

The stomach

The stomach is an elastic C-shaped sac capable of strong muscular contractions. The fundus or top of the stomach is situated just underneath the heart and the base joins the first part of the intestine.

The stomach wall is composed of four main layers:

- **The mucosa**, or lining of the stomach
- **The submucosa**, a layer of connective tissue beneath the mucosa
- **A mixed layer** of longitudinal, circular and oblique muscle, which create the waves of peristaltic action that moves food through the entire digestive tract
- **The serosa**, or outer coat.

Small amounts of water, salts and alcohol are absorbed through the mucosa of the stomach, but most absorption does not happen until a later stage of the digestive process. The stomach's main function is to break down the food and drink you have consumed into a digestible form. To do this, glands in the wall of the stomach secrete gastric juices. The flow of gastric juices begins even before food reaches the stomach due to the stimulation of the vagus nerve, which is activated by the sight, smell or taste of food. A strong circular muscle called the cardiac sphincter muscle, which is situated at the lower end of the oesophagus and guards the entrance to the stomach, prevents the highly acidic gastric juices from splashing up into the oesophagus.

Gastric juices consist of hydrochloric acid and enzymes. The hydrochloric acid kills bacteria and breaks down the connective tissues in meat. The main enzyme is pepsin, which starts protein digestion. A glycoprotein called the intrinsic factor, which is necessary for the absorption of vitamin B, is also secreted into the stomach.

The length of time that the stomach takes to digest its contents depends on the type of food eaten. A fatty meal remains in the stomach the longest.

Once food has been sufficiently digested in the stomach a strong muscular ring called the pyloric sphincter, which lies at the base of the stomach, relaxes and contracts to allow food to leave the stomach and enter the first part of the small intestine, the duodenum.

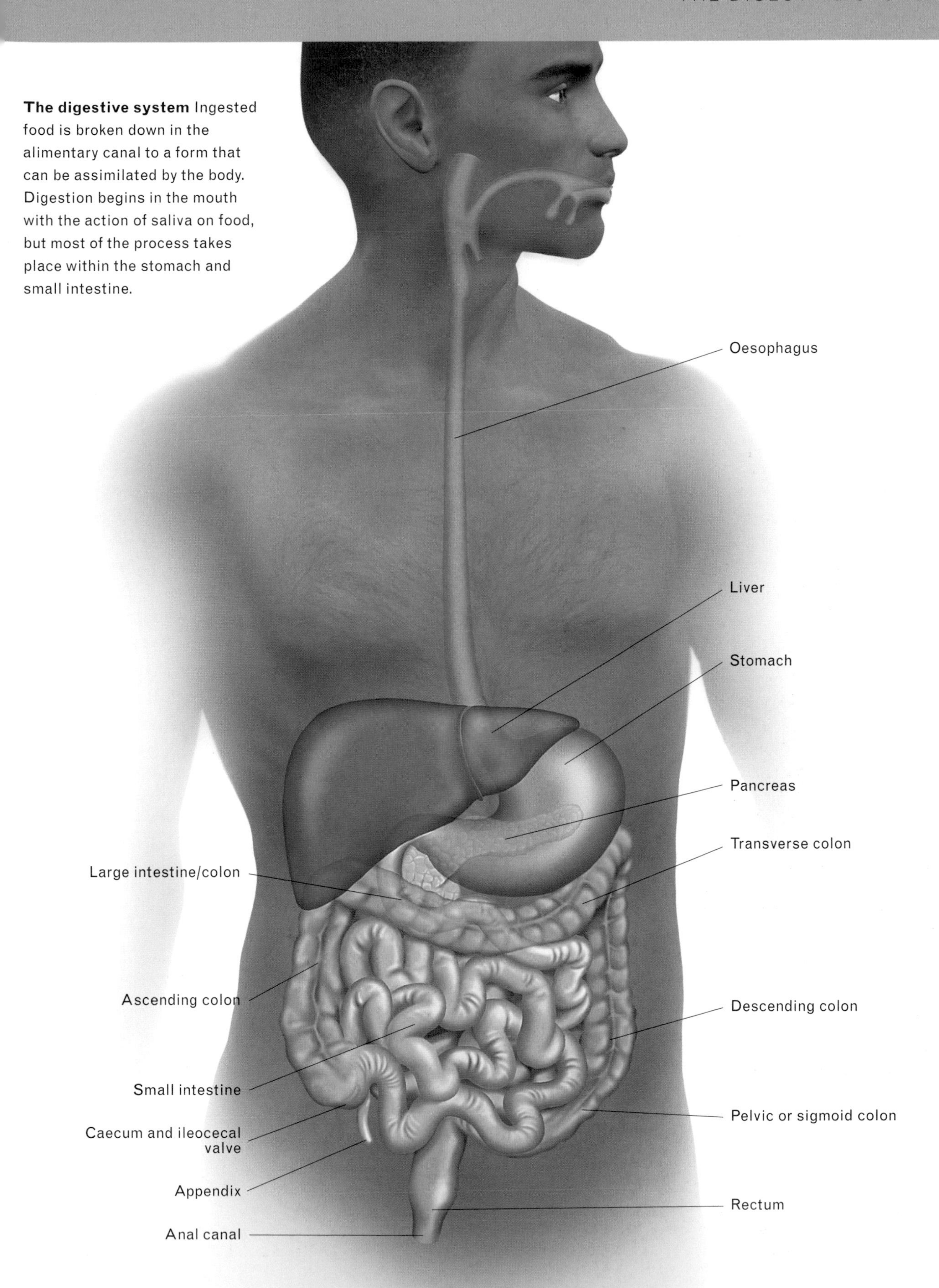

The digestive system Ingested food is broken down in the alimentary canal to a form that can be assimilated by the body. Digestion begins in the mouth with the action of saliva on food, but most of the process takes place within the stomach and small intestine.

The pancreas This gland is composed of cell clusters (acini) that secrete pancreatic juice containing a number of enzymes concerned in digestion. It also has an important role in the endocrine system, producing hormones such as insulin.

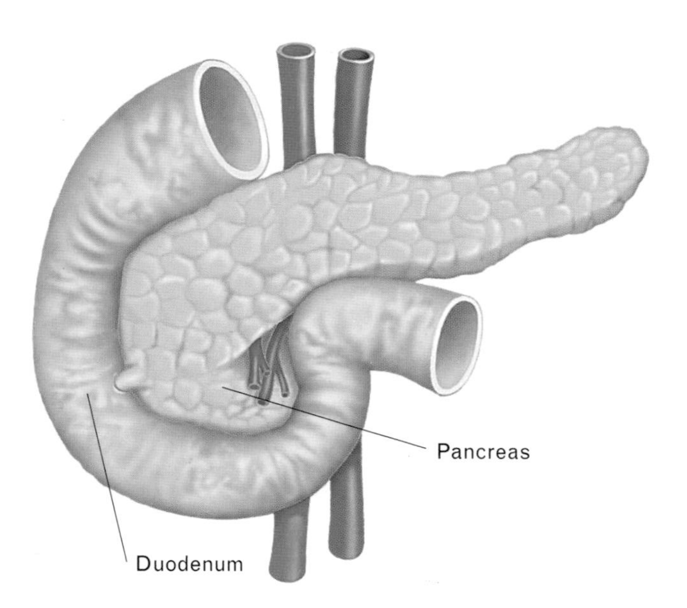

The liver A great detoxifier, the liver is particularly important in the digestive process. Harmful toxins that are not water-soluble are combined in the liver with natural enzymes, so they become water-soluble and can be passed to the kidneys or bowel for excretion.

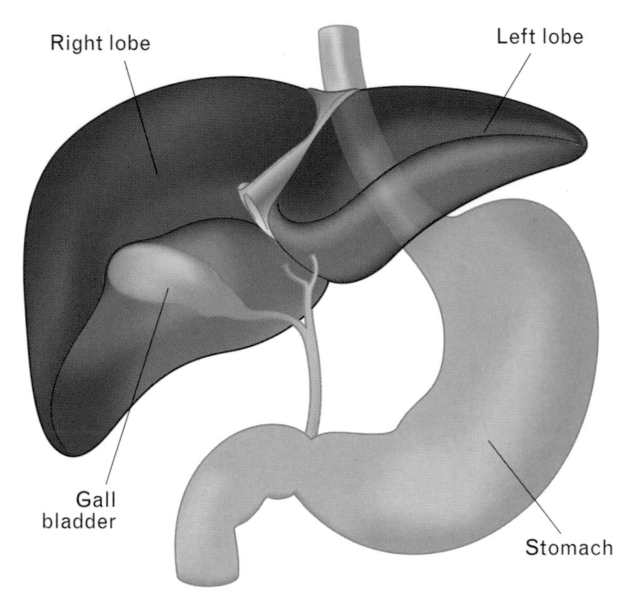

The pancreas

The pancreas and liver play an important part at this stage of the digestion process. The pancreas is a pale grey gland, about 12–15 cm (5–6 in) long, with a broad head, a body and a narrow tail. It lies behind the stomach with its head in the curve of the first part of the small intestine, the duodenum.

The pancreas produces enzymes secreted in an alkaline juice, which are released into the duodenum via the pancreatic duct and help in the digestion of carbohydrates, proteins and fats.

A further very important function of the pancreas is the production of hormones from its endocrine areas (see 'The endocrine system', page 98–101), called the islets of Langerhans. Here, the alpha cells secrete glucagon and the beta cells produce insulin. These hormones work in opposition to control the level of glucose sugar in the blood. Inadequate production of insulin results in diabetes mellitus.

The liver and gall bladder

The liver lies on the right-hand-side of the body and is one of the most important organs in the human body. It is wedge-shaped and has two lobes, the left lobe being smaller than the right. Its internal structure is formed of tiny tubes and billions of cells.

The liver has some amazing chemical processing abilities. It produces bile, cholesterol and vitamin B12, and stores vitamins A, D, E and K as well as iron, copper and some water-soluble vitamins such as folic acid, vitamin B, pyridoxine and niacin. It converts glucose to glucogen, and converts stored fat into a form that can be used by the body to provide energy and heat.

The liver deals efficiently with the detoxification of drugs and toxins and the ethanol found in alcohol. It also produces bile, which is vital to digestion, emulsifying fats and also providing lubrication for the bowel. Bile consists of water, bile pigment and bile salts, cholesterol, mineral salts and mucus. Up to 1,000 ml (1¾ pints) of bile is secreted by the liver daily and stored in the gall bladder.

The gall bladder is a small, pear-shaped sac about 10 cm (4 in) long, which lies just under the liver. As the muscular wall of the gall bladder contracts, bile is pushed through the bile duct into the duodenum.

The small intestine

The small intestine is really a continuation of the stomach. The first part, the duodenum, is about 25 cm (10 in) long

DETOX FOODS

Your body's digestive system, especially your liver, is an efficient natural detoxification system, but what you eat is also crucial for good health. You can help by reducing your intake of toxins such as alcohol, caffeine, nicotine, saturated and other bad fats and sugar) and by choosing foods that boost the detox process. These might include:

- **Apple** contains antioxidants quercetin and vitamin C, and pectin which helps excrete heavy metals.
- **Avocado** contains glutathione, an antioxidant that fights free radicals.
- **Beetroot** contains methionine, which helps purify natural waste products from the body.
- **Cruciferous vegetables** neutralize toxins and contain glucosinolates to boost enzyme production.
- **Kiwi fruit** contains the antioxidant vitamin C.
- **Prunes** are antioxidant and a natural laxative.
- **Seaweed** contains alginates that bind with heavy metals preparing them for excretion from the body.

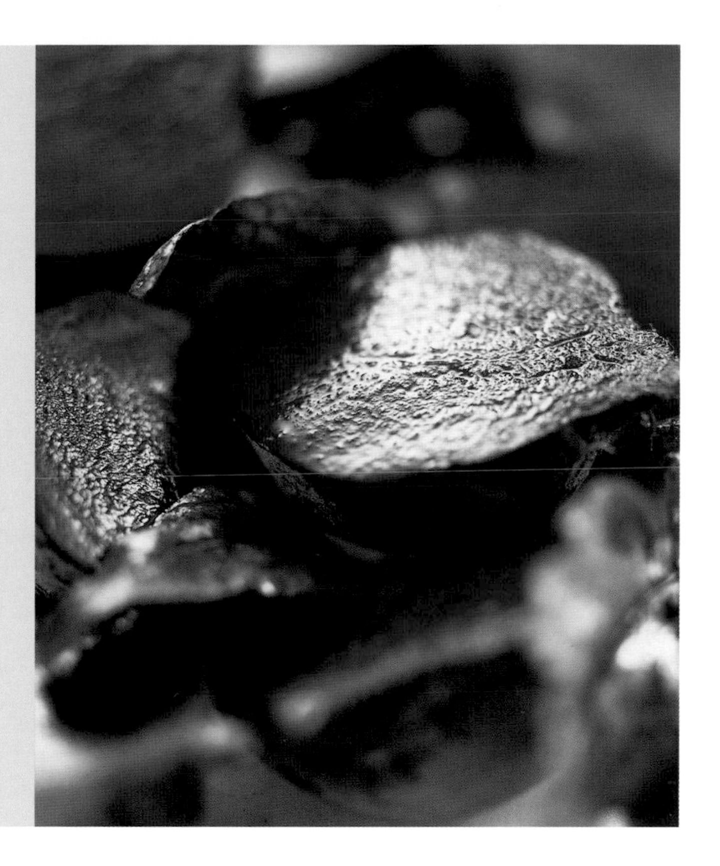

and encircles the head of the pancreas. The middle part, the jejunum, is about 2 metres (6 feet) long and the final section, the ileum is about 3 metres (10 feet) in length. The ileum ends at the ileocecal valve, which joins the small and large intestine. This little valve prevents backflow of waste material once it has left the small intestine.

Most of our food absorption goes on in the small intestine, which secretes intestinal fluid to help complete the chemical digestion of carbohydrates, protein and fats and then absorbs all the necessary nutrients through the intestinal walls.

The physical stretching of the intestine walls as semi-processed food passes through, together with hormonal triggers, stimulate the intestinal glands to secrete their digestive fluid, which also helps protect against the invasion of infection. Millions of projections in the lining of the small intestine, called villi, hugely increase the surface area, making the process of absorption of nutrients more efficient.

The large intestine, rectum and anal canal

The large intestine forms an arch around the small intestine and undergoes various name changes along its length: caecum, ascending colon, transverse colon, descending colon and pelvic or sigmoid colon (see the illustration of the digestive system on page 73). The total length of the large intestine is approximately 1.5 m (5 ft), but, although it is much shorter than the small intestine, the space it encloses is larger than that of the whole of the small intestine.

The lining of the large intestine lacks villi and produces no digestive enzymes. Its functions are to absorb sodium and water, incubate bacteria which produce vitamin K and some of the B complex vitamins, and eliminate waste in the form of undigested and unabsorbed food and bile pigments. Faecal matter moves through the large intestine at a slow speed, permitting the reabsorption of approximately 1.3 litres (2½ pints) of water every day.

Deep in the pelvis, the pelvic colon terminates in the rectum, a slightly dilated part of the colon about 12 cm (5 in) long, which in turn leads into the anal canal. The anal canal is only about 3.8 cm (1½ in) long in an adult, and transfers faecal matter to the exterior. Two sphincter muscles control the anus: the smooth muscle of the internal sphincter is under the control of the autonomic nervous system but the striated muscle of the external sphincter is under voluntary control.

Digestive disorders helped by reflexology

More than any other system in the human body, the digestive system makes us aware when all is working efficiently and, equally, we are soon informed when the system is upset and in need of attention.

Indigestion

Indigestion causes the stomach to feel (and sound) as if it is going into revolt as it rumbles and gurgles. Add to this an unpleasant acid reflux action and a bout of indigestion means that we really do feel completely out of sorts. Usually, such upset is the result of the stomach having to work overtime to digest extremely rich or spicy food which it is having difficulty in breaking down, or it may be trying to cope with a meal eaten very hurriedly. The stomach is also extremely sensitive to emotional upsets, so our mood and feelings affect the fine balance of the activity of this organ.

Constipation and intestinal problems

When waste food is kept in the body for far too long it can become compacted and difficult to pass, and the colon becomes constipated. The modern diet, with its abundance of processed foods high in fat, sugar and salt, such as white bread, cakes, biscuits and pies, does not encourage chewing and grinding of food and so even the first stage of digestion, in the mouth, does not work as it should. Constipation is a common sign that a diet is low in fibre. The trend towards a low-fibre, highly processed diet has been reflected in the increase over the last 30 years or so of bowel disorders and diseases, particularly bowel cancer. The longer waste material is left in the bowel, the more likelihood there is of disease occurring. A famous medical herbal college believes that 'death begins in the colon' – and so do all the cures!

Stress and lack of exercise also have a disastrous effect on the colon, and everyone in the medical world is seeing an increase in irritable bowel syndrome. This is not a straightforward disorder, but a collection of different symptoms that can have a variety of causes.

Food allergies

People who suffer from allergies have a more delicate constitution than others who can eat exactly what they like at any time without any adverse bodily reaction at all. I have remarked that some people have the constitution of a Mini and others of a Rolls Royce – and we all know that you can get far more performance from the latter.

Unfortunately, it can often be difficult to tell exactly what we are putting into our systems. Processed foods contain surprising amounts of chemicals to preserve them and give them colour and taste. Even fresh fruit and vegetables, unless organically grown, are raised in chemically treated soil and sprayed with strong insecticides to provide supermarkets with blemish-free fruit and vegetables. Chemicals have become part of the average diet.

There is evidence to show that when some infants are fed with cow's milk or wheat-based products, an allergic reaction can start up in the mucous membranes of the body. Those most likely to suffer from allergies are babies with a family history of allergic reactive illnesses. Reactions can take a number of forms, often seemingly far removed from the digestive system, such as migraine (80 per cent of migraine is caused by an allergy), hayfever, eczema, hives or other irritating rashes. Some babies are born with eczema that has been caused by a certain food or foods that the mother has been eating, maybe in excess. (Many pregnant mothers have strange cravings for all manner of foods, often the very ones to which they are allergic.)

The introduction of certain foods into the digestive system at too early an age can set up an inflammatory state in the body, placing stress on the stomach, pancreas, liver and intestines. A child may start suffering from ear infections, a constant running nose, sore throats or a rash. This is Mother Nature desperately trying to signal that all is not well in the child's body. We are all exactly what we eat and what we are exposed to. When an inflammatory condition occurs in the digestive system, normally because of food intolerances, the body tries to reduce the inflammation by producing mucus. All the excretory organs, including the skin, nose and bowel, are used to try to get rid of the infection.

When they see a child with repeated skin, ear, nose and throat inflammations, naturopathic doctors tend to examine the diet, believing the root cause of such problems to be in the digestive system. Breastfeeding is the best food for a baby. Breastfed babies do not suffer from constipation, and the quality of milk as well as the quantity changes with the demands of the baby as it grows. Nevertheless, there are some very good-quality formulas available now.

How reflexology can help

If a young baby is suffering from an acute ear infection, the mother will of course go to the doctor for help; earache is very painful and debilitating. The doctor will usually treat the infection by prescribing an antibiotic.

GOOD DIGESTION, GOOD HEALTH

Here are some tips to help you prevent indigestion, acid reflux, bloating and wind:

- Apple cider vinegar is packed full of minerals and vitamins. To aid digestion, slowly sip a glass of warm water with three teaspoons of apple cider vinegar, about half an hour before you eat.
- Do not drink during eating, as this will dilute the digestive enzymes in your stomach.
- Limit portion size. Chinese doctors say we should never eat more food than can be contained in the palms of our two hands, at any meal.
- Don't eat if you are stressed. Before you eat, try to achieve a calmer state by taking a brisk walk, meditating or listening to some relaxing music.
- Avoid eating fruit after fish or meat as this can cause fermentation in your stomach.
- Take your last meal no later than 7 o' clock to allow your body to digest the food before you go to bed.
- Avoid eating salty or very sweet foods during the evening, as salt and sugar stimulate the body.

Unfortunately, however, antibiotics have quite a disastrous effect on the digestive system as they destroy the friendly bacterial flora that keep the intestinal tract healthy. The danger is that this sets up a never-ending circle of problems: more ear infections, more antibiotics and more damage to the very area that was in a sensitive state to start with.

A naturopath or herbalist, on the other hand, would concentrate on helping the digestive system, perceiving the inflammation or congestion causing the earache to stem from a reaction to certain foods. The removal of these foods, most usually dairy and wheat products, would give the inflammation and congestion in the system time to heal and future allergic reaction to the food would be far less likely. Many children have an intolerance to cow's milk products, which create an excess of mucus in the body. Wheat can also have an inflammatory effect on the digestive system.

Reflexology follows the same course, which is why working the digestive system is such an important part of a treatment session.

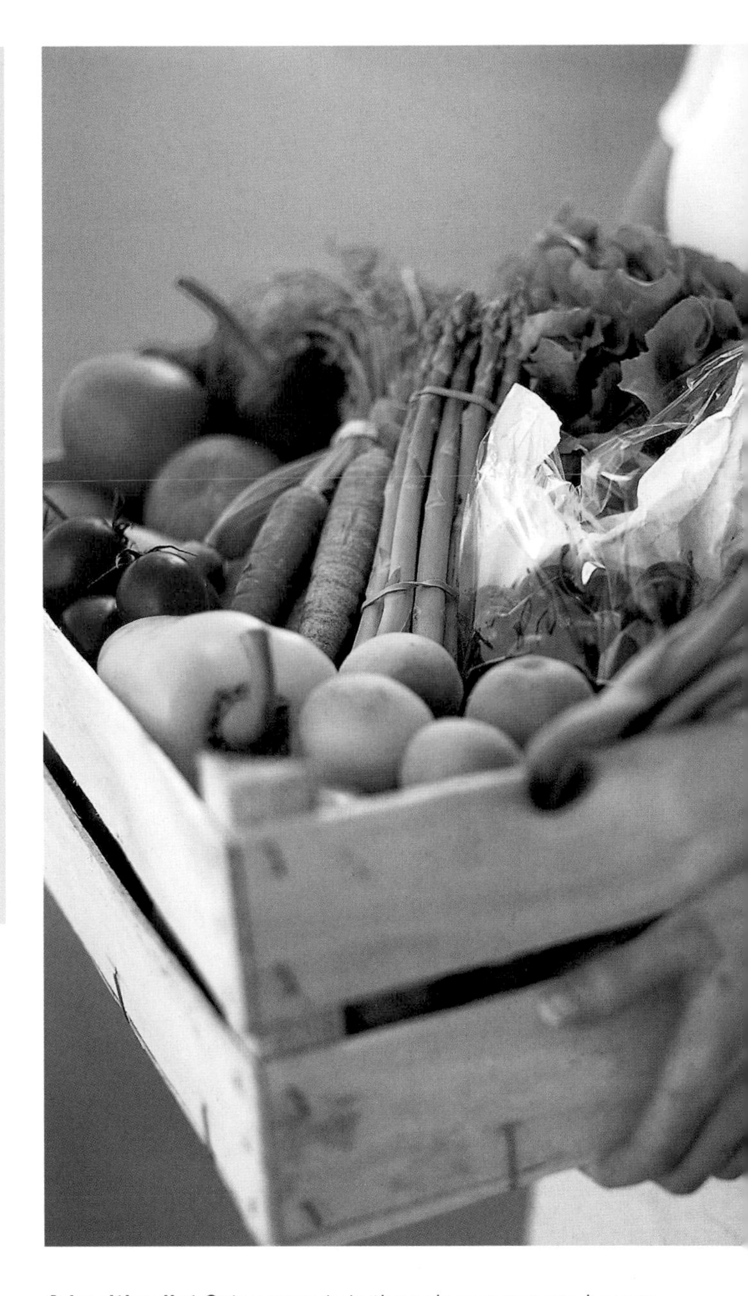

A healthy diet Going organic is the only way you can be sure that you are not ingesting allergy-causing pesticides along with the nutrients in your fruit and vegetables.

Working the associated reflex points

This routine focuses on the middle section of the foot, between the diaphragm line and the pelvic (heel) line, reflecting the concentration of digestive organs in the centre of the body. This includes the liver, stomach and intestine reflexes.

CASE STUDY

IRRITABLE BOWEL SYNDROME

CLIENT PROFILE

Malcolm was an executive in a large international company and had been experiencing trouble with his digestive system, causing him pain and discomfort. He complained of frequent bouts of either embarrassing diarrhoea or days of chronic constipation. This was interfering with his job, which involved a lot of travelling, both by air and driving long distances. Often, lunch would be a hurried sandwich instead of stopping for a much-earned proper break. He seemed extremely tense and said he had difficulty in sleeping, as he found it hard to switch off from work problems.

Malcolm's intestinal reflexes were extremely sensitive as would have been expected. He also had lots of reaction in the solar plexus region. This reflex area is usually over-sensitive in those in a very stressed state.

REGULARITY OF REFLEXOLOGY TREATMENT

Weekly for six weeks and then a further six months on a monthly basis.

REFLEXES

Main reflexes	Assistance
Entire intestinal areas	To alleviate irritable bowel
Stomach and pancreas	To strengthen digestive processes
Solar plexus	To help relieve stress

TREATMENT OUTCOMES

After his first treatment he said that he had not slept so well for many months and his bowel action the following day was normal. After eight sessions, Malcolm had normal bowel movements, was more relaxed and was able to sleep well for at least eight hours every night.

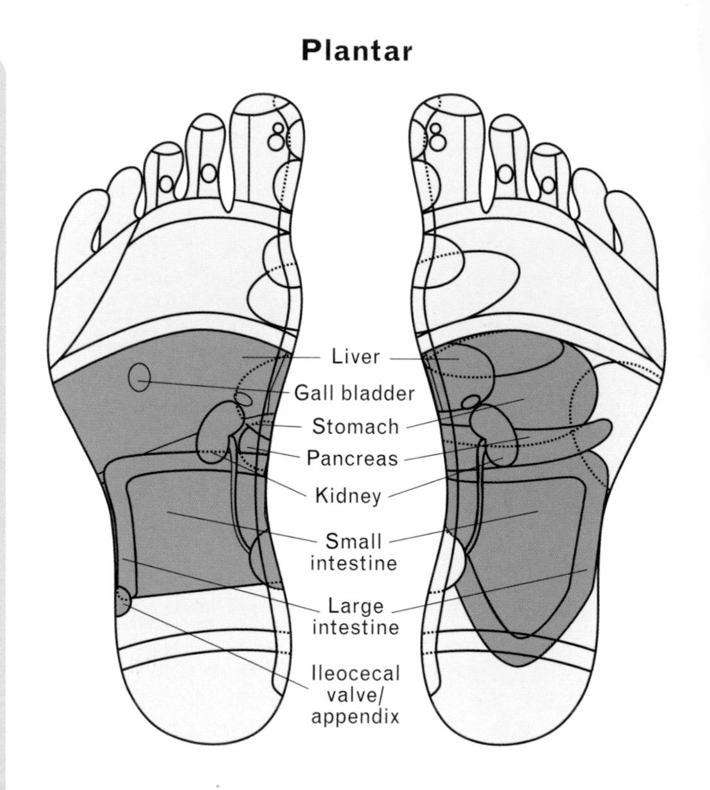

The liver area

Right foot – plantar
Medial to lateral – top support

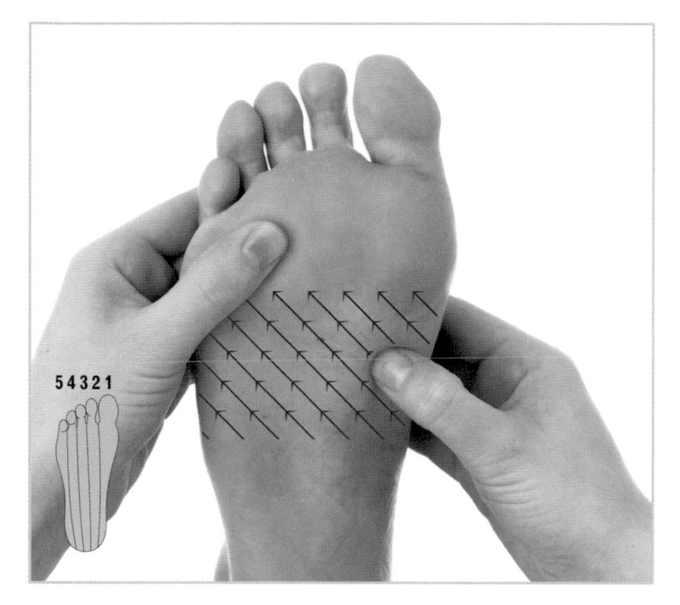

1 Support the right foot with your left hand and, using the right thumb, work out the entire area in a criss-cross direction from the medial to the lateral edge.

Right foot – plantar
Lateral to medial – top support

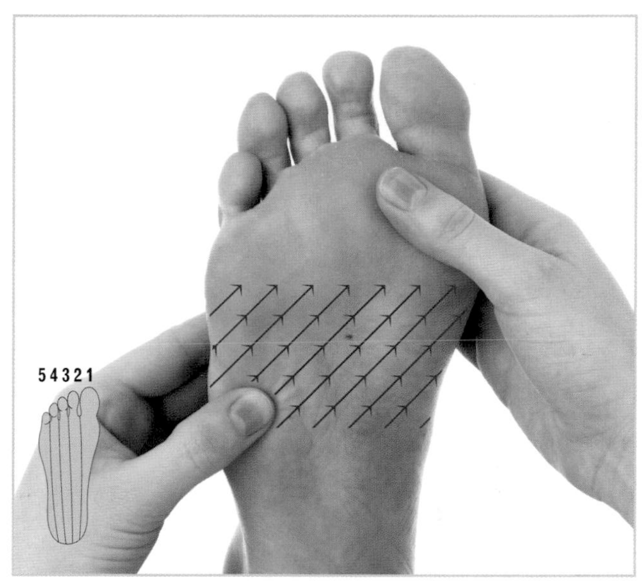

2 Support the right foot with your right hand and, using the left thumb, work out the entire area in a criss-cross direction from the lateral to the medial edge.

The stomach and pancreas areas

Left foot – plantar
Medial to lateral – top support

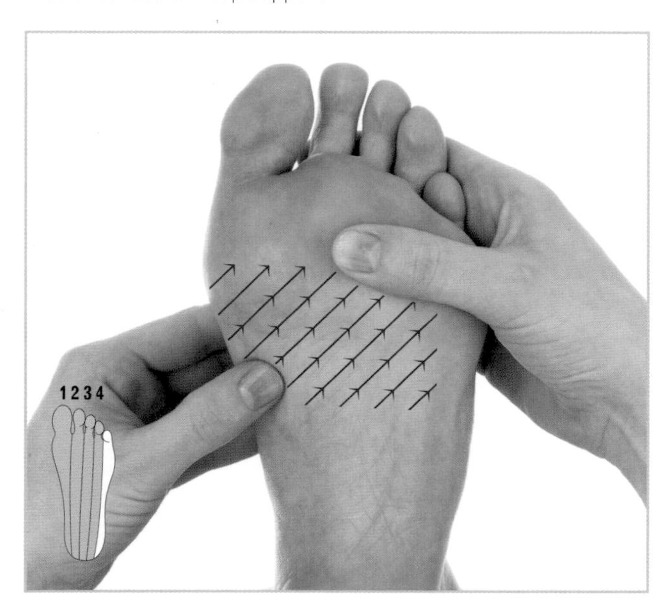

1 Support the left foot with your right hand and, using the left thumb, work out the area in a criss-cross direction from medial to lateral.

Left foot – plantar
Lateral to medial – top support

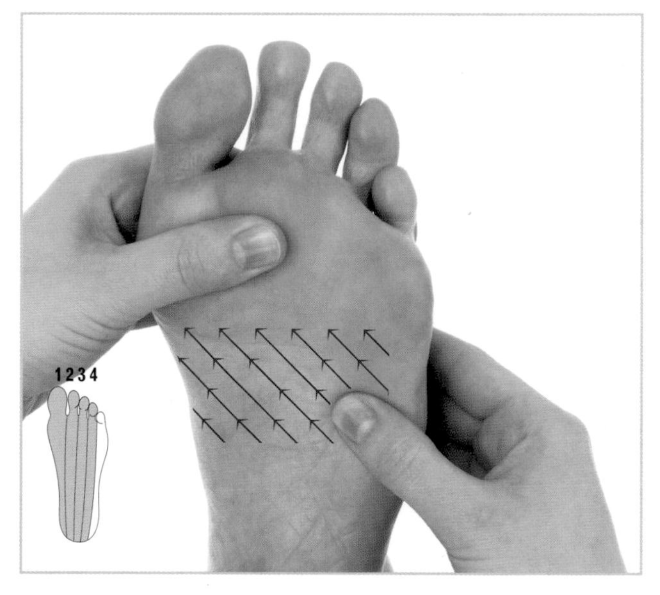

2 Support the left foot with your left hand and, using the right thumb, work out the area in a criss-cross direction from lateral to medial.

The ileocecal valve

Right foot – plantar
Lateral hooking out technique – heel support

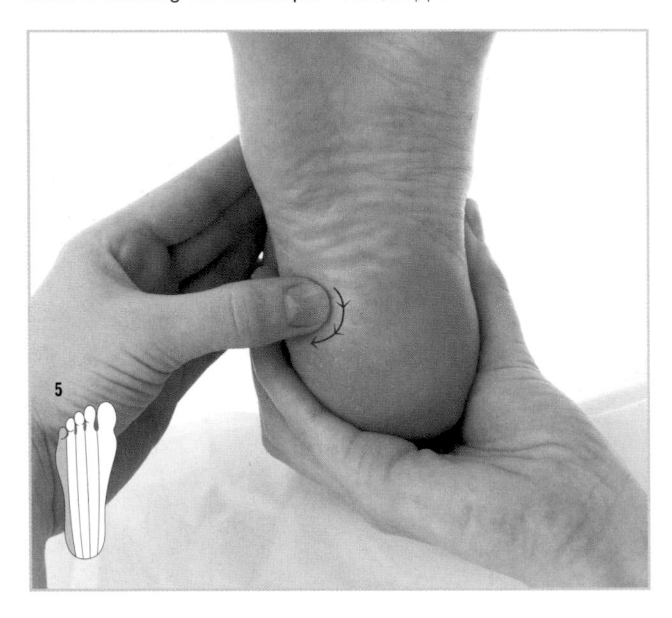

Support the right foot at the base of the heel with your right hand, place the left thumb on the heel line and use a 'hooking out' procedure.

WORKING ALL THE INTESTINAL REFLEXES

This routine works over the entire intestinal area, including the ascending, transverse and small intestines, and also the buttocks and the back of pelvis, which are situated below the heel line. Working Zone 3 on the left foot only has a particular application for the lower part of the large intestine.

Working the ileocecal reflex involves using the less usual 'hooking out' technique, which is described on page 53.

The intestinal area

Right foot – plantar
Medial to lateral – heel support

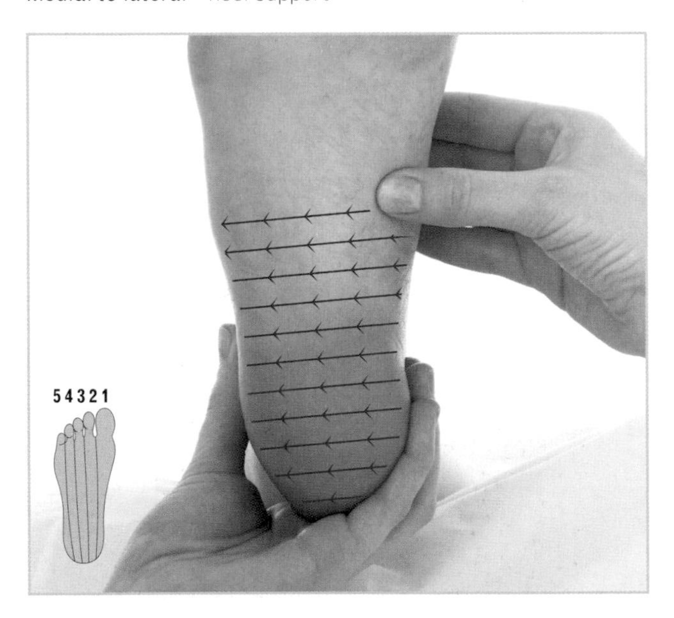

1 Support the right foot at the base with your left hand, use the right thumb and work in straight lines across the foot from medial to lateral.

Right foot – plantar
Lateral to medial – heel support

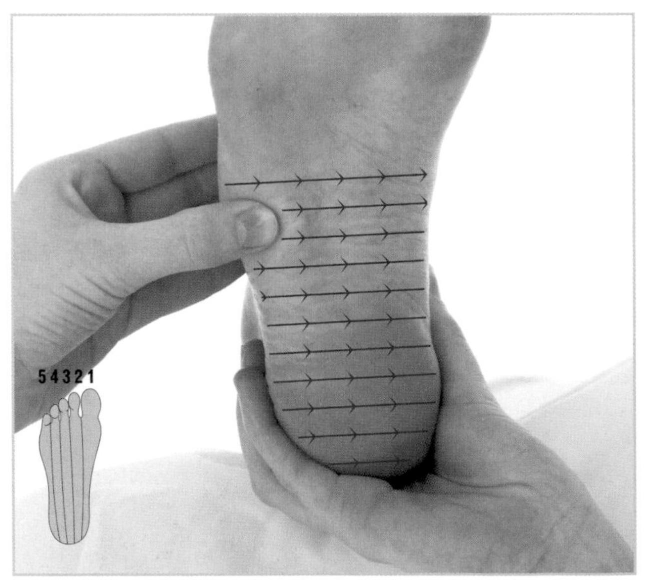

2 Supporting the right foot at the base with your right hand and using the left thumb, work out in straight lines from lateral to medial.

The intestinal area

Left foot – plantar
Medial to lateral – heel support

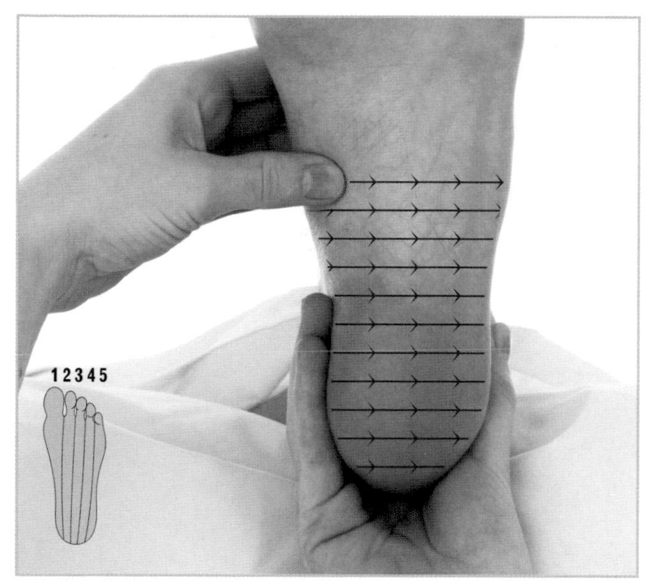

1 Support the left foot in your right hand at the base and, using the left thumb, work out in straight lines from medial to lateral.

Left foot – plantar
Lateral to medial – heel support

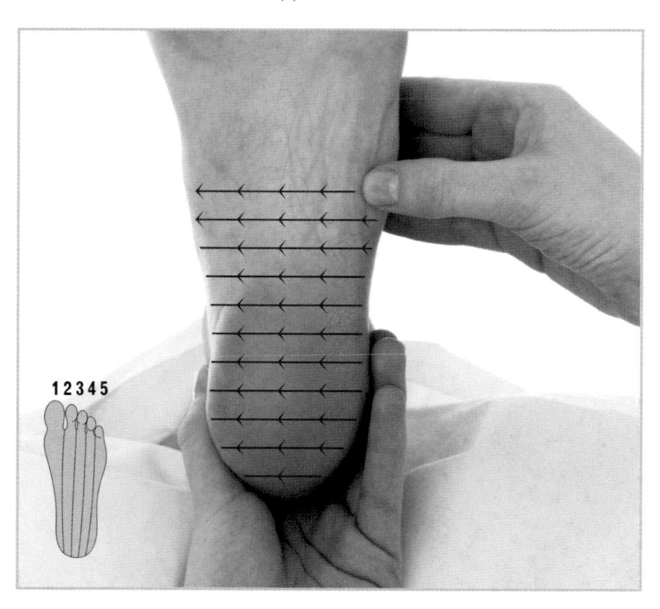

2 Support the left foot at the base with your left hand and, using your right thumb, work across in straight lines from lateral to medial.

The sigmoid or pelvic colon

Left foot – plantar
Mid to medial – heel support

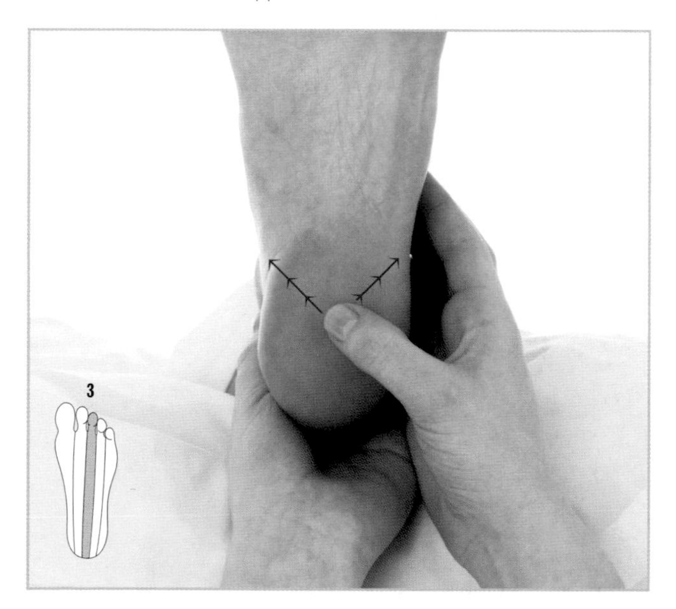

1 Support the left foot at the base with your left hand, place the right thumb on the mid point and work towards the medial edge and then the lateral edge as indicated.

Left foot – plantar
Mid to lateral – heel support

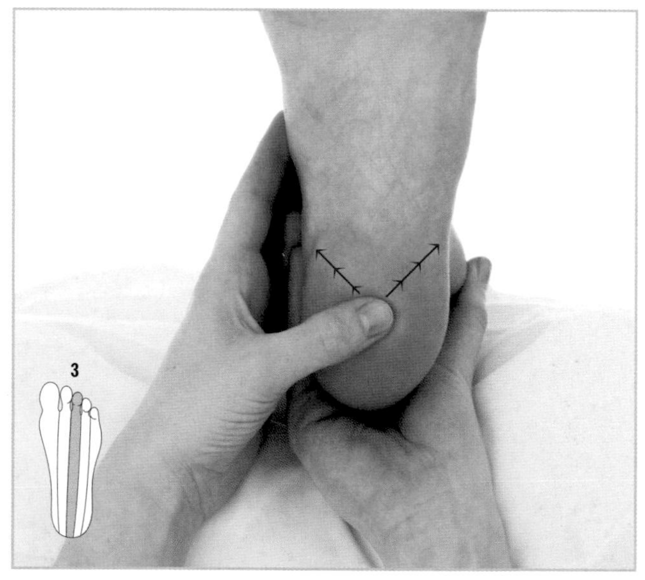

2 Support the left foot at the base with your right hand and work with the left thumb towards the lateral and then the medial edge as indicated.

The respiratory system

The lungs and heart provide the body with oxygenated blood, which is necessary for the survival of every single cell. As the body is unable to store oxygen, we need to breathe continuously for survival, so breathing is an automatic reflex, continuing even when we are asleep or unconscious.

The respiratory system comprises the nose, pharynx, larynx, trachea and the two lungs with their bronchi, bronchioles and alveoli. The ribs and diaphragmatic muscle are also integral parts of the breathing mechanism. The air we take in supplies all the cells of the body with oxygen. As we breathe out we expel waste carbon dioxide, which has been transported through the blood supply from these same cells to the lungs.

The nasal passages, pharynx and trachea

As we breathe in through the nose, our nasal passages warm up or cool down the air. Tiny hairs trap particles of dust and dirt that might irritate the lower airways.

At the back of the throat is an area that is shared by the digestive and respiratory tracts, making it possible to breathe through the mouth as well as the nose. This is necessary if your nose is blocked by a cold, but if you are a habitual mouth breather the incoming air bypasses the filtering system of the nasal passages, leaving you more open to sore throats. You will also probably snore.

During swallowing, a flap of tissue, the epiglottis, automatically closes off the larynx (voice box) preventing food from entering the respiratory system. From the pharynx the warmed air passes down the trachea through two bronchial tubes to the lungs.

The lungs

Each lung is cone-shaped, with a slightly concave base that sits on the diaphragm, the broad muscle that stretches across the body above the abdominal area. The lungs are protected by the rib cage which is quite flexible, with intercostal muscles between each rib space.

Surrounding each lung is the pleural membrane, filled with pleural fluid. This prevents friction building up as the lungs expand and relax.

The intricate network of air passages that supply the lungs resembles an inverted tree, with the trachea forming the trunk. The branches extend outwards and are called bronchi and bronchioles. Approximately 30,000 bronchioles are found in each lung. Bronchioles terminate in alveolar sacs, clusters of tiny chambers known as alveoli.

Alveoli are expandable, thin-walled structures that support a network of tiny blood-filled capillaries. Oxygen and carbon dioxide are exchanged through these thin walls. Oxygen from the inhaled air diffuses from the alveoli into the blood and carbon dioxide from the blood diffuses into the alveoli, to make the return journey up the bronchioles, bronchi and trachea in an exhaled breath.

Alveoli resemble bunches of small seedless grapes in shape. On their inner surfaces are white blood cells which ingest and destroy airborne irritants such as bacteria and grass pollen that have not yet been filtered out.

EVERY SOUND WE MAKE

Breathing out not only rids the lungs of carbon dioxide, it also allows us to speak and sing. Exhaled air flows through the larynx or voice box, a broad part of the upper windpipe protected by tough cartilage that forms the Adam's apple. Two bands of tissue, the vocal cords, form a V-shaped opening across the larynx. As we speak these tighten, narrowing the opening. Air passing across these cords vibrates them and produces sounds.

By almost infinite variations of positions of the tongue, lips and teeth we create the different sounds that make up speech and song. The volume of a voice is controlled by the force of the breath, the nasal cavities give resonance and the length of the vocal cords dictate the pitch: the longer the cords, the lower the pitch.

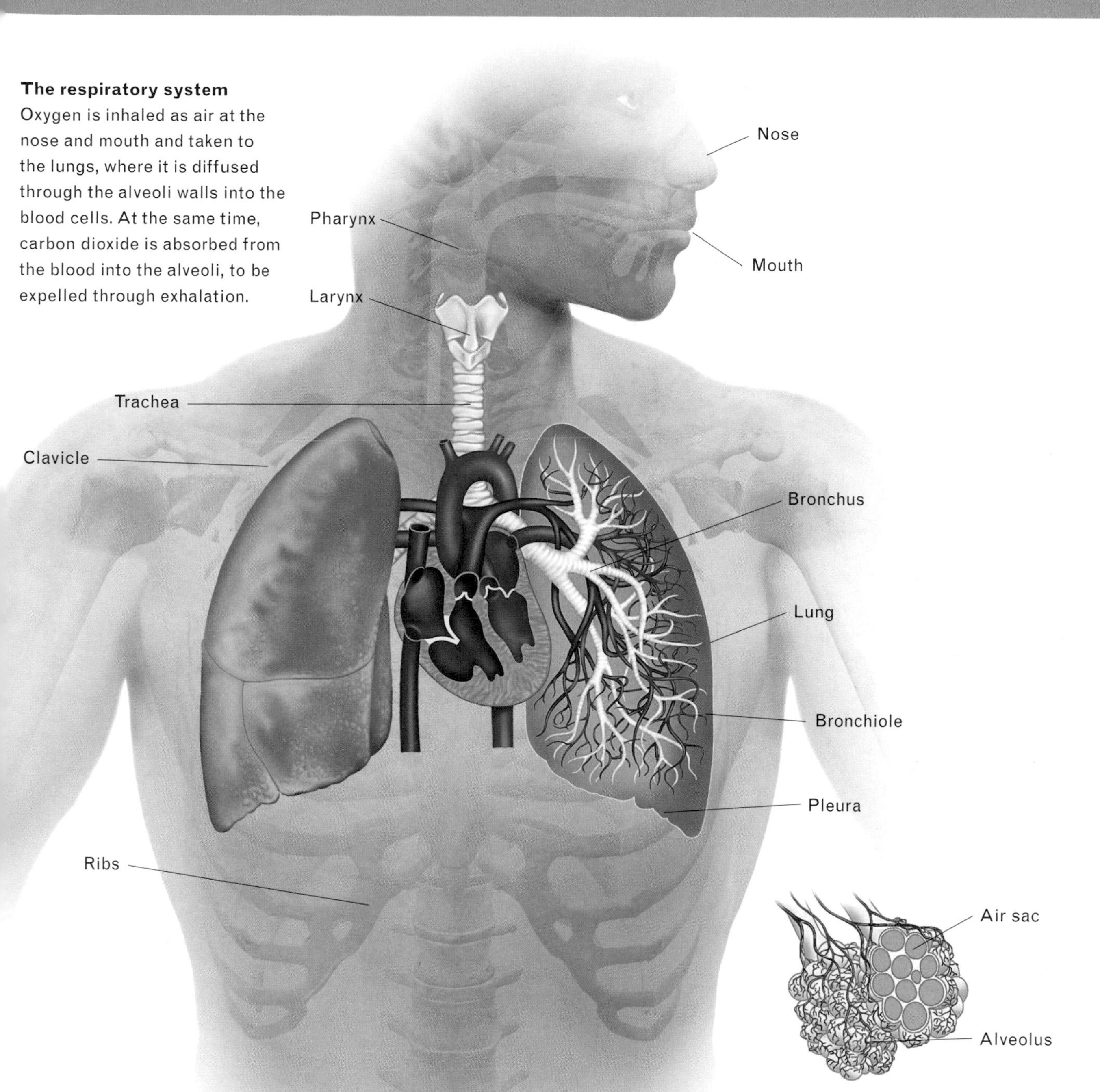

The respiratory system
Oxygen is inhaled as air at the nose and mouth and taken to the lungs, where it is diffused through the alveoli walls into the blood cells. At the same time, carbon dioxide is absorbed from the blood into the alveoli, to be expelled through exhalation.

Each alveolar sac is minute, but if they were all spread out the alveoli in a pair of lungs would cover half a tennis court. If disease destroys some alveoli, there is less surface area for gaseous exchange. This results in chronic breathlessness, which places a stress on the heart.

The mechanics of breathing

When we breathe in, the diaphragm (which stretches laterally across between the thoracic and abdominal cavities) descends and the rib cage expands, thanks to the intercostal muscles between each rib. The diaphragm acts like a bellows to the lungs, descending to help them expand and then rising to push out air on the out-breath. We normally breathe in and out about 10–17 times each minute, but the respiratory rate can vary enormously. It drops to a slow rate during sleep but can increase dramatically, to perhaps 80 times a minute, if we are running or climbing a mountain, when huge effort is needed and the whole body is demanding increased oxygen. The respiration rate can also become very fast if breathing is difficult, as the congested airways reduce the overall oxygen capacity.

Respiratory disorders helped by reflexology

When the respiratory system is affected by an irritant, whether a virus or dust or a toxic chemical, the mucous membrane reacts by becoming inflamed and secreting mucus. This manifests itself in a variety of disorders.

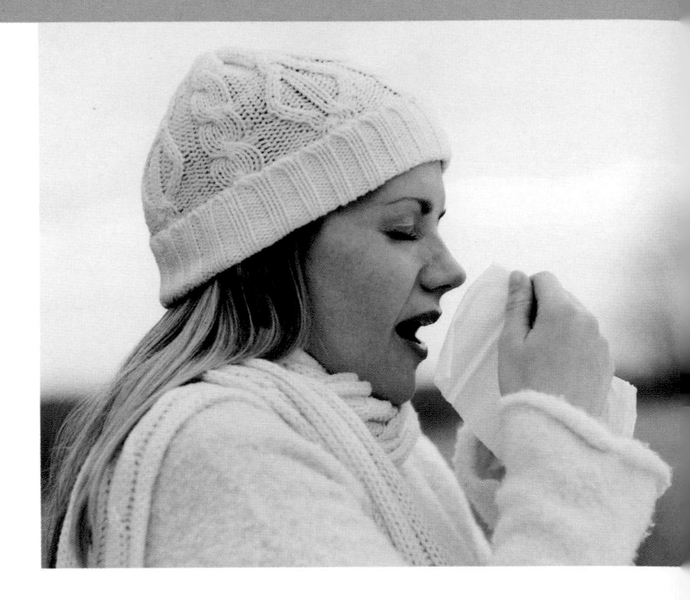

Let nature have her way Mucous discharge, coughs and sneezes are means by which the body rids itself of infection. Antibiotics that suppress symptoms should not be overused.

Lung diseases

Respiratory disorders are now very common throughout the world. Major causes are smoking and working in dusty environments. The lung tissue of chronic smokers and of those who work in dirty industries contains large areas blackened by carbon particles. This tissue does not expand and severely restricts the functioning of the lungs.

Until relatively recently, lung cancer was a male disease, but a growing number of women have become heavy smokers, and the incidence of smoking-related cancers in women is rising. If smoking were abolished, the cause of around 90 per cent of lung cancers would disappear. (While the nicotine is the substance that causes the addiction, it is the tar content and chemical mix in tobacco that causes cancers.) Quality of air is also an issue. Increased road and air traffic and the use of chemical sprays loads the air with toxins that pollute the delicate tissues of our respiratory system.

Asthma and bronchial difficulties

For a variety of reasons, the incidence of asthma in the Western world has doubled in the past two decades. Diet is a big factor (see box), and stress and air pollution are also key. The respiratory tract of young children is very susceptible to irritants and conventional treatments can exacerbate the underlying problem. One way of trying to alleviate infections is to remove the tonsils and adenoids. However, the tonsils and adenoids are lymphatic glands, the first line of defence in the body (see page 96). Their removal may help the ear, nose or throat infections, but with no adenoids or tonsils to absorb the bacteria, the next port of call will be the lungs.

It is probable that the child will then develop attacks of what doctors refer to as 'wheezy bronchitis'. Treatment will be more antibiotics, and if these do not help then various bronchial inhalers are used to expand the inflamed and infected bronchial tubes. These drugs can make a child tense and lead to behavioural problems, difficulty in sleeping or uncharacteristic aggressiveness. Such tension triggers asthmatic attacks.

THE DIGESTIVE–RESPIRATORY LINK

The mucous membranes lining the entire digestive system also line the respiratory system. A common cause of an allergic reaction is food (see page 76) and so, if the digestive system's mucous membranes are trying to fight off reaction to an allergic substance, the mucous membrane of the respiratory system is likely to react as well, which is why difficulties with breathing can be one result of an allergic reaction. In fact, poor functioning in the respiratory system often has its root cause in digestion.

How reflexology can help

The types of respiratory condition that the reflexologist will be able to relieve and assist are bronchitis, asthma, emphysema and all the other respiratory tract infections. (It is not advisable to stop taking any prescribed bronchodilating drugs without first consulting your doctor.) Reflexology addresses the underlying causes of respiratory diseases as well as treating respiratory areas such as the lungs directly. It is important to remember that the digestive system of person with a respiratory condition needs to be worked just as much as the respiratory areas (see page 76).

Working the associated reflex points

Lung reflexes are found on the plantar foot between the shoulder and diaphragm lines and in the same area on the dorsal side.

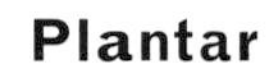

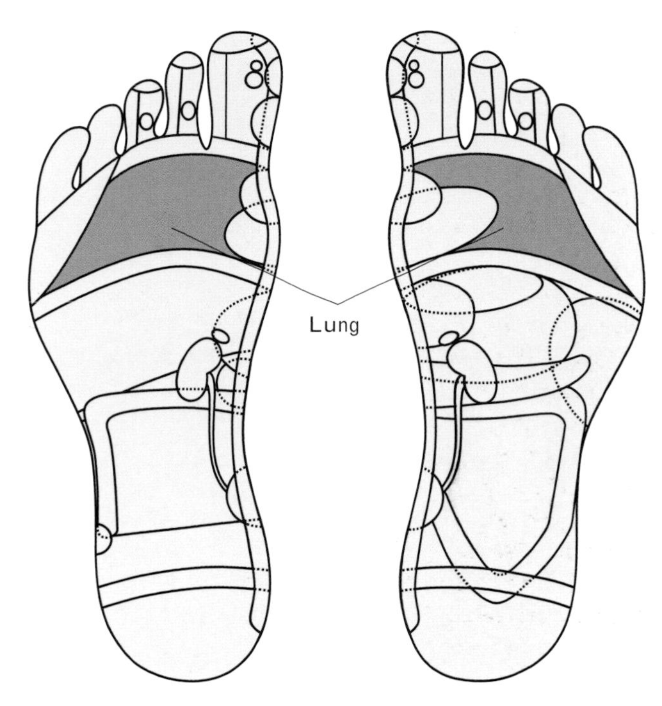

Dorsal

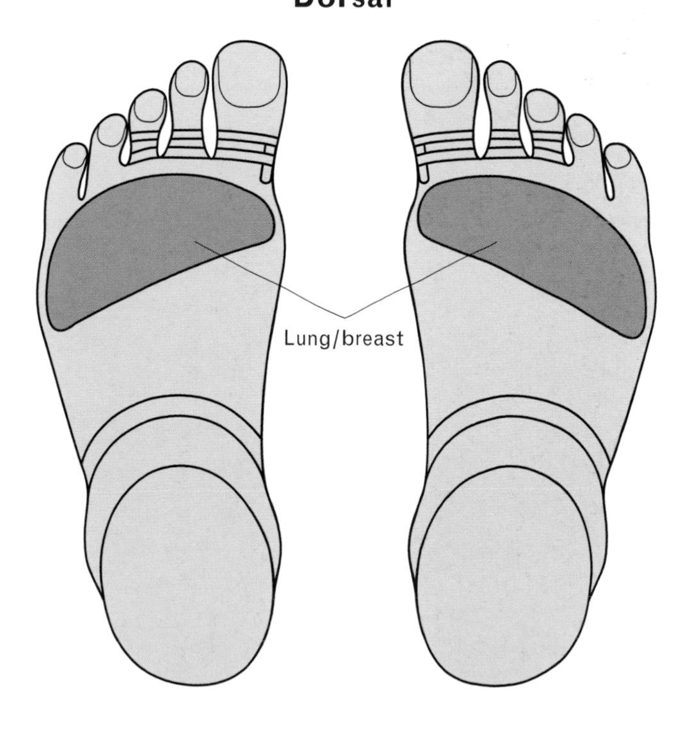

CASE STUDY **ASTHMA**

CLIENT PROFILE

Jane was eight years old when her mother brought her to me with a history of severe asthmatic attacks. On several occasions her breathing had been so laboured that she had been admitted to hospital. Her asthma began when she was three, following a bout of bronchitis. She had been on a variety of inhalers and medication, which all relieved the attacks, but her mother was concerned that her daughter was so dependent on medication. Jane was a very shy child, who had been unable to join in with school sports and other activities for so long that she had lost her self-confidence.

Most respiratory conditions begin in the digestive system in the form of food allergies (see page 76). The aim was to improve Jane's breathing and to strengthen her digestive system, to help the body cope with allergies. I also advised her mother to exclude dairy products and food colourings from her diet.

REGULARITY OF REFLEXOLOGY TREATMENT

Jane had regular weekly reflexology treatments for three months and then one session a month for a year.

REFLEXES

Main reflexes	Assistance
Stomach and intestinal areas	To help with potential food allergies
Lung	To improve respiration
Ribs/thoracic spine	To help posture and improve breathing
Solar plexus	To aid relaxation

TREATMENT OUTCOMES

After three months, the results were encouraging. Jane's attacks were far less severe, she was more physically active and her use of inhalers had been reduced.

The lung area

Right foot – plantar
Medial to lateral – top support

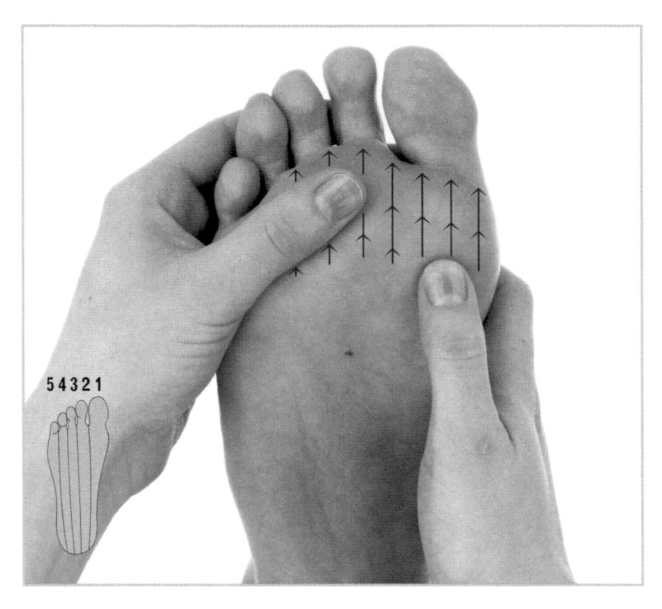

1 Support the right foot with your left hand and, using the right thumb, work up the foot in straight lines from medial to lateral.

Right foot – plantar
Lateral to medial – top support

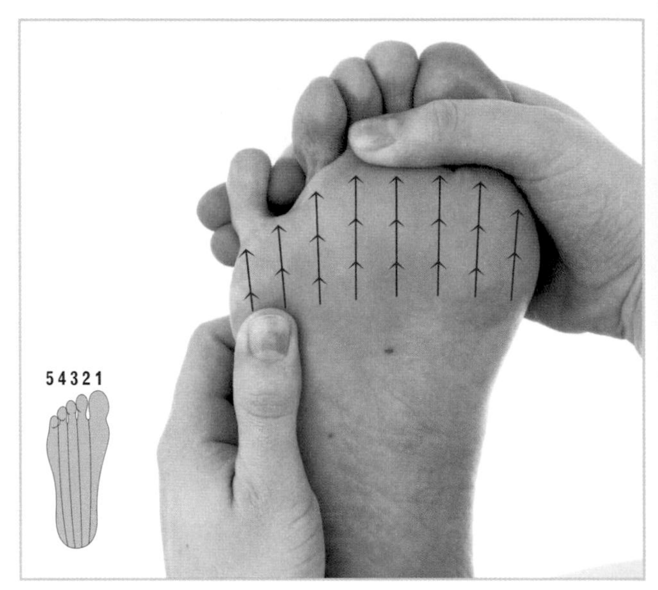

2 Support the right foot with your right hand and, using the left thumb, work up the foot in straight lines from lateral to medial. Separate each toe as you proceed.

The lung/breast area

Right foot – dorsal
Medial to lateral – top support

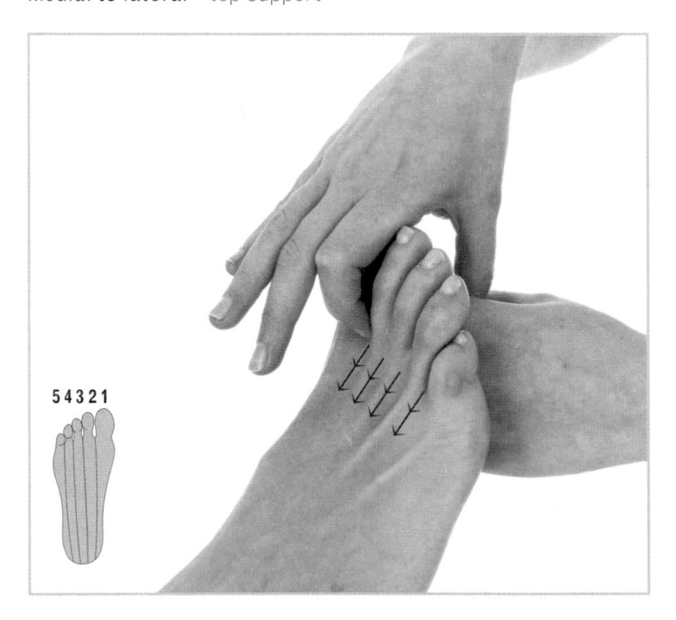

1 Support the right foot with your left fist and, using the right index finger, proceed downwards from medial to lateral.

Right foot – dorsal
Lateral to medial – top support

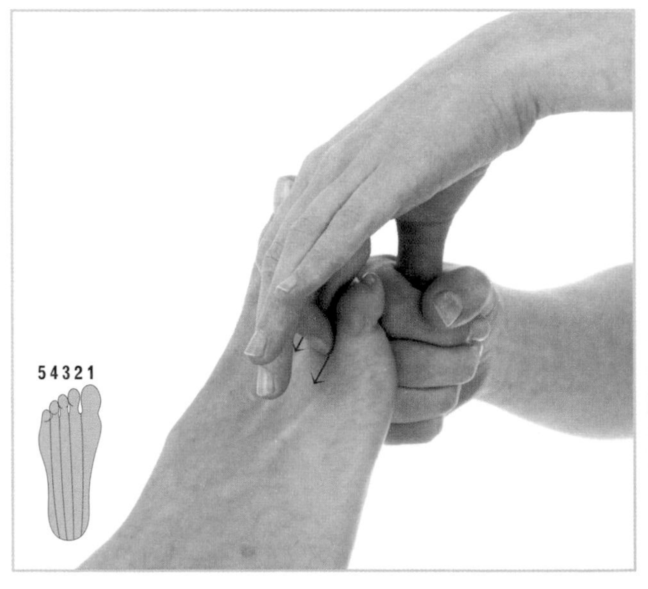

2 Support the right foot with your right fist and, using the left index finger, proceed downwards from lateral to medial.

The lung area

Left foot – plantar
Medial to lateral – top support

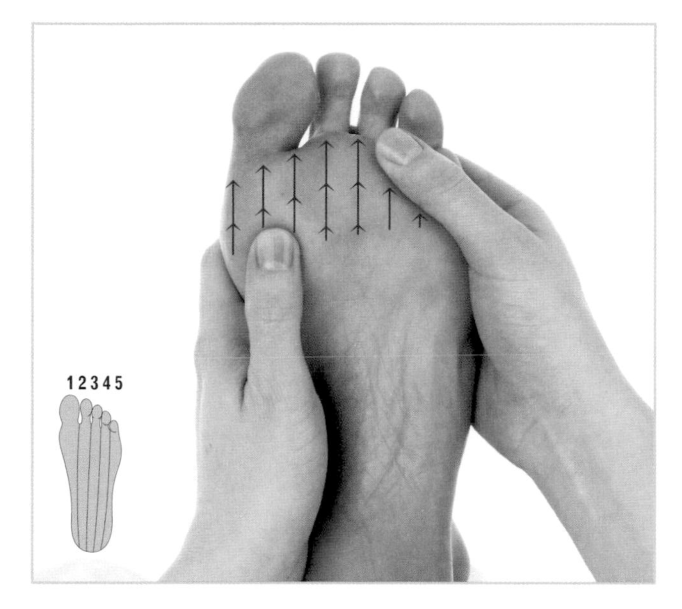

1 Support the left foot with the right hand and, using the left thumb, work up the foot in straight lines from medial to lateral.

Left foot – plantar
Lateral to medial – top support

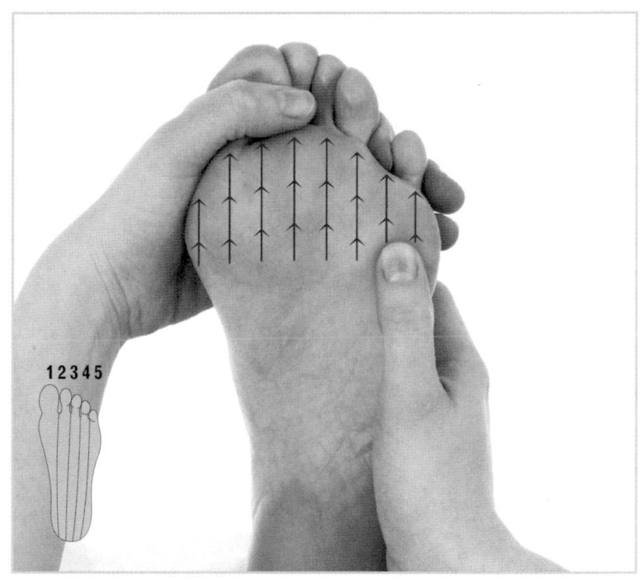

2 Support the left foot with the left hand and, using the right thumb, work up the foot in straight lines from lateral to medial. Separate each toe as you proceed.

The lung/breast area

Left foot – dorsal
Medial to lateral – top support

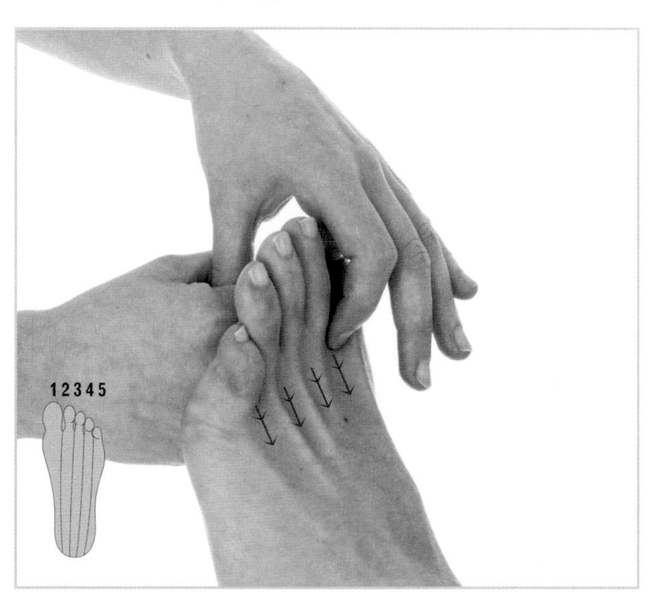

1 Support the left foot with your right fist and, using the left index finger, proceed downwards from medial to lateral.

Left foot – dorsal
Lateral to medial – top support

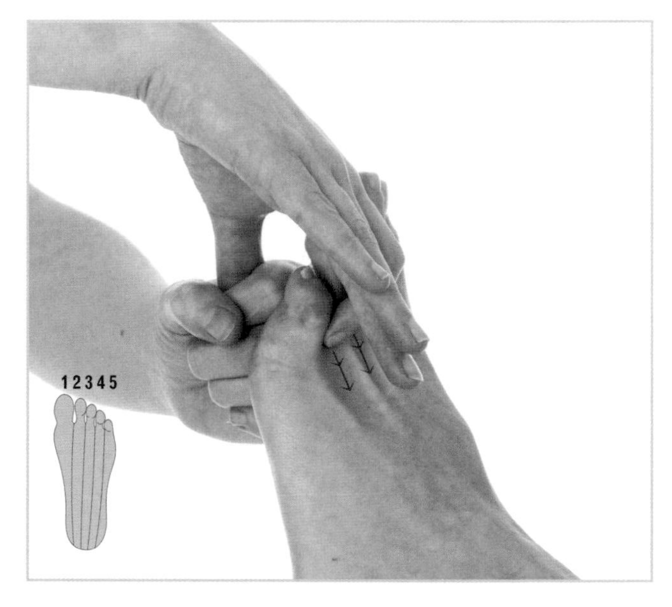

2 Support the left foot with your left fist and, using the right index finger, proceed downwards, from lateral to medial.

The circulatory system

As a dynamic pump, the heart is an amazingly sophisticated piece of equipment. No manufactured pump can work so tirelessly, efficiently and silently as the human heart, which may go on performing its duties for 100 years or even more without any form of servicing or attention.

Blood carries oxygen and vital energy to every part of the human body and transports waste matter to where it can either be purified, as in the liver, or expelled via the lungs or kidneys. The heart pumps this life-giving blood around the body through a network of blood vessels, including arteries, veins and capillaries, whose combined length would circle the earth nearly two and a half times!

The heart

The heart starts its life in the fetus as two beating tubes that can be detected on sophisticated monitoring equipment as early as the 16th day after conception. It develops into a cone-shaped organ, about the size of its owner's fist, which lies in the thoracic cavity between the lungs, a little more to the left than the right.

The wall of the heart consists of three layers. From the inside out, these are the endocardium (the smooth lining), the myocardium (heart muscle) and pericardium (the strong sac enveloping the heart).

The term myocardium derives from the Greek *muos*, 'muscle', and *kardia*, 'heart'. This is a specialized muscle that controls the beating of the heart. The myocardium can continue working tirelessly over the course of a long lifetime without requiring any medical intervention.

The heart is a double pump, with the right and left sides completely separated by a wall or septum. Each half is divided into an upper and lower chamber. The upper two chambers are called the atria (atrium in the singular) and the two lower chambers are the ventricles.

The atrium and ventricle of each half are separated by a valve, which opens and closes according to the changes of pressure in the chambers, allowing blood to flow in one direction only. The valve between the right atrium and the right ventricle is called the tricuspid valve. The valve on the left side is the bicuspid valve.

Valves also guard the exits from the ventricles into the principal artery or vein. Between the left ventricle and the aorta is the aortic valve, and between the right ventricle and the pulmonary artery is the pulmonary valve. Again, these valves only allow the blood to flow in one direction.

Arteries, veins and capillaries

Arteries carry blood from the heart to every part of the body through a complicated network. Because they are carrying blood under pressure they have thick, strong walls that can expand to absorb the surge of blood and then contract until the next heart beat. If an artery is cut open blood will spurt out at high pressure.

The smallest arteries (arterioles) branch into minute vessels called capillaries. Their walls consist of a single layer of cells, so are very fragile. Their construction, rather like a tea-bag, permits the nutrients and oxygen in the blood to diffuse easily into the surrounding tissue.

In exchange, the capillaries take up carbon dioxide and other waste products from the tissues and transport them away into venules, the smallest branches on an equally vast network of veins that leads back to the heart.

Deoxygenated blood returning to the heart through the veins is at low pressure: if a vein is cut or punctured, blood will seep out in a slow, steady flow. Blood is helped through the veins by a succession of one-way valves that prevent backflow. Valves are in abundance in the veins of the lower limbs, where blood must flow a considerable distance against the force of gravity.

BLOOD SUPPLY TO THE BRAIN

Branches of the internal carotid arteries and the basilar artery form a circle of arteries at the base of the brain known as the circle of Willis. From here, blood vessels provide the brain with oxygenated blood.

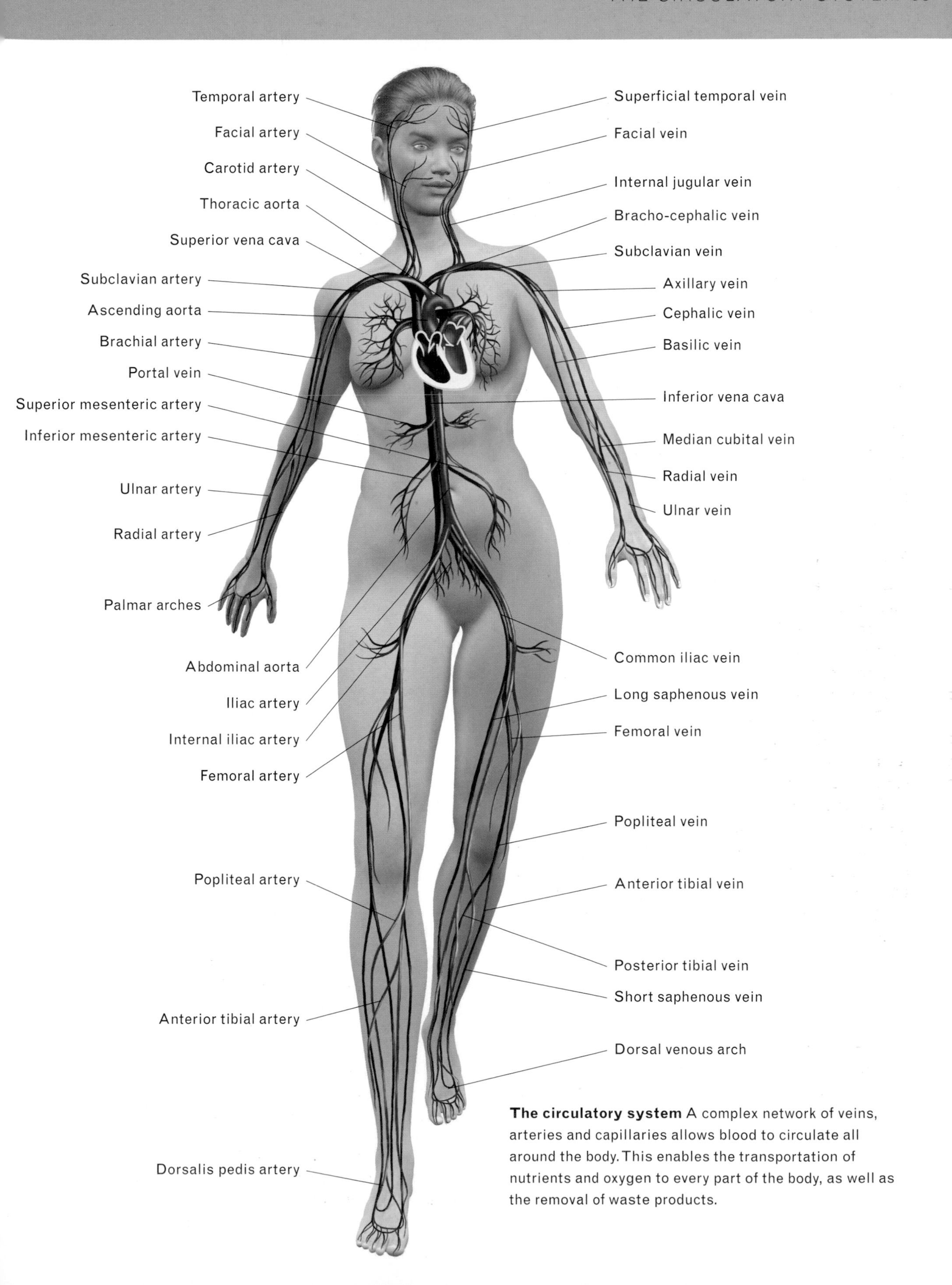

The circulatory system A complex network of veins, arteries and capillaries allows blood to circulate all around the body. This enables the transportation of nutrients and oxygen to every part of the body, as well as the removal of waste products.

Circulation

With each heart beat, oxygenated blood is pumped to every part of the body and de-oxygenated blood is pumped from the heart into the lungs to be re-oxygenated. The two largest veins of the body are the superior and inferior venae cavae. They empty their contents (de-oxygenated blood that has come from the body) into the right atrium. The atrioventricular (tricuspid) valve then opens, triggered by the increase in pressure in the right atrium, and the blood passes through into the right ventricle.

From the right ventricle the blood is pumped into the pulmonary artery, the only artery in the body that carries de-oxygenated blood. This divides into the left and right pulmonary arteries to carry blood to the lungs. Here an exchange of gases takes place and inhaled oxygen diffuses into the blood. (This is explained in more detail in 'The respiratory system', page 82.)

Two pulmonary veins, one arising from each lung, carry the freshly oxygenated blood to the left atrium of the heart. This stage, from the right ventricle of the heart to the lungs and back to the left atrium, is called the pulmonary circulation.

The arrival of blood in the left atrium opens the left atrioventricular (bicuspid) valve into the left ventricle. From here the blood is pumped directly into the aorta, which is the largest artery in the body. This is the first artery of general circulation and it descends behind the heart through the thoracic cavity, behind the diaphragm and into the abdominal cavity. It then divides to form the right and left iliac arteries and then continues throughout the body in what is called systemic circulation.

The speed at which the heart beats is controlled by the vagus nerve. The resting rate is usually about 70 beats per minute, but this increases dramatically during exercise or in times of stress. A healthy heart will have an even beat and both parts of the heart will pump out the same amount of blood after each beat and take in the same amount as they pump out.

RED BLOOD CELLS

Red blood cells (or erythrocytes) carry the oxygen content of blood and are responsible for its red colour. The life span of a red blood cell is about 120 days and new cells are continually being produced in the bone marrow to replace dead cells. This ensures that sufficient red blood cells are produced to carry a constant supply of oxygenated blood. A deficiency of red blood cells results in anaemia, which, if left untreated, causes tiredness and creates a strain on the heart.

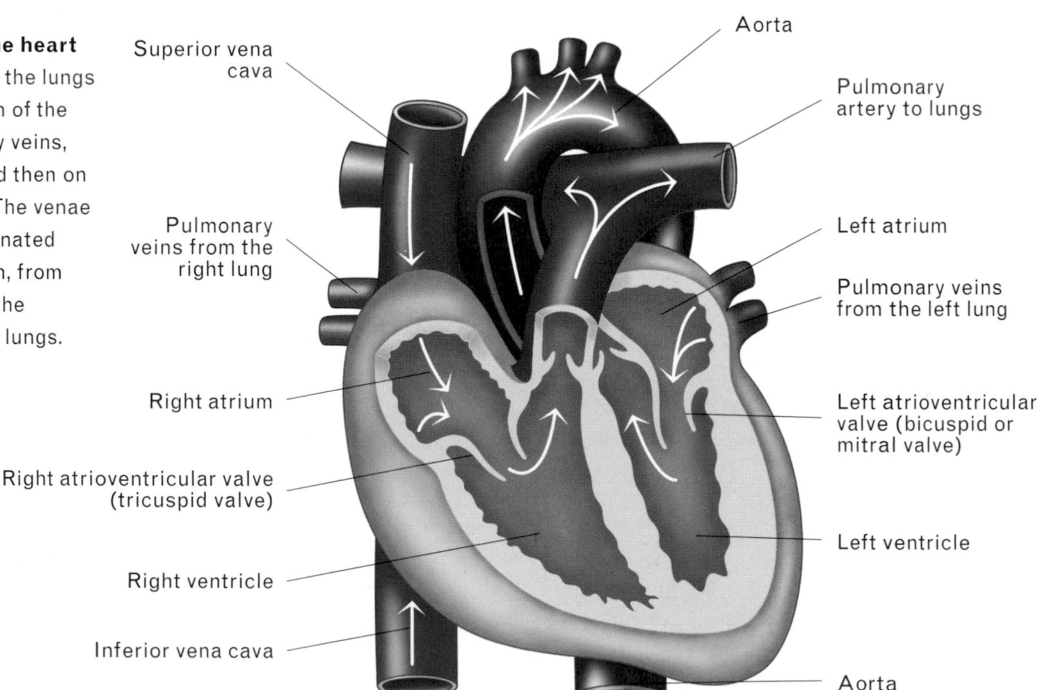

Blood flow through the heart Oxygenated blood from the lungs arrives in the left atrium of the heart via two pulmonary veins, passing to the aorta and then on to the rest of the body. The venae cavae deposit de-oxygenated blood in the right atrium, from where it is pumped via the pulmonary artery to the lungs.

Circulatory disorders helped by reflexology

The heart is so efficient it is often taken for granted, but when it lapses the repercussions for body are severe.

Coronary heart disease

Heart disease is a major killer in the Western world today, caused by poor diet, smoking, an excess of alcohol, a sedentary lifestyle and stress. Genetics is also a factor, in which case lifestyle changes are even more important.

Coronary heart disease is caused by narrowing of the coronary arteries that supply the heart with oxygen. Fatty deposits build up in the artery walls (atherosclerosis) and restrict the blood flow to the heart muscle, depriving the myocardium of oxygen. The heart receives insufficient oxygen and also cannot get rid of its waste products, so pain and discomfort are experienced in the chest, neck, arm or sometimes around the bottom of the diaphragm.

If fatty deposits become detached from the artery wall, a clot can form in the artery, causing an obstruction in the blood flow and depriving the heart of its fuel. A blocked artery can lead to a heart attack (myocardial infarction).

Coronary heart disease is three to six times more common in men than in women because the female hormone oestrogen offers the artery walls protection. Oestrogen also assists in avoiding hardening of the peripheral arteries. Despite this, the gender gap is narrowing as more women smoke and drink too much.

Arrhythmia

Although heart *rate* (beats per minute) varies, being slow at rest but increasing when physical or emotional demands are put on it, heart *beat* usually remains regular. Sometimes, however, it can develop an irregularity, such as unexpected quickening (tachycardia) or slowing (bradycardia). Arrhythmia can cause ectopic (extra) beats or fibrillation (weak contractions). While most of us have experienced such palpitations from time to time (the heart racing from too much caffeine, for example), an unsteady rhythm may be indicative that something is wrong, perhaps with the heart muscle or with a valve.

Hypertension (high blood pressure)

Blood pressure is determined by the force at which blood flows through the arteries, the elasticity of the arteries and the volume of blood in the body. A haemorrhage (severe bleeding) lowers the pressure, whereas poor renal function, for example, raises it. High blood pressure, 'the silent killer', can remain undetected for years. A person with high blood pressure is at increased risk of heart disease, stroke and other serious conditions.

Stroke

A stroke is a blockage or bursting of a blood vessel in the brain, usually associated with high blood pressure. The arteries in the brain are not as strong as other arteries. Eventually, the constant pressure leads to a clot or a bulge in the artery wall that bursts and creates a 'bleed in the brain', affecting the nerve supply to the body. A typical result would be paralysis (permanent or temporary) of an arm and leg, and loss of speech.

Aneurysm

An aneurysm is an abnormal swelling in a weakened arterial wall, which forms due to injury or disease. If it bursts, haemorrhaging will occur and frequently leads to death. Risk factors for aneurysm include diabetes, obesity, high blood pressure and smoking.

How reflexology can help

Reflexology can be of great support in the post-operative care of heart-attack patients and also helps alleviate symptoms such as angina and irregular heart beat. Treating heart conditions with reflexology is safe and effective; remember that the heart is a muscle that is similar to other organs and muscles.

Reflexology has proved very successful in helping people after a stroke, provided the treatment is given just as soon after the incident as is possible. Treatment must be given on a daily basis to get the maximum benefit.

Any form of circulatory malfunction can be improved with reflexology. Many patients report an improvement in circulation and cold feet often become a thing of the past.

REFLEXOLOGY AND DIABETES

People with diabetes often tend to have increased problems with circulatory disease in their later years. It is quite common for someone with diabetes eventually to suffer coronary conditions. The blood supply to their legs is often severely diminished and many suffer from ulceration and gangrene. Diabetes is also associated with stroke, renal failure and loss of sight. Reflexology is of great value in warding off these effects and is highly recommended for people of all age groups with diabetes.

Working the associated reflex points

In heart conditions, the main areas to work are obviously the heart and the lung reflexes. Diaphragm relaxation is of the utmost importance. It is also of great benefit to work the whole of the thoracic spine many times in order to stimulate the nerve supply to the thoracic cavity. Working on the liver is also very beneficial.

CASE STUDY **HEART ATTACK**

CLIENT PROFILE

John, who was 55, awoke one night with severe chest pains and within an hour was rushed into hospital as an emergency. Tests confirmed that he had suffered a heart attack. He said that, looking back, he had had odd sharp pains in his chest from time to time and noticed that when he walked up hills he become breathless, but had dismissed these symptoms as being due to the fact that he was getting older.

After discharge from hospital he was very frightened by the experience and anxious to do all he could to avoid another episode. A couple of years previously he had had reflexology to help him with a back condition so was well aware of the benefits of the treatment and felt that reflexology could now aid the healing process and help him back to recovery.

REGULARITY OF REFLEXOLOGY TREATMENT

Weekly for three months, then recommended to have regular monthly treatments to maintain his health.

REFLEXES

Main reflexes	Assistance
Heart	To aid the healing process of the heart
Lungs	To aid general respiration
Liver	To detoxify the blood
Solar plexus	To help stress levels

TREATMENT OUTCOMES

After three months of weekly treatment John returned to hospital for a check up, and his blood pressure, blood tests and ECGs were fine and the consultant was extremely pleased with his progress.

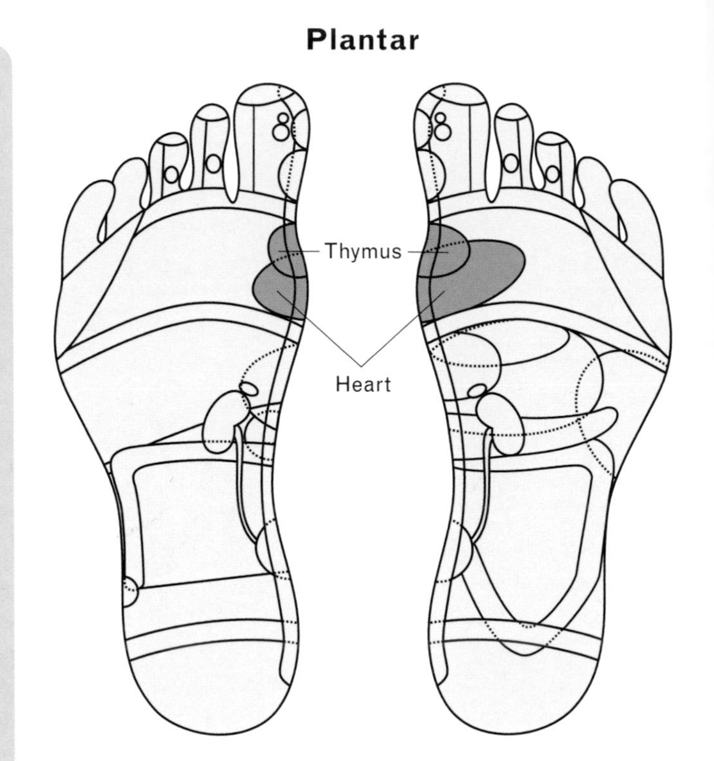

The heart area

Left foot – plantar
Medial to lateral – top support

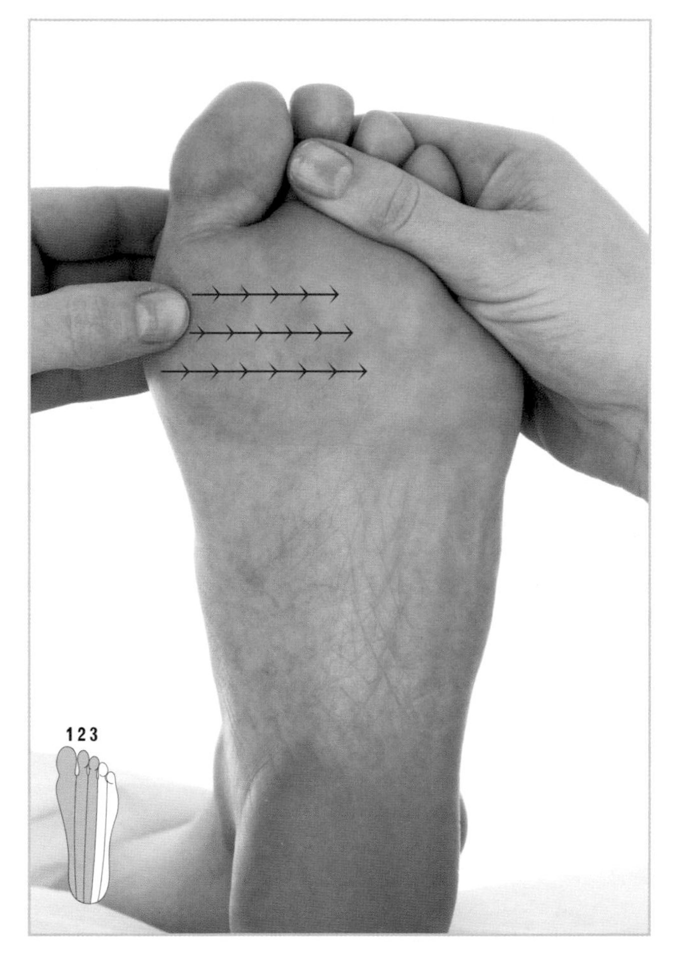

Support the left foot with your right hand and, using the left thumb, work in horizontal lines across the foot from medial to lateral. As the heart will already have been worked out thoroughly within the respiratory area, we do not overwork this area and therefore need only to proceed in one direction. (Just as organs and functions overlap in the human body, so reflex points overlap on the foot.)

BACK AND HEART CONDITIONS

In his book *The Heart Revolution*, Dr Paul Sherwood discusses the strong link between back conditions and heart problems. This has been a very welcome finding for me personally. During my long years as a practitioner, I have been involved in treating heart conditions on many occasions and I have been confused at finding intense sensitivity in the thoracic spine in those suffering from angina, coronary artery disease and the like.

There have been many occasions when people have been admitted into hospital after suffering a massive heart attack, when tests, even ECGs, have been completely normal. In these cases, if a clot had caused the coronary blockage it would still be present, shutting off the blood supply to the heart muscle, which would ultimately cause much damage. (When a muscle is damaged some of it dies and filaments from the dead muscle are released into the bloodstream as proteinous deposits.) If no clot is detected, the reason for the attack must have been a spasm in the coronary artery caused by inflammation and tension in the muscles, nerves and ligaments in the thoracic and cervical spinal areas.

As 'structure governs function' it is not difficult to understand how a long-term back condition could be associated with a heart attack: the attack being caused not by diseased arteries alone but by muscular spasms. When the thoracic and spinal areas were examined in a study of patients who had suffered one or more heart attacks, evidence of considerable tension in the paravertebral muscles in the area was found.

The lymphatic system

The lymphatic system works in conjunction with the blood's circulatory system but has its own network of vessels. It absorbs fat from the digestive system, helps to regulate body fluid and provides the body with its vital natural defences against disease.

When blood being pumped through the arteries reaches the smallest capillaries to deliver oxygen and nutrients to the surrounding tissues (see 'The circulatory system', page 88), not all the fluid that passes through the capillary walls drains back into the network of veins for the return journey to the heart. Instead, some 10 per cent of it remains behind in the tissue and enters the lymphatic system. Once the fluid enters the vessels of the lymphatic system it becomes known as lymph. It is a salty, straw-coloured liquid, like the fluid part of blood but containing less protein.

Lymph flow

The lymphatic system can be described as the body's secondary circulatory system, in which lymphatic fluid is moved around the body. Lymphatic fluid is not pumped by the heart, but encouraged to flow by the pulsation of arteries, the pressure difference in the thorax created by breathing, peristaltic movements of the intestine and contractions in the lymph vessels themselves. Its flow is also stimulated by muscular activity and movement, particularly walking. Many cup-shaped valves in the vessels ensure that the lymph flows in one direction only, towards the thorax.

Lymph is transported through a network of vessels, the outer walls of which are about the same thickness as small veins. These vessels drain into lymph nodes. The largest of all the lymphatic system's vessels is the thoracic duct, which runs up the body in front of the spine. Lymphatic vessels from all over the body, except the upper right quadrant, drain into it. The lymphatic vessels in the upper right quadrant of the body drain into the right lymphatic duct.

From these two main ducts, lymph returns to the bloodstream: the thoracic duct drains into the left subclavian vein near the left shoulder and the right lymphatic duct drains into the right subclavian vein near the right shoulder.

The spleen

The spleen, a spongy, fist-sized, purplish organ, is the largest organ in the lymphatic system and plays an important part in circulation and combating infection. It is located just in front of the spine, below the diaphragm and to the left of and behind the stomach. Entering and leaving the spleen are the splenic artery, splenic vein, lymphatic vessels and nerves.

As blood flows through the spleen, worn-out red and white blood cells are removed by large scavenger cells, and bacteria and parasites are destroyed. The spleen produces antibodies and protein to attack viruses and other agents of infection. In addition, the spleen also manufactures some of the blood formed in the fetus before birth.

Fluid retention and fat absorption

Lymph glands are found in all parts of the body, except for the central nervous system, teeth, cartilage and bone. The lymphatic system is probably best known for its role in the body's defence system. However, this system also provides two other important functions: it controls the fluid levels in body tissue and it absorbs fat from the digestive system.

Before fluid enters the lymphatic system as lymph it bathes the tissue cells throughout the body, when it is called interstitial fluid. This fluid is drawn off by the lymphatic system, which purifies it and returns it to the blood at a rate of about 3 litres (5 pints) daily. If this process is blocked or interrupted at any point, fluid builds up and leads to swelling, or oedema.

The lining of the small intestine has a high concentration of lymph vessels, called lacteals. These absorb the fat and fat-soluble vitamins from digested food as it passes through the small intestine. The fluid, which is so fat-laden that it has a milky appearance (which also explains the name of 'lacteal' for the initiating vessels), is called chyle.

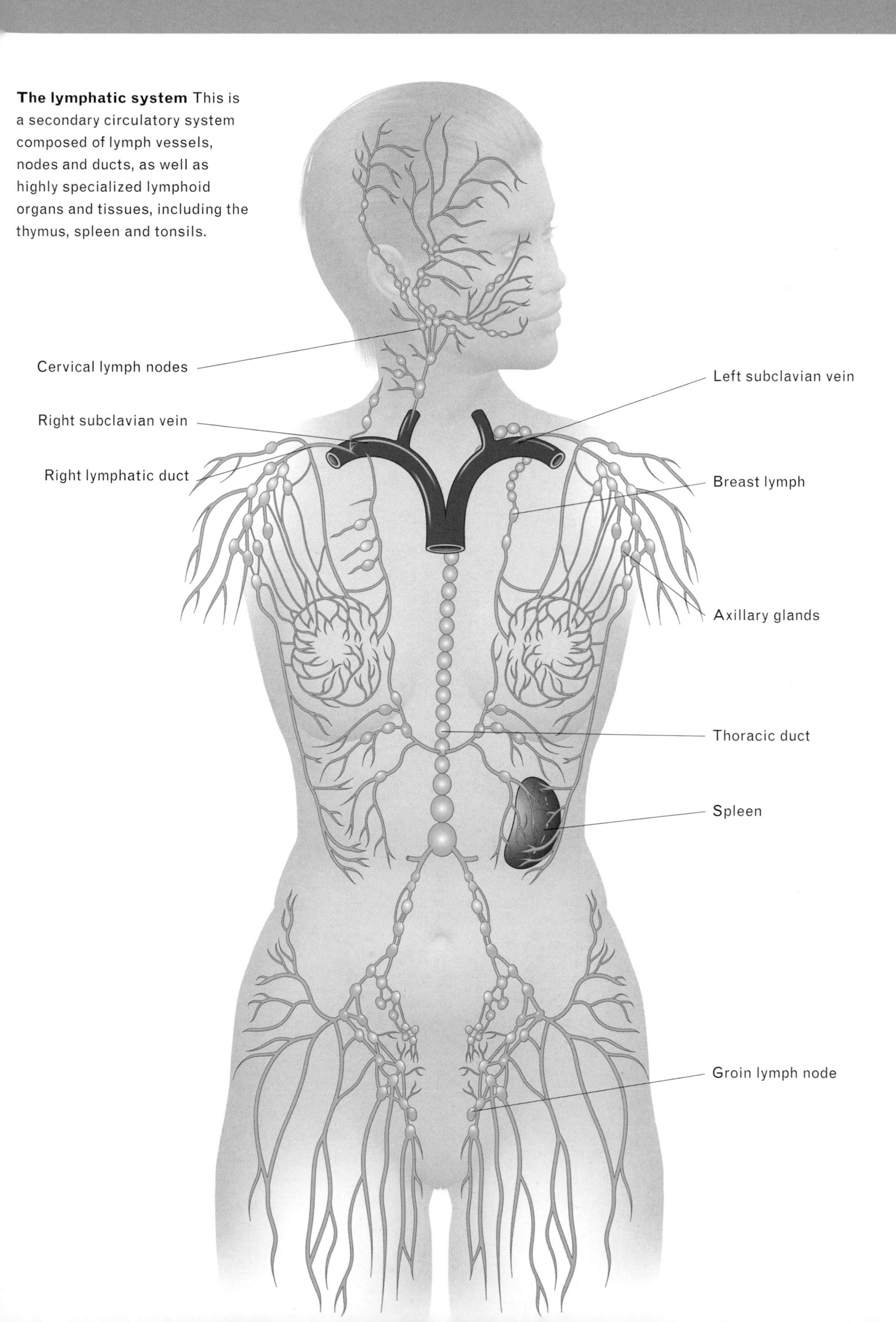

The lymphatic system This is a secondary circulatory system composed of lymph vessels, nodes and ducts, as well as highly specialized lymphoid organs and tissues, including the thymus, spleen and tonsils.

The lymphatic as a defence system

The body has two types of defence: non-specific and specific. Non-specific defences include, for example, the hairs in the nose that filter out foreign particles in inhaled air and the acid and enzymes in the stomach that destroy unwelcome bacteria in food or drink. The skin is important in this first line of defence. Specific defence is the job of the lymphatic system.

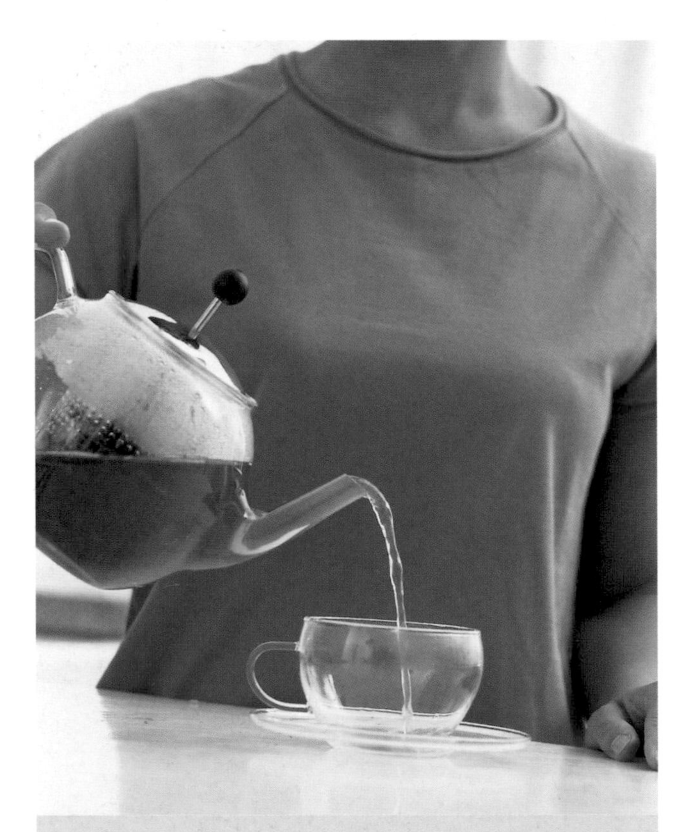

BOOSTING LYMPHATIC CIRCULATION

Reflexology aids the natural flow of lymph around the body. You can also boost lymph flow by:

- Drinking dandelion or fennel tea (natural diuretics), if you have a tendency to fluid retention.
- Circling your ankles and walking about after a long period of sitting, such as a long flight or car journey.
- Avoiding alcohol, especially on extended journeys in a confined space, as alcohol causes dehydration and increased swelling.
- Taking up exercise. Activities such as cycling, swimming and skipping will all boost lymph flow.

Strung along the network of lymphatic vessels are the lymph nodes. These are scattered throughout the body, but are found in large quantities in areas where there is a rich arterial supply: under the armpits, in the intestines and in the breast and groin areas. Some nodes are the size of a pinhead, others the size of an olive. Their function is to filter from the lymph any potentially hazardous microorganisms that have found their way into the body.

To fight off bacteria and other harmful substances, lymph nodes contain specialized white blood cells, notably lymphocytes. These respond to invaders in two principal ways: lymphocyte T cells attack an alien organism directly, while lymphocyte B cells produce protein compounds called antibodies.

Thymus gland

Located in the upper thorax, the thymus plays a key role in the body's immune process. One of the roles of the thymus gland is to secrete the hormone thymosin, which stimulates the development of T cells (B cells originate in bone marrow). B cells work in tandem with T cells, producing antibodies designed to eliminate and destroy threatening organisms when prompted by T cells. Importantly, though, it is B cells that hold the 'memory' of any previous battle against an antigen, allowing the body to react extremely swiftly when it recognizes a threat it has encountered before.

How reflexology can help

When infection attacks the body, the lymph nodes swell at strategic points: the neck, armpit, liver, intestines, groin and knee. If you have an acute attack of tonsillitis, for example, the lymph nodes around your neck and throat will swell in an attempt to prevent the infection rising into the brain. A healthy body can defend itself against most types of disease-causing organisms. Unfortunately, there are many aspects of modern everyday living that cause the lymphatic system to become depressed. 'The immune system' (pages 190–193) looks in more detail at how a weakened immune system leaves the body open to infection and illness, and how reflexology can be used to boost its powers.

One way in which reflexology can help the lymphatic system is by ridding the body of the excess fluid that can build up in many parts, especially the legs, feet, fingers and hands. Fluid can build up because lymphatic fluid is circulated not by the heart but by the movement of muscles, so if we sit still for too long a period the lymphatic fluid may pool in the legs and cause the legs and feet to swell.

Working the associated reflex points

As the lymphatic system is distributed throughout the body, we do not need to isolate specific areas on the feet. The whole lymphatic system is treated as we work on the entire body. The thoracic duct, for example, runs in front of the spine in the rib cage area, so working out the thoracic area of the spine would stimulate this area and assist drainage of the lymphatic system.

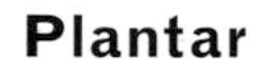

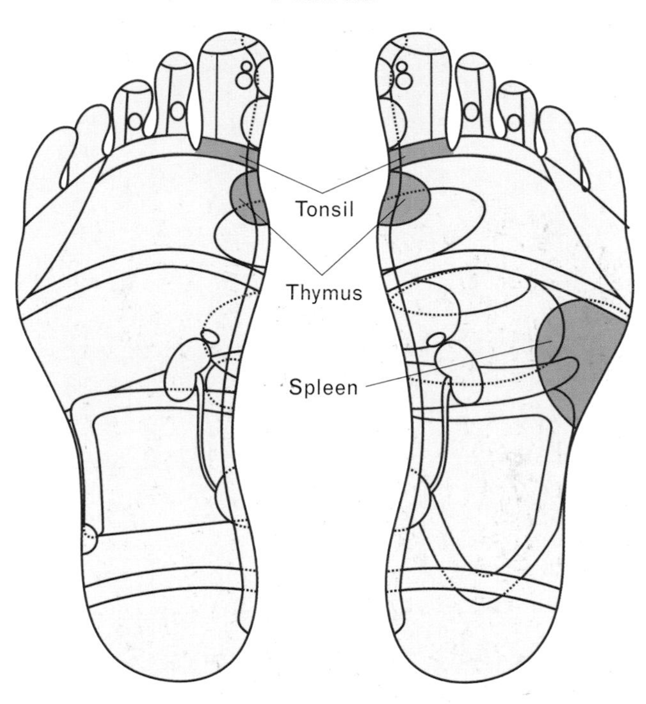

Dorsal

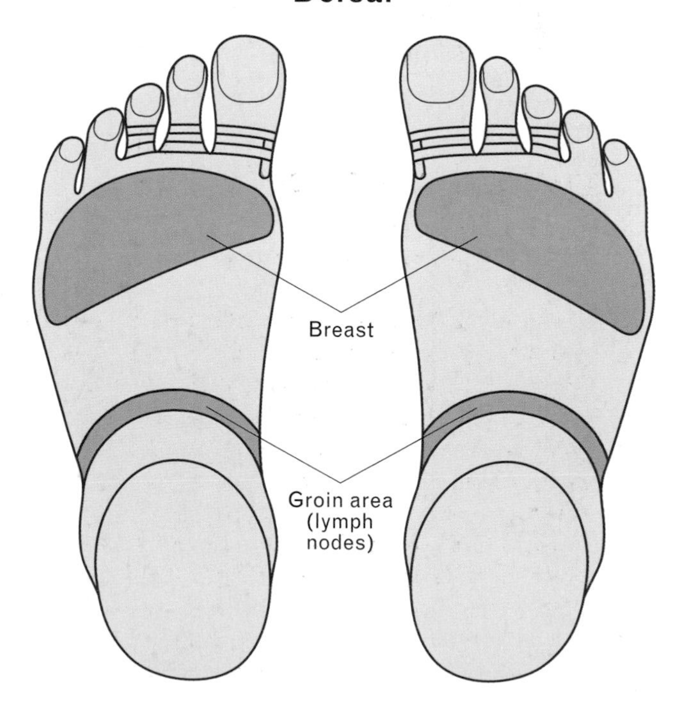

CASE STUDY **BREAST CANCER**

CLIENT PROFILE

Mary had come for treatment following a mastectomy of her right breast. She was feeling depressed and anxious about her diagnosis and was suffering from pain and swelling of her right arm following removal of lymph nodes from her armpit.

REGULARITY OF REFLEXOLOGY TREATMENT

Twice weekly in the first three weeks and then a further six treatments on a weekly basis.

REFLEXES

Main reflexes	Assistance
Breast and lymphatic areas	To help reduce pain and swelling
Spleen	To help general immunity
Entire endocrine system	To help the hormonal system and balance the body

TREATMENT OUTCOMES

Mary's feet were extremely sensitive in the breast area on the right side, which was to be expected following surgery. Following her first treatment she reported that she felt relaxed and had slept well. After three sessions she was quite amazed that she was able to lift her arm with greater ease. At the end of her treatment sessions the mobility in her right arm was almost back to normal, the pain level had reduced and she felt more relaxed and able to cope with life again. Mary continued with reflexology on a regular basis to help her general health.

The endocrine system

The endocrine system consists of glands and tissues in various parts of the body that produce hormones. Since hormones regulate many of the body's internal systems and cycles, many aspects of our physical and mental health are reliant on the endocrine system functioning well.

The glands and tissues of the endocrine system are the:

- Hypothalamus
- Pituitary gland
- Pineal gland
- Thyroid gland
- Four parathyroid glands
- Thymus
- Two adrenal glands
- Islets of Langerhans in the pancreas
- Two ovaries in the female and testes in the male.

The endocrine system works with the nervous system to maintain the body in a steady state. It does this through the secretion of hormones or monitoring the rate of hormonal secretion. Hormones are chemical messengers that carry information concerning the speed at which glands and organs work. Hormones are themselves mostly controlled by a mechanism called 'feedback'. When a gland is working overtime, the hormonal system reduces the power, rather like a thermostat. If the activity of a gland becomes sluggish and malfunctions, the hormonal system gives it a boost and increases the power. In this way the endocrine system regulates the metabolism, the use of nutrients by cells, salt and fluid balance, and growth and reproduction, and it also helps the body to cope in times of stress.

The pituitary gland and the hypothalamus

Endocrine activity is controlled by an area of the brain called the hypothalamus, acting in conjunction with the pituitary gland. The hypothalamus has a direct controlling effect on the pituitary gland and an indirect effect on many other aspects: it links the nervous and endocrine systems.

The pituitary gland lies between the eyes and behind the nose, protected by a very strong arch of bone called the sella turcica (Turkish saddle). The gland regulates the activity of most of the other endocrine glands and is referred to as 'the conductor of the orchestra'.

The pituitary has an anterior and a posterior lobe. The anterior lobe secretes the following tropic hormones (so-called because they stimulate other endocrine glands):

- **Thyroid stimulating hormone (TSH)**: This activates the thyroid gland.
- **Adrenocorticotropic hormone (ACTH)**: Responsible for stimulating the adrenal glands.
- **Gonadotropic hormones**: In a woman, these stimulate the development and release of an egg from the ovaries each month. In a man, they stimulate the production of spermatozoa and testosterone. (See page 146 for more on hormones in the reproductive system.)

The anterior lobe also secretes two non-tropic hormones:

- **Growth hormone**: This promotes growth of the skeleton, muscles, connective tissue and organs.
- **Prolactin**: This stimulates the cells of the mammary glands to secrete milk.

Two other hormones are secreted by the hypothalamus, stored in the posterior lobe of the pituitary and released when required:

- **Oxytocin**: This promotes contraction of uterine muscles and contraction of the cells of the lactating breast, squeezing milk into the large ducts behind the nipple. In late pregnancy the uterus becomes very sensitive to oxytocin. The amount secreted will be increased just before and during labour as well as when the baby is suckling.
- **Antidiuretic hormone (ADH)**: This regulates fluid balance and indirectly controls blood pressure. ADH helps the body conserve water by increasing water reabsorption from the kidneys' collecting ducts.

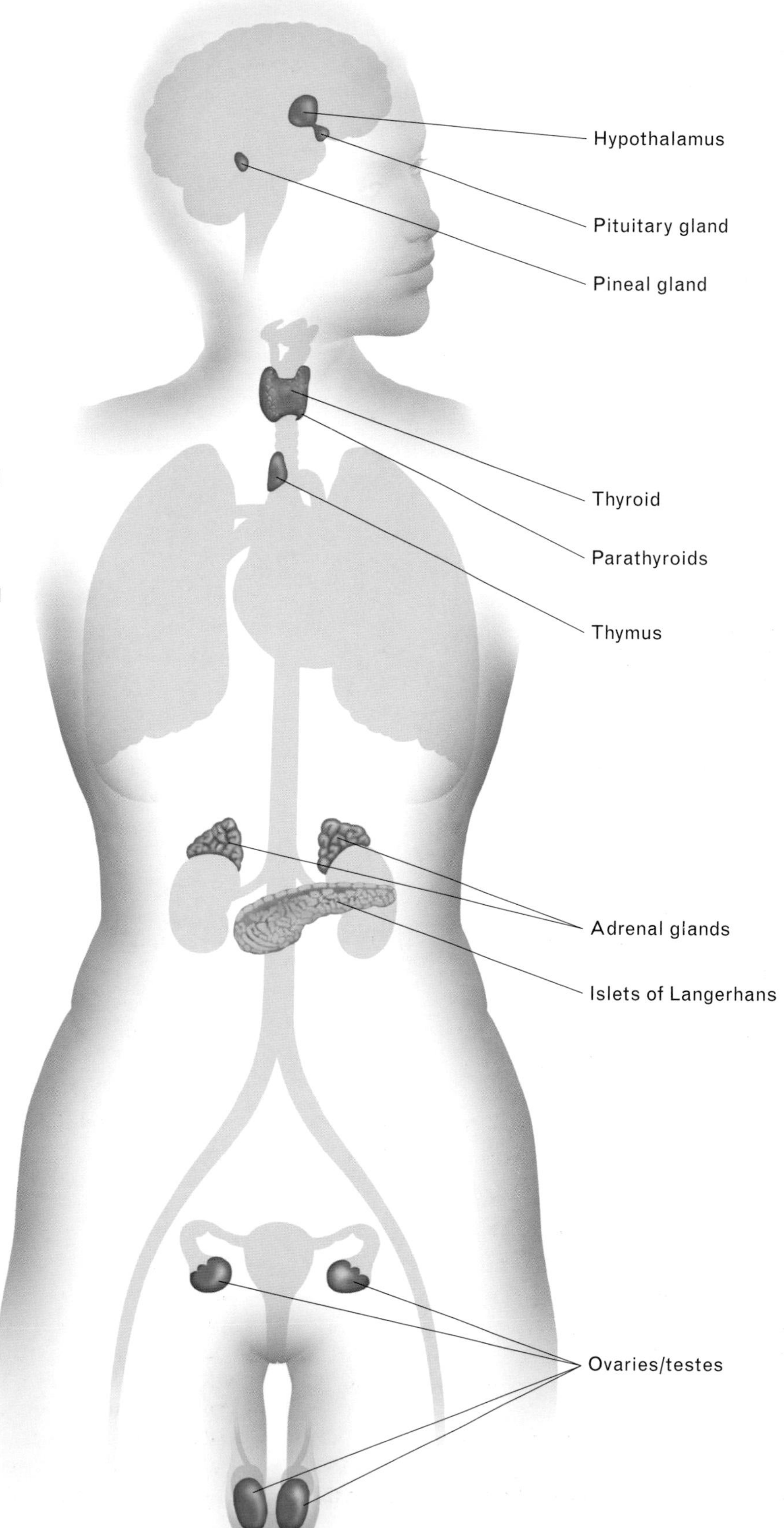

The endocrine system The endocrine glands and tissues produce hormones, the 'chemical messengers', and release them into the bloodstream. Endocrine glands and tissues include the pituitary, thyroid, parathyroid and adrenal glands, as well as the ovaries, the testes, part of the pancreas and the placenta.

THE ULTRAVIOLET EFFECT

For a long period through the winter, the people of the Arctic circle have to live in semi-twilight. During this time displays of uncharacteristic behavioural patterns, such as manic depression, hysteria and paranoia, are common. In extreme cases, people have been known to lose the use of a limb or limbs; this is often referred to as 'hysterical paralysis'.

Psychologists and psychiatrists studying the people of Greenland concluded that such behaviour patterns resulted from extreme climatic conditions and lack of sunlight. When patients with mental difficulties were given a daily dose of ultraviolet rays in the area of the pineal gland for 20 minutes over the period of a month, the results were outstanding: 90 per cent of sufferers regained their normal mental state.

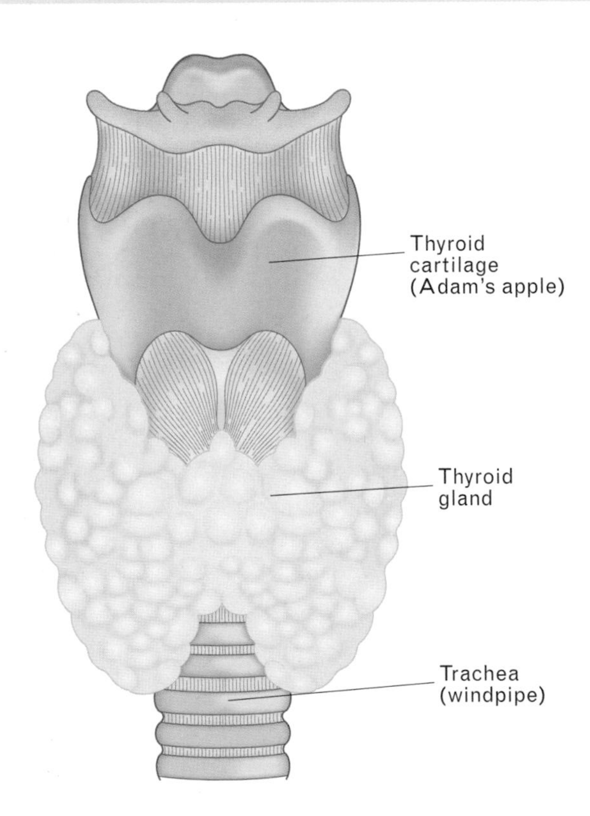

The thyroid gland One of the largest endocrine glands, the butterfly-shaped thyroid gland has many functions including regulating growth, metabolism and the body's sensitivities to other hormones. It also controls fertility, as hypothyroidism can inhibit conception.

The pineal gland

This little gland is situated in the forebrain and resembles a pine cone in shape, hence the name. It is connected to the brain by a short stalk containing nerves, many of which terminate in the hypothalamus. It is about 10 mm (just under ½ in) long, reddish brown in colour and surrounded by a capsule.

The pineal gland secretes a hormone called melatonin in response to low light levels. This helps us to feel sleepy in the late evening. Secretion levels are at their peak in the middle of the night and then gradually fall. Increased light inhibits production of melatonin, which encourages us to awaken from sleep in the morning.

There is a direct association between the pineal gland and moods and behaviour patterns. Many people find that during the autumn and winter months they tend to mimic the behavioural pattern of animals: they gain body weight, become less active and find that their mental activities become reduced. This behavioural change continues until spring when the hours of daylight lengthen and the earth and life itself become vital again.

In countries that have long seasons with little sunlight, seasonal affective disorder, often referred to as SAD, is quite common. The main reason for its depressive symptoms is lack of sunlight. Many people find that exposure to ultraviolet light has a direct effect on mood and it is now felt that the pineal gland has some reflecting effect upon the brain that is transmitted via the optic nerve (see box).

Although most of us would agree that it is far better to look out on a sunny day than a grey dismal one, SAD is more than just an emotional response; it is a basic physiological fact that we need sun to keep us in good mental health. That is probably the reason why the intake into psychiatric hospitals during the autumn and winter months is so high.

The thyroid and parathyroid glands

The thyroid, situated in the neck, is one of the larger endocrine glands and is responsible for stimulating growth and development. It extracts iodine from the blood in order to produce hormones including thyroxine and calcitonin.

The thyroid is also responsible for the metabolism of the body and influences the heart rate. An overactive thyroid can result in unpleasant heart palpitations. Other symptoms include greasy skin and hair and an increased appetite but with a paradoxical loss of weight. The body is running in a very high gear, so the ability to relax becomes impossible, insomnia becomes a problem and anxiety levels increase.

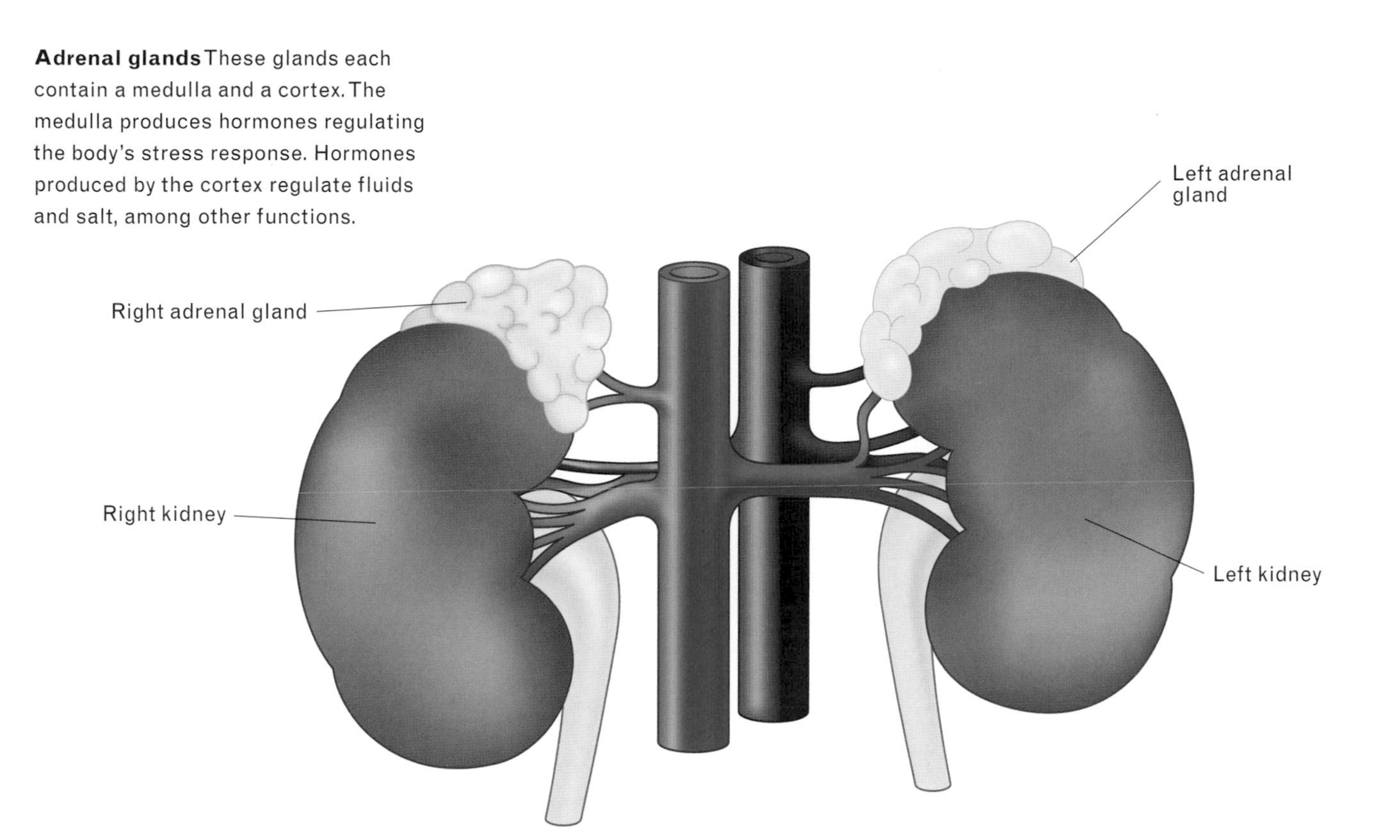

Adrenal glands These glands each contain a medulla and a cortex. The medulla produces hormones regulating the body's stress response. Hormones produced by the cortex regulate fluids and salt, among other functions.

If the thyroid gland is underactive, the opposite signs are apparent: an increase in weight, dry and scaly skin, thin, dry hair, lethargy, muscle weakness and reduced mental abilities (a child born with a malfunction of the thyroid would be mentally impaired).

The parathyroid glands lie embedded in the thyroid gland and secrete parathyroid hormone, a small protein that regulates the calcium level of the blood and tissue fluid. The thyroid and parathyroids work together to regulate blood calcium levels.

The thymus

This pink-grey gland lies just behind the sternum at the base of the throat. The function of the thymus changes as we develop: from before birth until puberty it produces the immune system's T cells (see 'The lymphatic system', page 96). It is very large in children as it is their main organ of immunity, but it reduces in size as they become young adults, when the spleen matures and takes over this function.

The adrenal glands

The adrenal glands are found above the kidneys. Each one has an inner medulla surrounded by an outer cortex, both of which secrete several different hormones. The medulla secretes epinephrine (adrenaline) and norepinephrine (noradrenaline). Noradrenaline raises heart rate and blood pressure and both hormones affect the body during stress (see page 102). The cortex secretes hormones that regulate fluid and salts, such as aldosterone, which maintains a sodium and phosphate balance, and cortisol, which helps the body cope with stress and inflammatory conditions and controls how the body uses carbohydrates, fat and protein.

In addition, the adrenal glands secrete very small amounts of the sex hormones androgen (masculinizing effect) and oestrogen (feminizing effect). These hormones, released in both sexes, are so small that they have little effect on the body.

The islets of Langerhans

These are found within the pancreas and regulate the sugar levels in the blood. Their function and the link with diabetes are described in greater detail in 'The digestive system', on page 74.

The ovaries and testes

The female ovaries and male testes produce hormones that control sexual development and secondary sexual characteristics (see 'The reproductive system', page 146).

Endocrine disorders helped by reflexology

Stress and the endocrine system are closely linked, and so the endocrine conditions for which reflexology can achieve the best results are tension states.

Stress is, in the main, not destructive; in fact we all need to be stressed at times to be able to achieve anything. It is how the body copes with stress that is all important.

Some individuals thrive on stressful situations. They often go through life creating situations to activate stress levels in the body, because they perform better when in an emotionally charged state.

Stress-related problems

It is when we are tense all the time that troubles in our health begin. We hold tension in our neck and shoulders, hence the phrase 'He's a real pain in the neck'. How stress manifests itself through the body varies from person to person, but the following are just a few of the common symptoms (see also page 196):

- Migraine
- Indigestion
- Angina
- Colitis
- Asthma
- Back pain

When we are in a tense, anxious condition, our immune system becomes depressed; too much nervous energy has been burnt up and so the general vitality of the body is affected, leaving us wide open to the onset of illness. It is not surprising to find great sensitivity in the big toe area of those suffering from depression, anxiety and other stress-related conditions.

Our adrenal glands are very receptive to emotions and feelings. The days when we all lived in caves and caught wild animals to survive have long passed, but our adrenal glands have not evolved and still react to excitement, alarm or danger as if we literally had to run or fight for our lives (see below).

Racing through life at the speed of light, having little time to 'stand and stare' has a destructive effect. People who meditate or practise relaxation techniques generally enjoy better health than those who do not, which is proof enough that relaxation and good feelings about oneself benefit the body. The greatest benefit we can ever achieve with reflexology is relaxation of the body, mind and spirit.

Tension, anxiety and fright

It's worth looking at what actually happens when we are tense, anxious or frightened and comparing the body processes with those experienced by our cave-dwelling ancestors. As he stalked his prey the hunter's nerves would be quivering and alert to any movement or sound, glucose and fats would be released from his liver to give him extra energy and power; his bronchial tubes would dilate to enable him to take in more oxygen; his heart would beat faster to distribute the oxygen around his body, preparing him to attack or run for his life. His blood was already thickening in his veins so that it would be able to clot faster if he were wounded and he probably had a great desire to urinate frequently or have a bowel movement. His pupils were dilated to enable him to see better and even his hearing was more acute as he watched and listened.

All these bodily changes resulted from the release of enormous amounts of adrenaline. And what a life-saving hormone it was, for a lack of strength or speed or alertness at a crucial moment might mean either no food or becoming the prey instead of the predator.

The energy used in the hunt was enormous and afterwards he would sleep for many hours to recover from the emotional and physical experience. This is exactly how the human machine was meant to perform and how adrenaline is intended to serve us.

Today, although we live in a totally different world, our bodies react to fear, alarm and tension in exactly the same way. We're unlikely to have to face a wild boar, but we might have a patronizing and difficult boss to contend with, who releases in us all sorts of emotions from anger to utter despair. We live in fear of redundancy. We fight through traffic jams and worry about the future of our children in a world of so much violence.

In response to these modern-day anxieties, fears and tensions, our bodies produce the same symptoms and hormones as a caveman's. (That urgent desire to urinate or empty the bowels when confronting an alarming situation, such as taking an examination or facing an audience, is a remnant left over from the time when you had to carry as little weight as possible in order to escape!) The big problem is that we seldom have the opportunity to run for our life or burn off, by extreme physical exercise, the excess of adrenaline. So our body retains the excess of fats, glucose and adrenaline in our system, clogging up our arteries and causing the cardiovascular diseases that are so prevalent today.

We need more exercise and relaxation, a balance of both. What better way to achieve total relaxation than through reflexology?

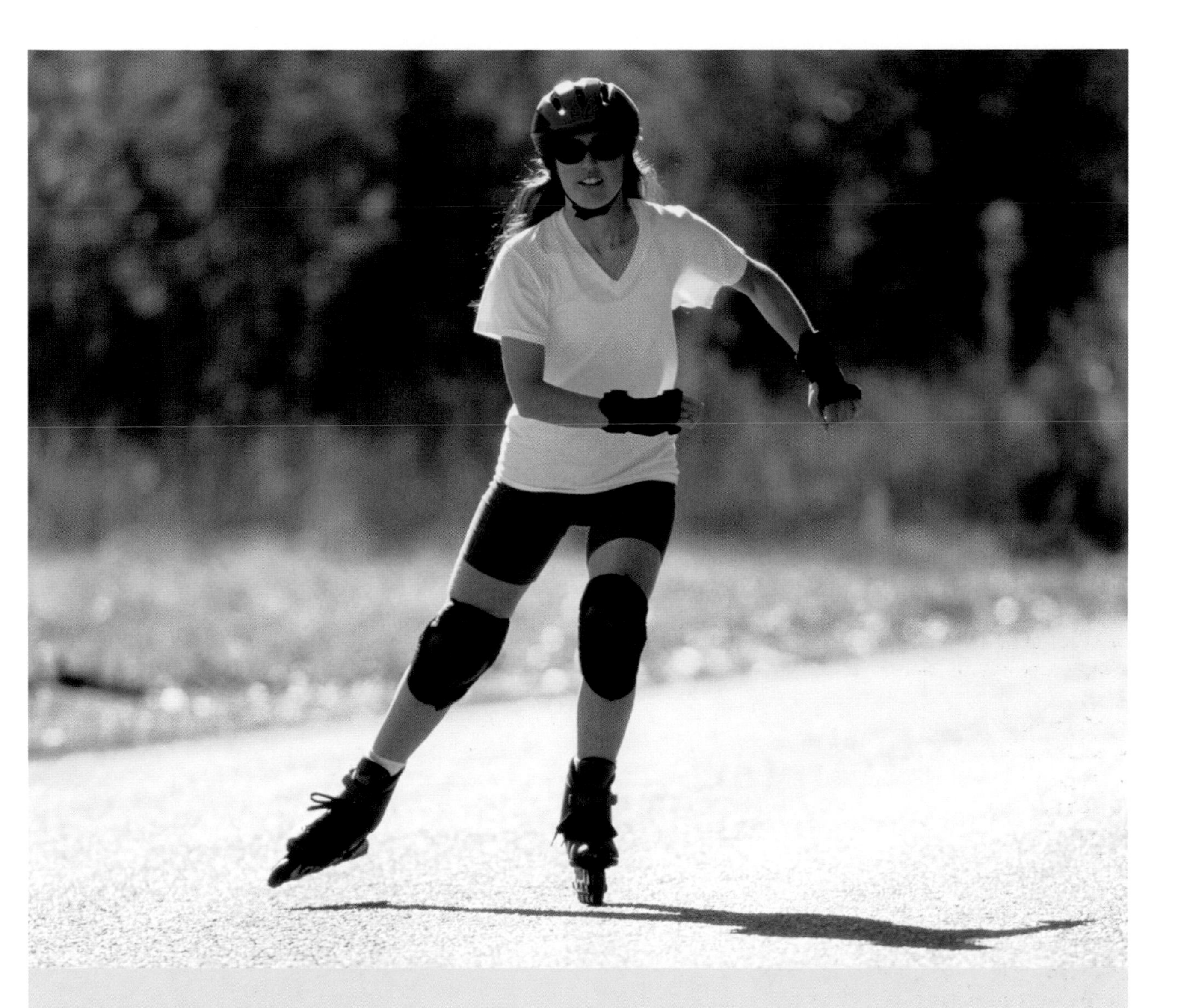

STRESS-BUSTING ACTIVITIES

When we feel we have to 'run for our life', the glands of the endocrine system release adrenaline to stimulate heart beat and speed up the body's functioning. Too much adrenaline can have a negative effect, causing us to feel stressed and anxious, with symptoms like a racing heart, excessive perspiration, diarrhoea and rapid shallow breathing. Exercise is the very best way of dealing with surplus adrenaline, so here are some tips for making the most of your physical activity:

- Go for a run, cycle or work out at the gym. Aerobic activity will burn up the adrenaline in your bloodstream and make you feel instantly better.
- Don't exercise straight after eating as the increase in blood sugar levels can make exercise uncomfortable. You can eat a light snack about an hour beforehand.
- Remember to eat after exercise. Consuming some carbohydrates within 30 minutes of strenuous exercise will replace fuel stores and help your body to recover.
- Keep it varied. If you find yourself becoming bored with your exercise regime, then try out a new activity. Alternatively, set yourself a target, such as training for a race.

Working the associated reflex points

The reflexes relating to the brain and thyroid areas are found in the toes, the adrenal and pancreatic reflexes are in the central plantar area and the reflexes of the reproductive organs are on the heel.

CASE STUDY

IRREGULAR MENSTRUAL CYCLE

CLIENT PROFILE

At 35 years of age, Pauline had for many years had a very erratic and painful menstrual cycle. Her periods would sometimes have a gap of 45–50 days and at other times would arrive within 21 days. As she was having trouble conceiving, she wanted to see if reflexology could regulate her cycle and improve her pain levels, before taking synthetic hormones (which she wanted to avoid).

REGULARITY OF REFLEXOLOGY TREATMENT

Weekly for three months.

REFLEXES

Main reflexes	Assistance
Pituitary/hypothalamus	To stimulate hormonal activities
Thyroid	To aid metabolism
Ovaries and uterus	To improve their function

TREATMENT OUTCOMES

Pauline's entire reproductive system was very sensitive. On her first visit her right ovary reflex in particular had a sharp reaction (when ovulation is imminent, the egg-producing ovary will express a sharp reaction in the foot). In view of this sensitivity I considered that Pauline was about to ovulate. Her thyroid gland was also sensitive.

The day after her first session she felt very active and a week later her period arrived and was pain-free, much to her delight. After three months of treatment her menstrual cycle was much more regular – between 28 and 30 days. It is hoped that conception will become possible now that her cycle has become more regular.

Plantar

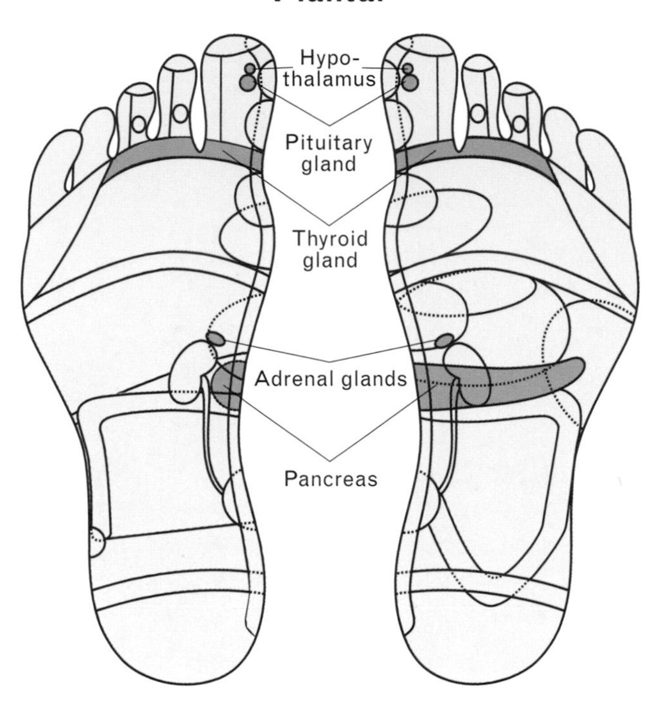

Lateral

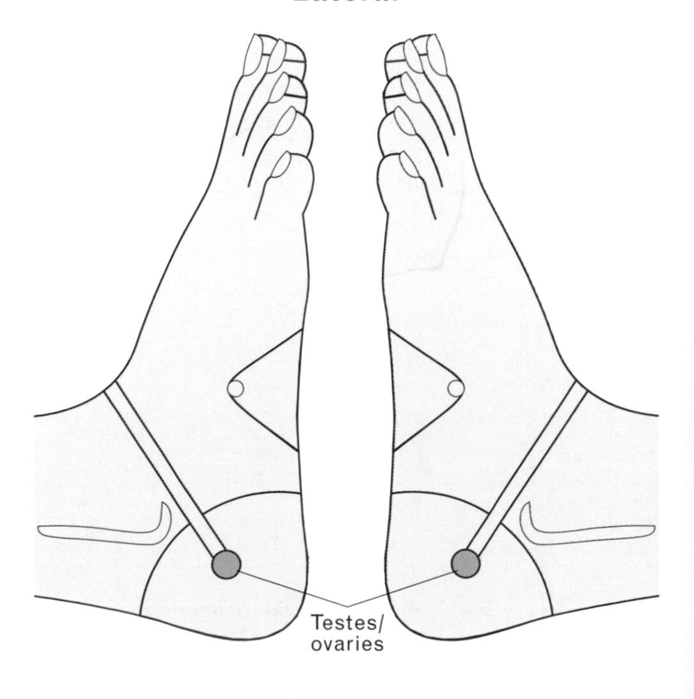

The pituitary, hypothalamus and pineal areas

Right foot – plantar
Medial – top support

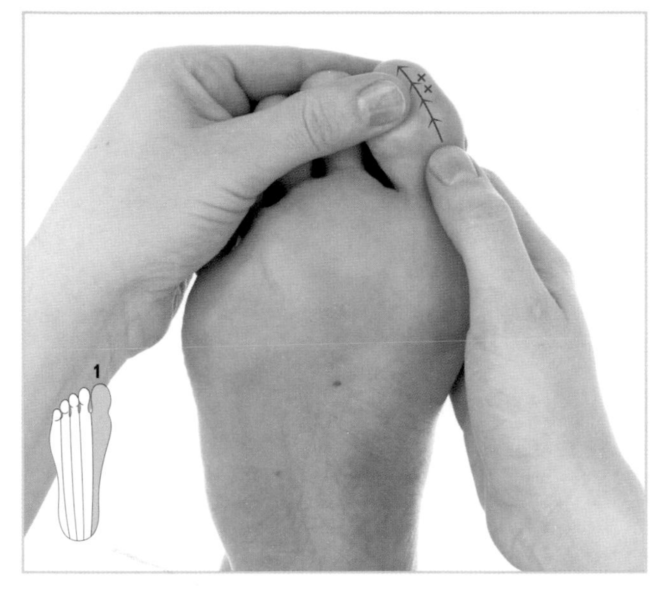

1 Support the right foot at the top with your left hand and, using the right thumb, work three times up the medial side of the big toe.

Left foot – plantar
Medial – top support

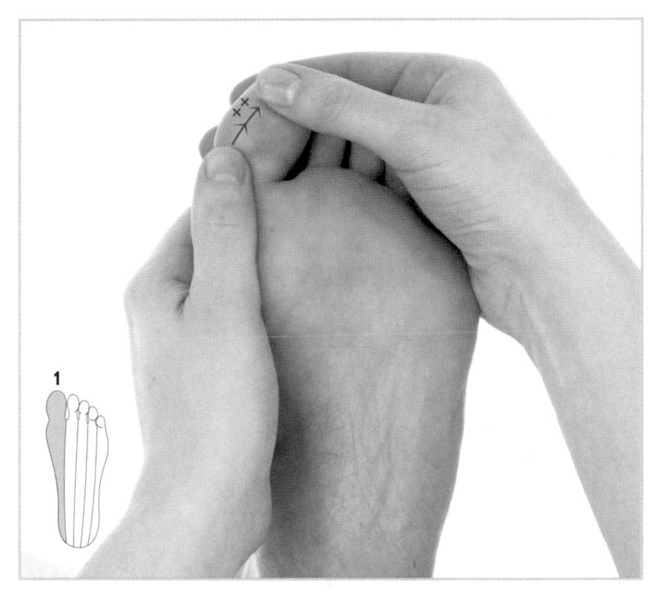

2 Support the left foot at the top with your right hand and, using the left thumb, work three times up the medial side of the big toe.

The thyroid/neck area

Right foot – plantar
Medial to lateral – top support

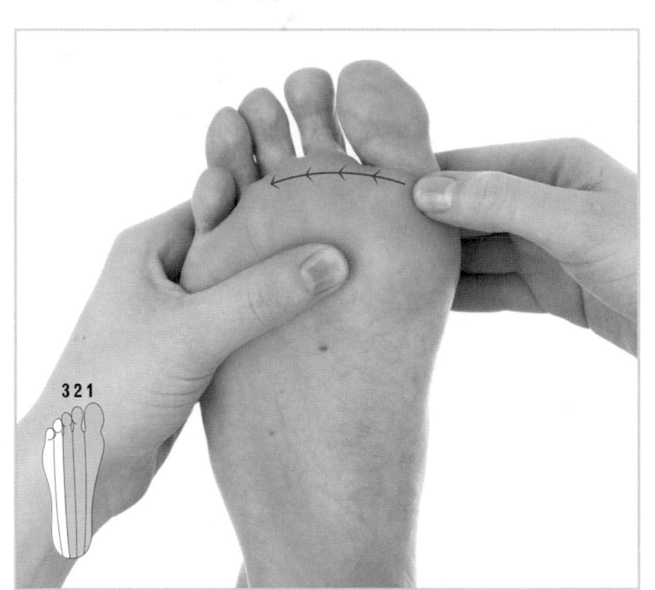

1 Support the right foot at the top with your left hand and, using the right thumb, work across the base of the three toes three times.

Right foot – dorsal
Medial to lateral – top support

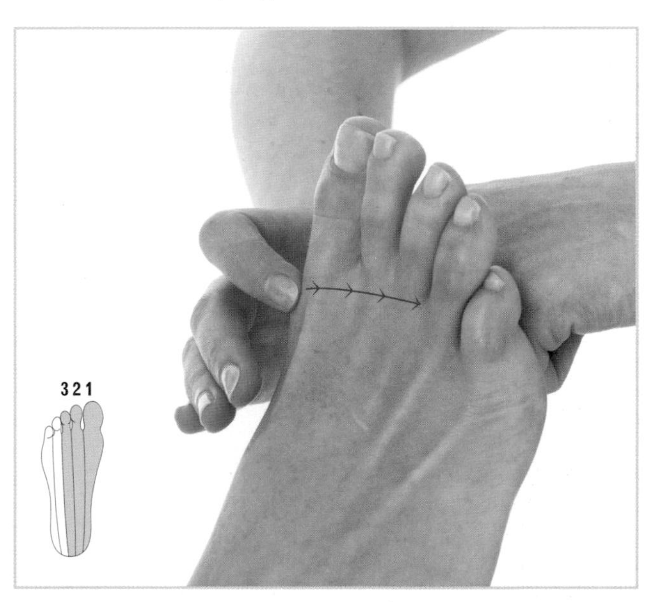

2 Support the right foot with your left fist and, using the right index finger, work across the join of the three toes three times.

The thyroid/neck area

Left foot – plantar
Medial to lateral – top support

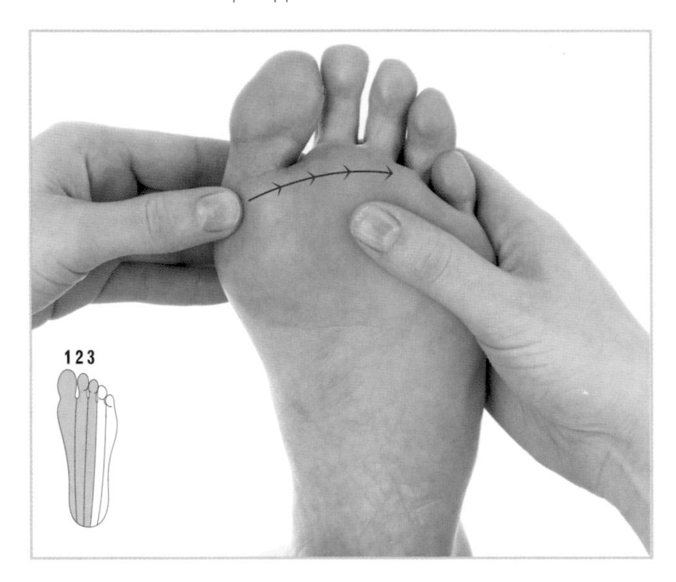

1 Support the left foot at the top with your right hand and, using the left thumb, work across the base of the three toes three times.

Left foot – dorsal
Medial to lateral – top support

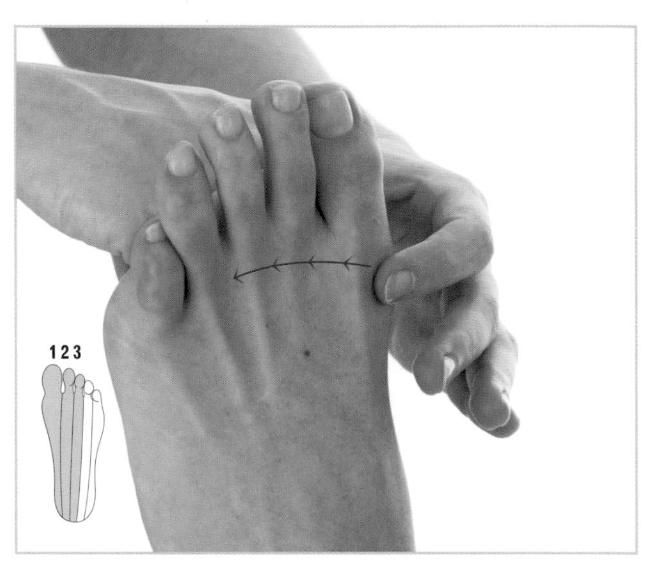

2 Supporting the left foot with your right fist and using the left index finger, work across the join of the three toes three times.

The adrenal glands

Right foot – plantar
Medial to lateral – top support

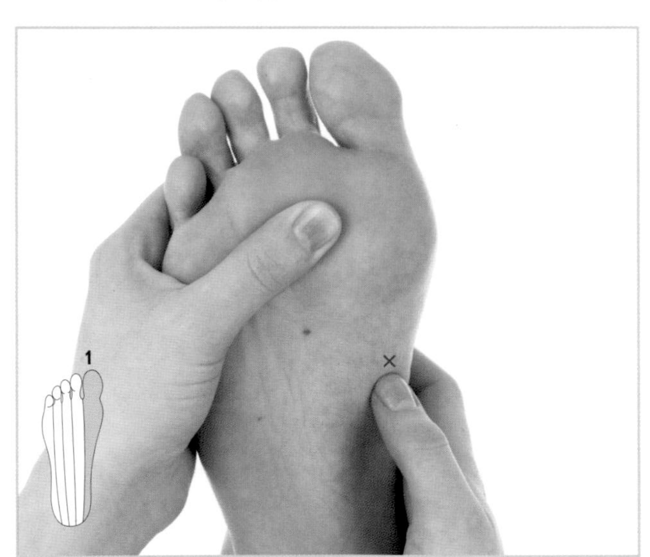

1 The adrenals are worked at the same time as the stomach and liver (see page 79). The cross indicates the precise reflex area. As you work upwards, apply pressure to the point with your thumb, turning the foot in an inward rotating direction while maintaining the pressure.

Left foot – plantar
Medial to lateral – top support

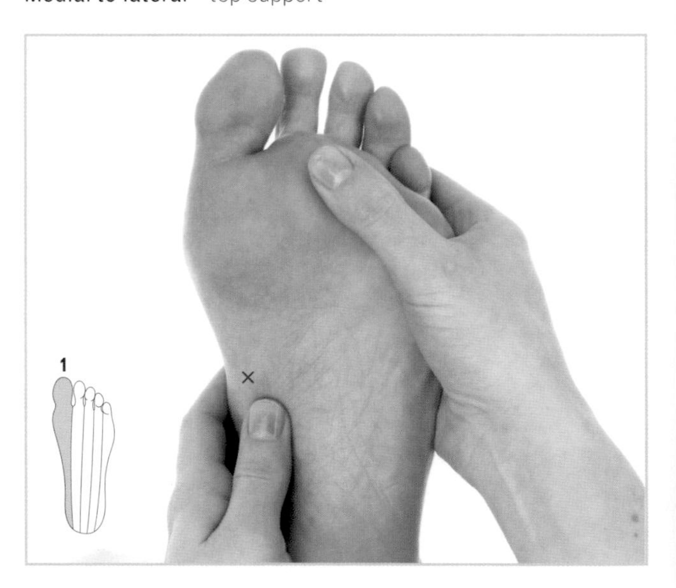

2 Support the left foot with your right hand and work upwards, applying pressure to the reflex point with your thumb. As you work, turn the foot in an inward rotating direction while maintaining the pressure.

The pancreas

Left foot – plantar
Medial to lateral – top support

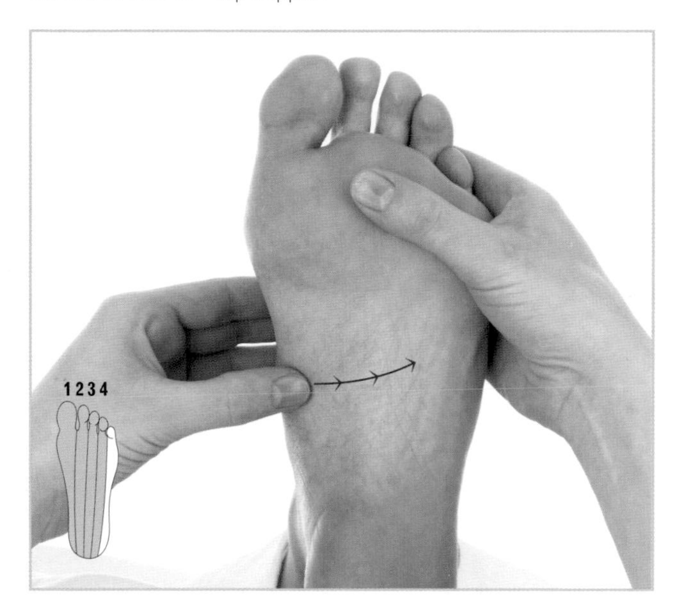

Supporting the left foot with your right hand, work across the area of the pancreas with your left thumb. Repeat this several times. The pancreas is mainly found on the left foot.

THE FEMALE REPRODUCTIVE CYCLE

Generally speaking, reflexology is of great benefit in the relief of menstrual discomforts and it has also proved to be of value in helping infertility. I have had two patients who were unable to conceive due to infrequent ovulation. Within three months both patients had regulated their ovulation cycle and conceived. They both now proclaim the virtues of reflexology. Many practitioners I know throughout the world have had similar results.

Reflexology can also bring relief during the menopause, when the body is undergoing another great hormonal upheaval. This is covered in more detail on pages 216–219.

The ovaries/testes

Right foot – lateral and top support

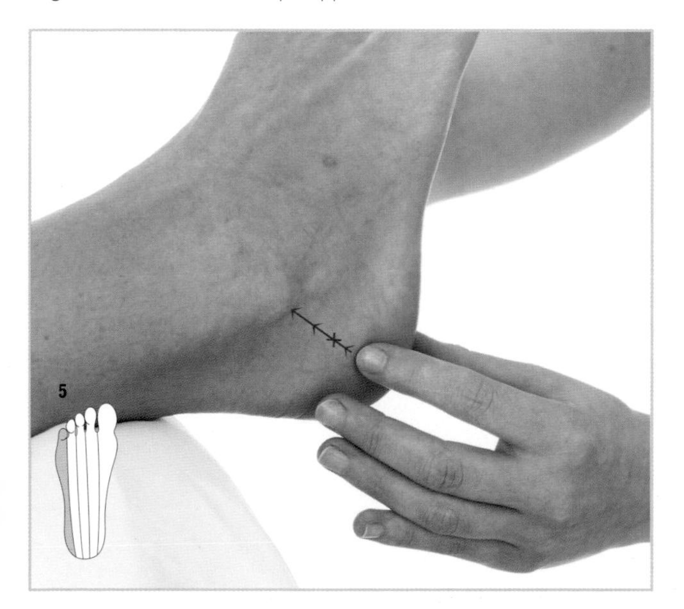

1 Support the right foot with your right hand and, using the left index finger, work over the area several time. The cross indicates the exact position for the ovary/testis on the right foot.

Left foot – lateral and top support

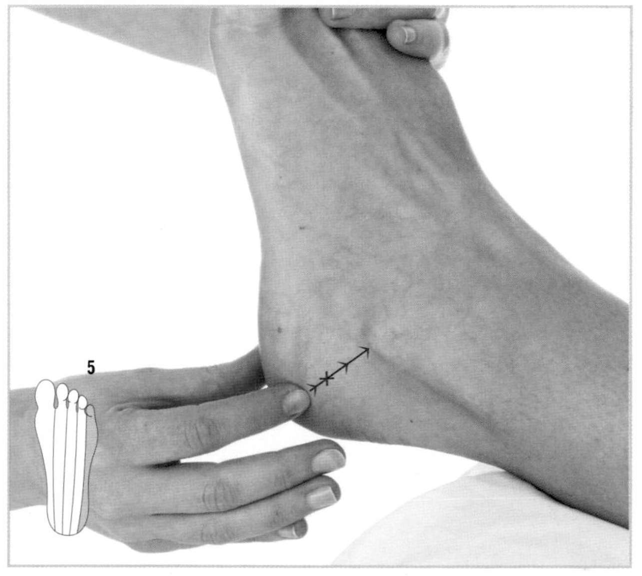

2 Support the left foot with your right hand and, using the left index finger, work over the area several time. The cross indicates the exact position for the ovary/testis on the left foot.

The solar plexus

Plexus means 'a grouping together of nerves'. The body has several such concentrations, but probably the best known is the solar plexus. Solar (of the sun) refers to the solar plexus's central location.

The solar plexus lies behind the stomach wall. Its tightly packed network of nerves and ganglia forms the largest autonomic nerve centre in the abdomen, and it has control over many important functions in that area, including the secretion of adrenaline from the adrenal glands (which sit on top of the kidneys) and muscular contractions of the intestinal walls. When you feel 'butterflies' in the stomach, perhaps caused by nervousness over an impending interview or at hearing sad or exciting news, they are vibratory signals initiated by the solar plexus.

How reflexology can help

In some Eastern belief systems the solar plexus chakra, also called the manipura chakra, is thought to be an important seat of the emotions. The solar plexus reflex is certainly a very good identifier of extreme stress in a patient, a barometer of emotional health. It provides an illustration of the way in which our physical health is intimately affected by our mental and spiritual health. Tension, especially persistent anxiety, has repercussions throughout the body, and can show itself in many ways (see 'Stress', pages 194–197), including nervousness and digestive disturbances. An adrenaline rush and 'butterflies' keep us on our toes and help us give a top performance when they are short-lived, but if they become a chronic state they can result in a variety of physical manifestations, including ulcers and irritable bowel syndrome. (For more on the multiple effects of adrenaline, see pages 102–103.)

Working the solar plexus area creates a feeling of wellbeing and has a relaxing effect upon the body.

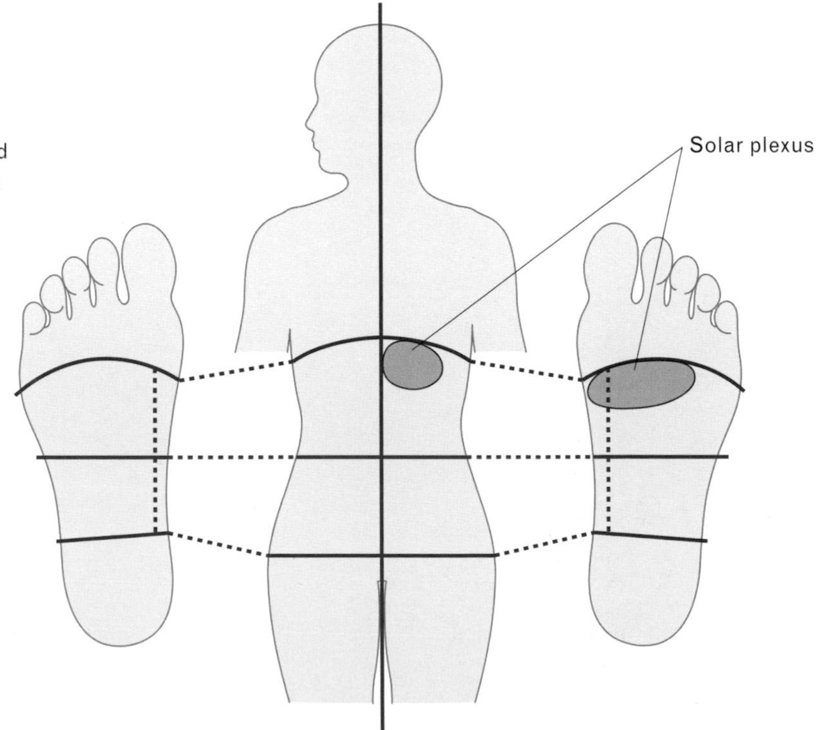

The solar plexus This configuration of sympathetic nerves and ganglia lies behind the stomach. The solar plexus is particularly responsive to emotions and feelings.

Working the associated reflex points

If you are treating patients who are under severe emotional stress and suffering from anxiety, perhaps going through a traumatic period in their lives, it is quite usual to pick up sensitivity when applying pressure in the solar plexus area.

It is not usually necessary to work out the area of the solar plexus separately, as it lies on the left foot behind the stomach area, just below the diaphragm line, and so it is automatically worked on at the same time as the stomach area. It is not possible to separate the solar plexus reflex entirely from the stomach reflex. However, if the patient is undergoing a stressful time, working both the solar plexus and stomach areas at the same time will be beneficial in releasing anxiety.

Plantar

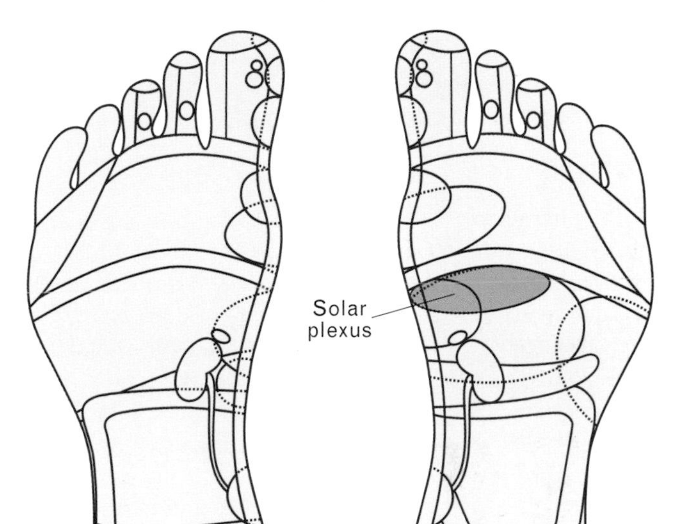

The solar plexus

Left foot – plantar
Medial to lateral – top support

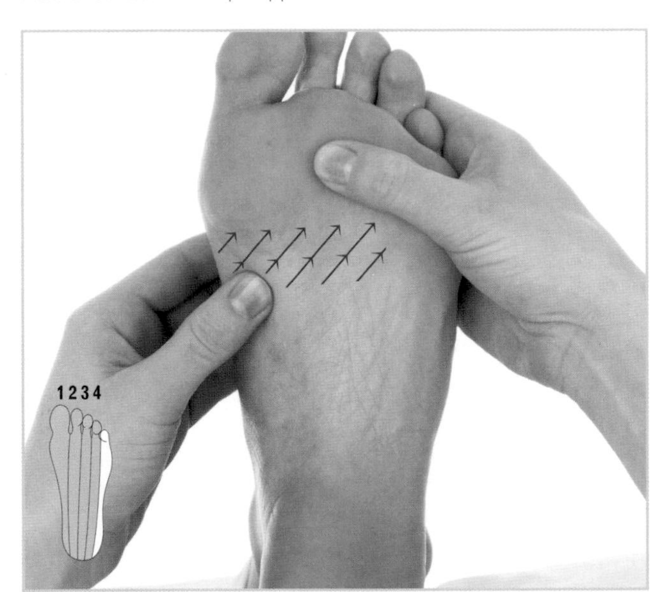

1 Support the left foot with your right hand and, using the left thumb, work out the area in a criss-cross direction from medial to lateral.

Left foot – plantar
Lateral to medial – top support

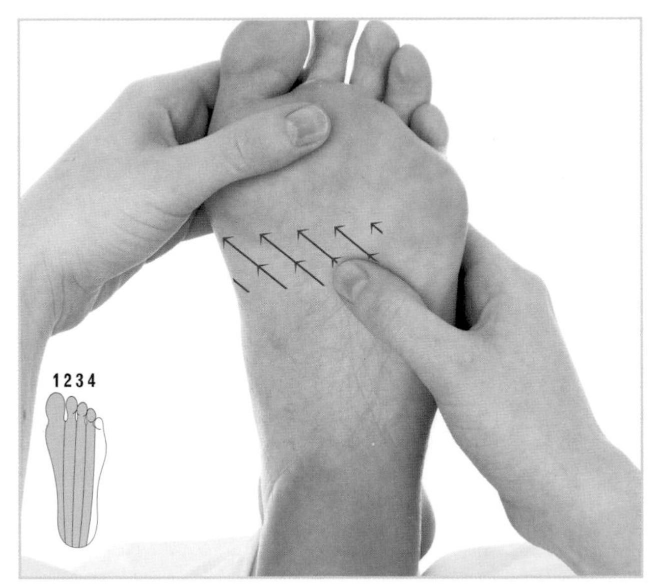

2 Support the left foot with your left hand and, using the right thumb, work out the area in a criss-cross direction from lateral to medial.

The nervous system

The nervous system consists of the central nervous system. comprising the brain and spinal cord, and the peripheral nervous system, the sensory and motor nerves throughout the body that relay information to and from the central system.

The brain

The brain, which looks like a giant wrinkled walnut, contains over 25 billion neurons and supporting glial cells, but weighs less than 1.4 kg (3 lb). With the spinal cord, the brain monitors and regulates many unconscious bodily processes, such as heart rate, and coordinates most voluntary movements. It is the site of consciousness, and from it arise all the different intellectual functions that allow human beings to think, learn and create.

The main parts of the brain are the cerebrum, the cerebellum and the brainstem. The cerebrum is partially divided into two halves, the right and left hemispheres, by a deep groove called the longitudinal fissure. The entire area of the cerebrum is covered by a layer of grey matter, the cerebral cortex, beneath which lies the brain's white matter. Different areas of the brain, the lobes (illustrated below), specialize in specific functions.

The limbic lobe is the ring of cortex and associated structures surrounding the ventricles of the cerebrum and is thought to be a link between emotional and thought processes.

Between the cerebrum and midbrain (part of the brainstem) is an area called the diencephalon, which includes the thalamus and the hypothalamus. The thalamus acts as an information centre, relaying important information, while the hypothalamus is closely linked with the limbic lobe and has overall control of autonomic bodily processes (see page 98 in 'The endocrine system').

The cerebellum, the second largest part of the brain, is responsible for coordination of movement.

The brainstem, made up of the medulla, pons and midbrain, controls centres that are vital for survival, such as respiration, blood pressure, heart beat and digestion.

Lobes of the brain The frontal lobe controls personality, judgement, planning and aspects of speech and movement. The temporal lobe recognizes sound and memory. The parietal lobe deals with stimuli like temperature and pain. The occipital lobe interprets visual imagining.

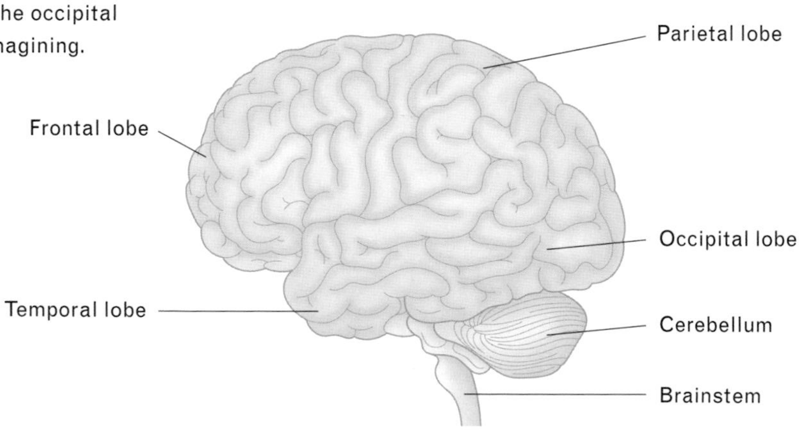

Parietal lobe
Frontal lobe
Occipital lobe
Temporal lobe
Cerebellum
Brainstem

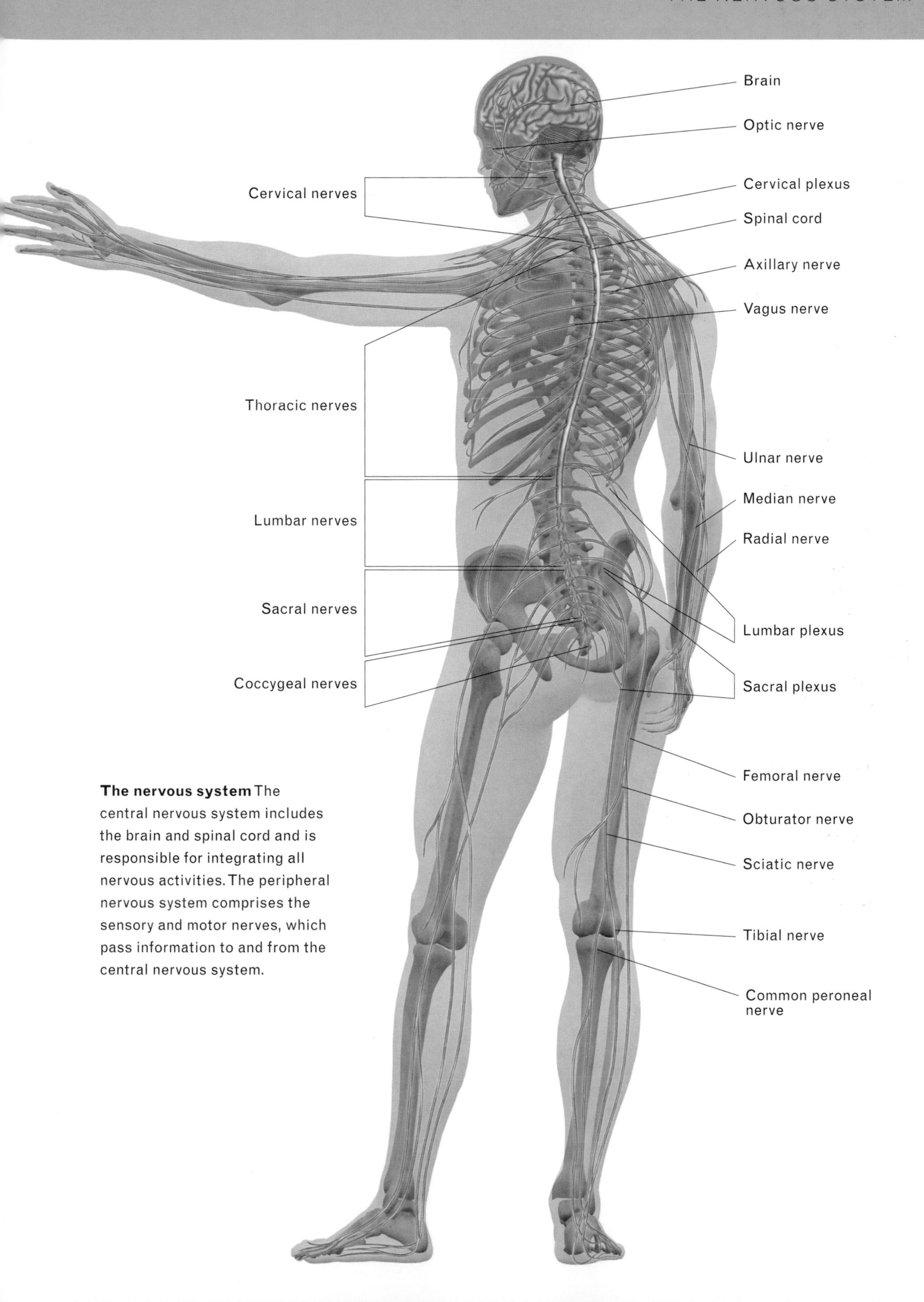

The nervous system The central nervous system includes the brain and spinal cord and is responsible for integrating all nervous activities. The peripheral nervous system comprises the sensory and motor nerves, which pass information to and from the central nervous system.

Cerebrospinal fluid

Cerebrospinal fluid (CSF) fills the ventricles (cavities within the brain) and the spaces between the meninges in the brain and spinal cord. The fluid has several functions. It acts as a cushion and shock absorber between the brain and bones of the skull; it protects and nourishes the brain and spine; and, most important of all, it contains lymphocytes to protect the brain against infection, the most dangerous of which is meningitis.

CSF consists of mineral salts, water, glucose, plasma proteins, creatinine and urea. Analysis of it is useful in the diagnosis of diseases such as polio, meningitis and multiple sclerosis.

CSF is secreted continuously into each ventricle of the brain through the choroid plexuses. These consist of areas where the lining membrane of the ventricle walls is fragile and contains quantities of blood capillaries. The fluid passes back into the blood through tiny diverticula of arachnoid mater.

The brain has an immense network of capillaries supplying it with blood containing life-supporting oxygen and glucose. Without these elements, brain function deteriorates rapidly (see also page 91).

The spinal cord

The spinal cord is just like a flex of wire approximately 43 cm (17 in) long. It descends from the brainstem to the edge of the second lumbar vertebra and is about as wide as your little finger. The cord is protected by the bony segments of the vertebral column and by enveloping meninges. Out of it arise the spinal nerves. Information received from these nerves stimulates impulses throughout the entire body.

The peripheral nervous system

The peripheral nerves convey information to and from the brain and spinal cord. Sensory nerves receive information from the skin and the internal organs, while motor nerves initiate the action of various parts of our body.

The peripheral nervous system (PNS) consists of 12 pairs of cranial nerves from under the surface of the brain and 31 pairs of spinal nerves emanating from the

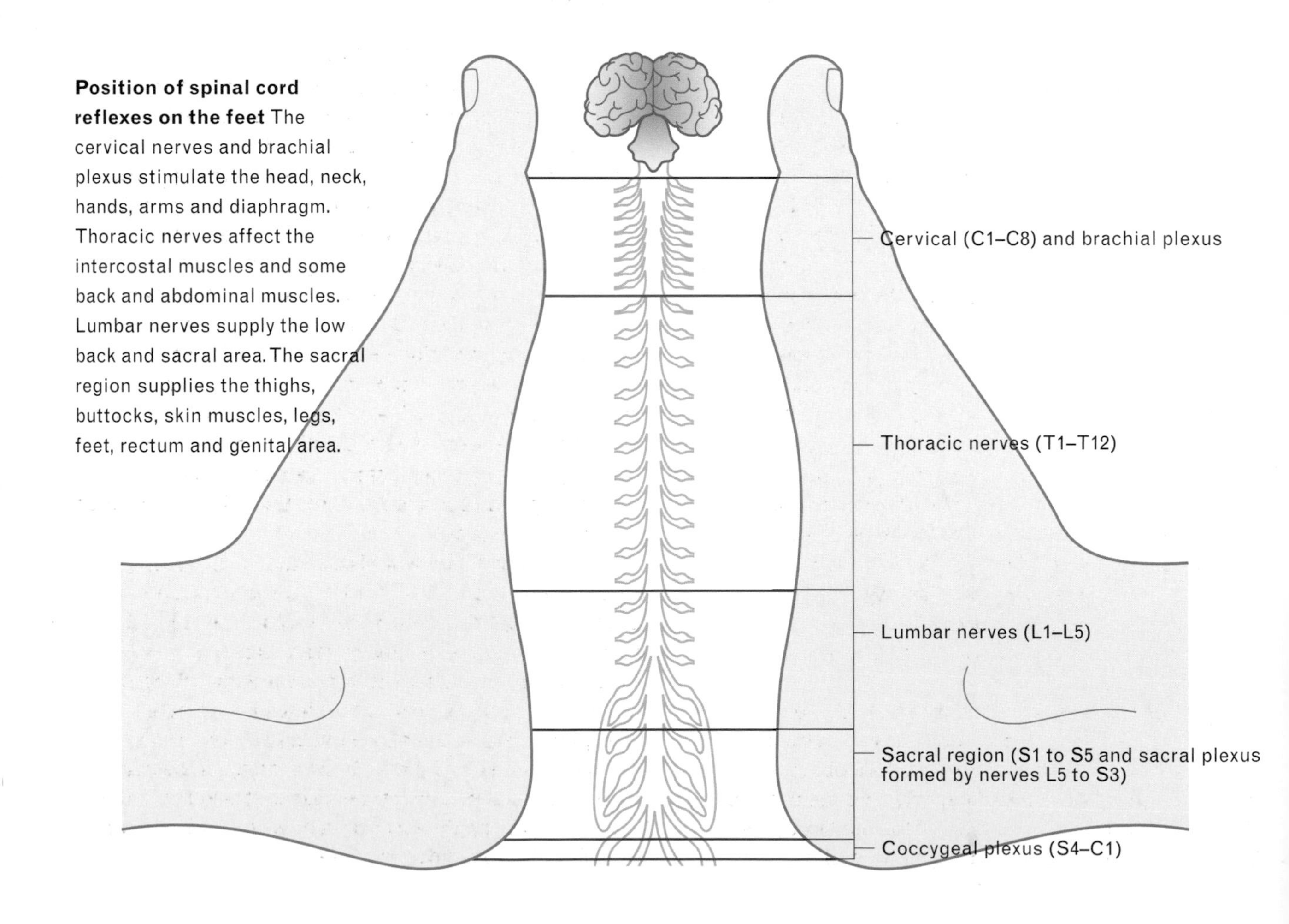

Position of spinal cord reflexes on the feet The cervical nerves and brachial plexus stimulate the head, neck, hands, arms and diaphragm. Thoracic nerves affect the intercostal muscles and some back and abdominal muscles. Lumbar nerves supply the low back and sacral area. The sacral region supplies the thighs, buttocks, skin muscles, legs, feet, rectum and genital area.

spinal cord. These pairs of spinal nerves leave the vertebral canal by passing between adjacent vertebrae. They are named and grouped according to the vertebrae with which they are associated:

- 8 cervical nerves
- 12 thoracic nerves
- 5 lumbar nerves
- 5 sacral nerves
- 1 coccygeal nerve.

Although we only have seven cervical vertebrae in our neck, we have eight pairs of nerves. The first to seventh cervical nerves (C1 to C7) exit from the vertebral canal above the respective cervical vertebrae (C1 above the first and C2 above the second, and so forth). The C8 spinal nerve is the exception to this rule because it exits below the seventh cervical vertebra.

The coccygeal, sacral and lumbar nerves leave the spinal cord near its termination (at the level between the first and second lumbar vertebrae) and then extend downwards, forming a group of nerves that resembles the tail of a horse (hence its name, cauda equina).

The autonomic nervous system

The autonomic nervous system works to maintain a steady state within the internal environment of the body by means of sensory fibres running through cranial and spinal nerves. The motor portion is divided into sympathetic and parasympathetic systems that are also part of some spinal and cranial nerves. The sympathetic system is responsible for preparing the body for action, while the parasympathetic system is most active during periods of calm and rest: it conserves and restores energy. When a stressful situation has passed, the parasympathetic nerves take over and help the function of the organs to return to normal.

Many organs function using both sympathetic and parasympathetic nerves. In the heart, for example, the sympathetic nerves increase heart rate while the parasympathetic (vagus) nerves slow it down. The digestive system is mainly under parasympathetic control: once food has been swallowed, the peristaltic muscular contractions take over and the food is no longer under your direct control.

The vagus nerves have more of an extensive distribution than any other cranial nerves, because they arise from nerve cells in the medulla oblongata and pass through the neck into the thorax and the abdomen. The vagus has branches to most of the major organs, including the heart, lungs and digestive system.

Neurological disorders helped by reflexology

Paralysis or weakness of various areas in the body results from damage to the motor areas of the brain or nerve pathways of the spinal cord. Damage to the middle or lower area of the spinal cord can cause paralysis of the legs and trunk (paraplegia). and damage to the motor areas on one side of the brain causes paralysis to the opposite side of the body. Quadriplegia results from damage in the area C1 to T4 (if damage occurs between C1 and C2, survival is unlikely).

As well as destroying muscle function and limiting movement, other functions such as breathing and bladder and bowel function may also be affected, depending on the area of damage.

Multiple sclerosis, epilepsy, Parkinson's disease and Alzheimer's disease are all further conditions that affect the nervous system. It is well worth while treating these conditions, particularly in the early stages, and good responses have been obtained.

How reflexology can help

The central nervous system and brain are the most important areas to work in reflexology. If you only have 20 minutes to work on your best friend who, perhaps, is feeling tired, has a headache or menstrual cramps, you can stimulate the entire body simply by working on the central nervous system via the feet. Nerve impulses arising from the spine serve all organs, functions and parts of the human body, so as you work on the spinal area you are giving vital stimulation to the whole body.

When you are treating people for a particular condition, concentrate on working extensively on whichever part of the spinal area supports the ailing part. Constant reference to the information in this section will soon acquaint you with an understanding of the nerve supply to specific parts of the body. You will find that your results improve rapidly.

As an example, you would get outstanding results when treating a patient suffering the effects of a heart attack or angina if you worked the area of the thoracic spinal nerves, as well as the heart and lung.

Remember, reflexology is not just about working on the spine to help back pain or the intestines to help constipation; it involves a true understanding of the working of the entire human body. A study of the nerve supply, where to contact these delicate structures in the feet and how to apply the correct pressure and technique will help achieve the desired result.

Working the associated reflex points

Zone 1 is the most powerful zone in the body as within this zone falls the brain (containing the influential pituitary, hypothalamus and pineal area), the spinal cord and vertebral column. It is not unusual, therefore, to find that most people have a sensitivity in this zone.

CASE STUDY **MULTIPLE SCLEROSIS**

CLIENT PROFILE

Following the birth of her first child, Amy began to suffer from muscle weakness in her legs, and as the years went by she experienced increasing weakness and poor coordination in various parts of her body. Eventually multiple sclerosis was diagnosed. Amy was only 29.

Amy found it hard to cope with the painful leg spasms and the various medications from her doctor all gave her unpleasant side-effects. She had received physiotherapy, but felt there might be more help in the complementary medical field, particularly reflexology.

REGULARITY OF REFLEXOLOGY TREATMENT

Weekly for eight weeks and then, as recommended, monthly attendance.

REFLEXES

Main reflexes	Assistance
Entire spine and brain areas	To stimulate central nervous system
Adrenals	To stimulate more vitality in the body
Solar plexus	To help general stress

TREATMENT OUTCOMES

When working on the spine/central nervous system, Amy's feet were extremely sensitive. In fact, as I worked on them both legs went into spasm. By persevering with many relaxation techniques her legs soon became relaxed. After several weeks of treatment Amy reported that her painful leg spasms had reduced considerably and she felt a little stronger. As Amy spent a lot of time sitting in a chair I showed her how to work the nervous system by working on her own hands and recommended that she did this several times a day.

Plantar

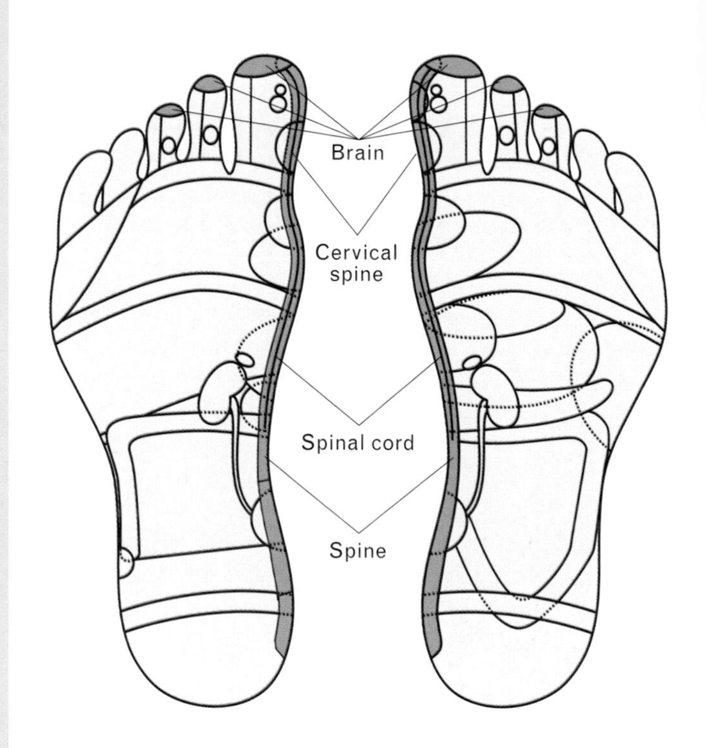

The vertebral column, cervical spine and brain

Right foot – medial
Top support

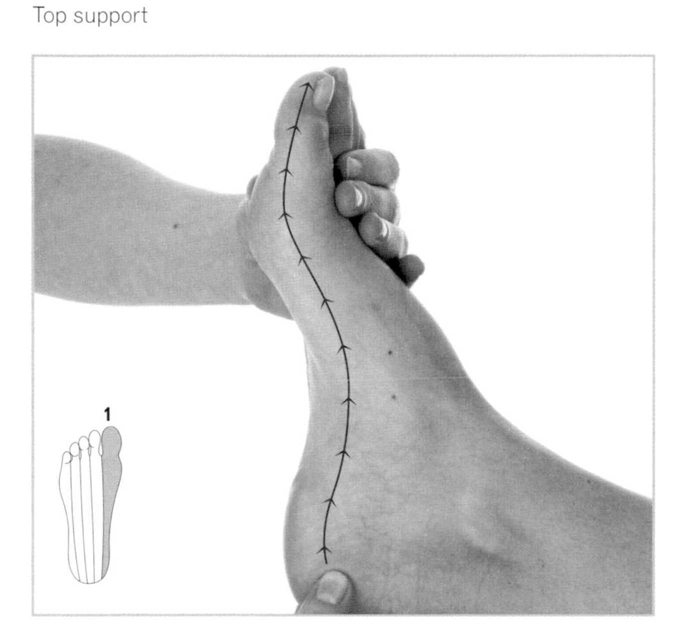

1 Support the right foot at the top with your left hand and, using the right thumb, proceed to work up the vertebral column.

Right foot – medial
Top support

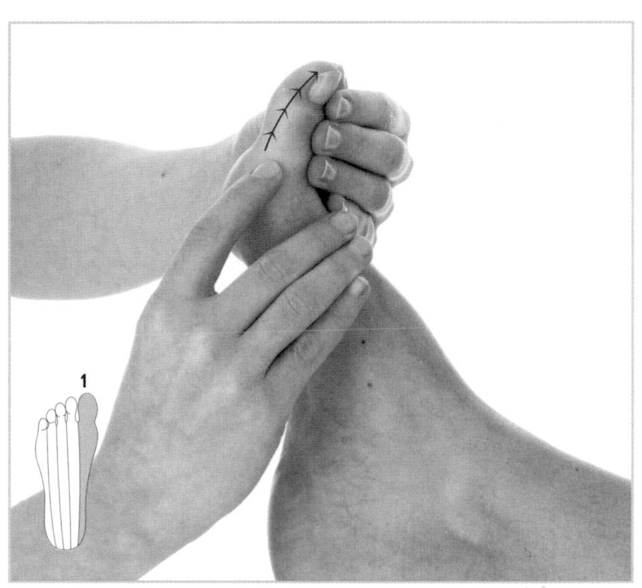

2 Using the right index finger, proceed to work up the very fine area of the cervical spine. (A better result will be achieved with the index finger.)

Right foot – medial
Top support

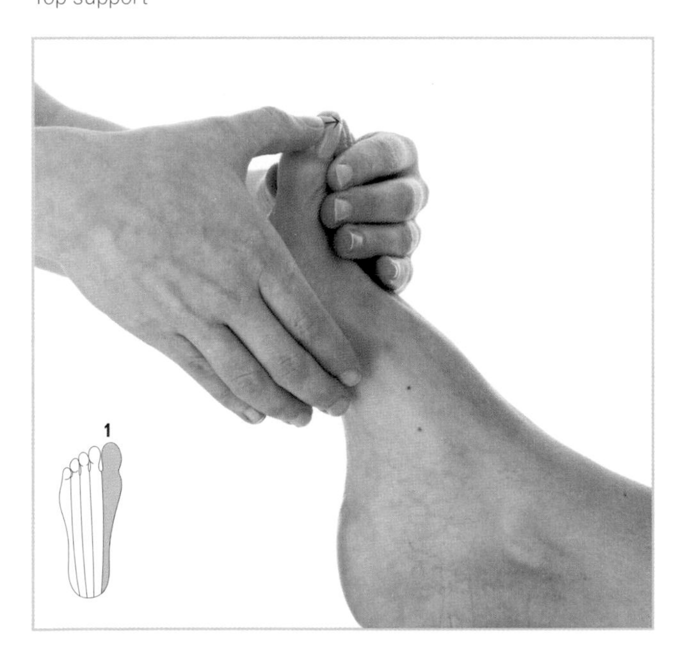

3 As you move into the brain area at the top of the toe, switch back to your right thumb. Continue supporting the foot with your left hand at the top.

Right foot – medial
Top support

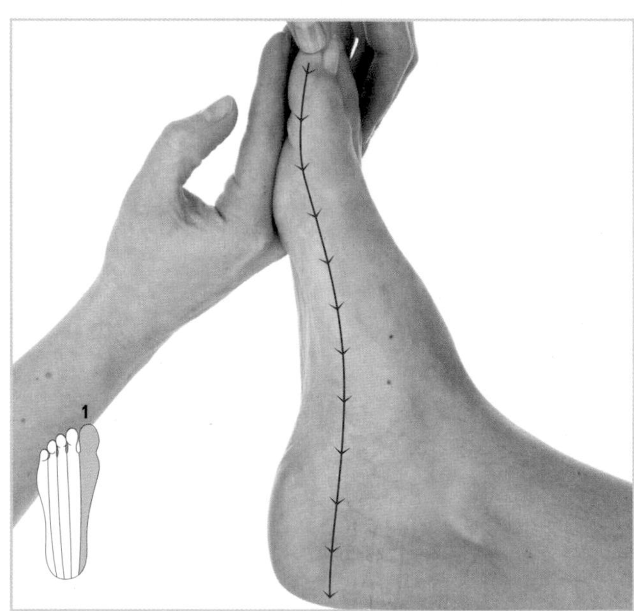

4 Support the foot with the back of your right hand as you work down the spine line with your left thumb.

The vertebral column, cervical spine and brain

Left foot – medial
Top support

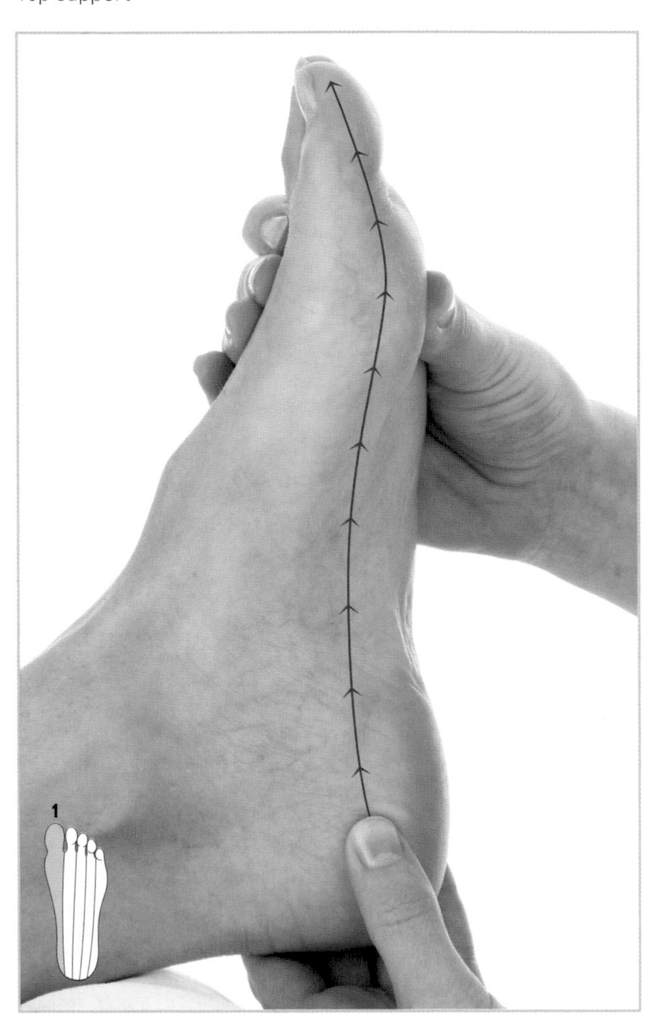

1 Support the left foot with your right hand and, using the left thumb, proceed to work up the vertebral column.

Left foot – medial
Top support

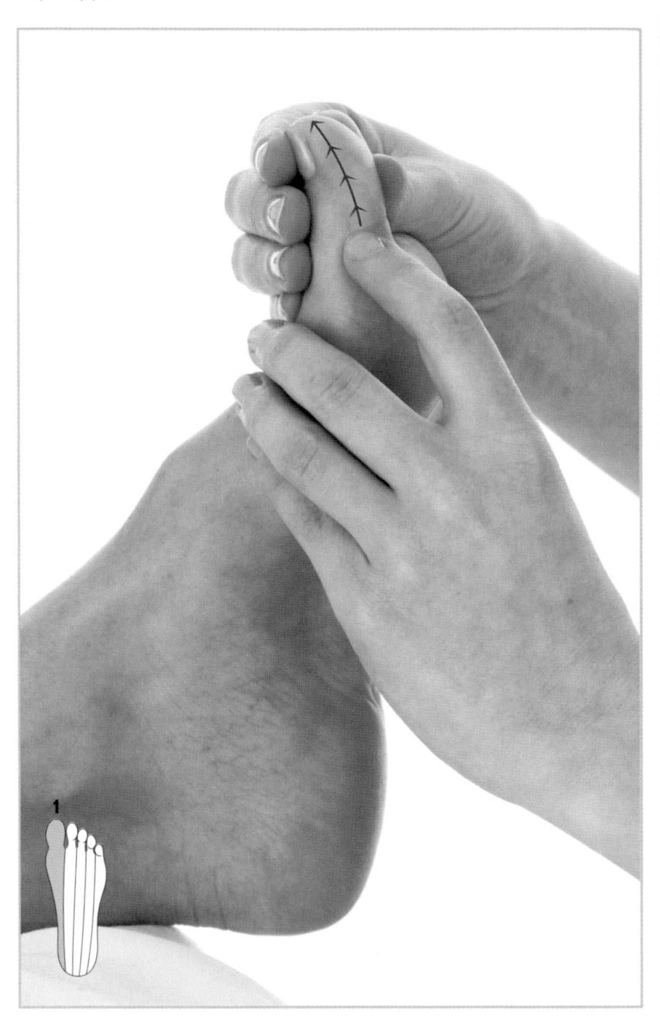

2 Using the left index finger, proceed to work up the very fine area of the cervical spine. (A better result will be achieved with the index finger.)

Left foot – medial
Top support

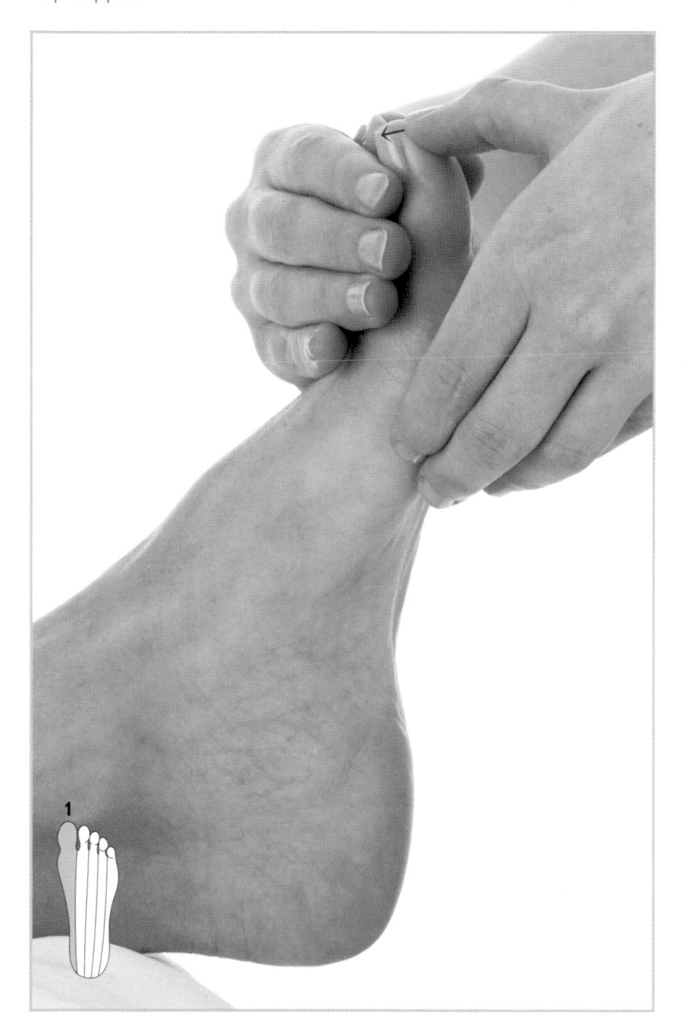

3 As you move into the brain area at the top of the toe, switch back to your left thumb. Continue supporting the foot with your right hand at the top.

Left foot – medial
Top support

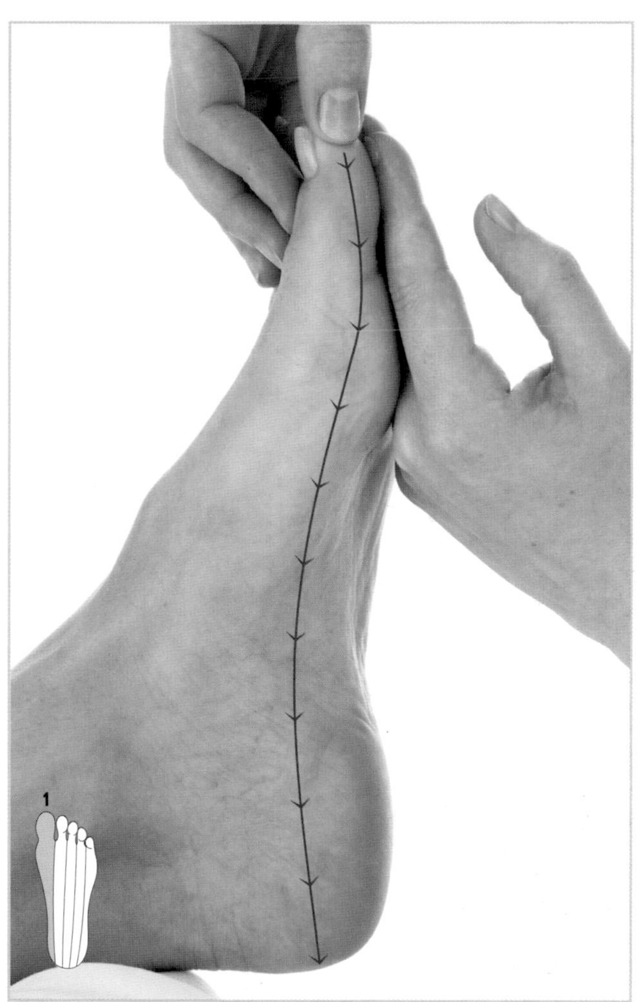

4 Support the foot with the back of your left hand as you work down the spine line with your right thumb.

The ears, eyes and face

Much of how we perceive and experience the world comes to us via our eyes and ears, and a dulling of or interference with any of our senses diminishes our feeling of wellbeing. Also included in this section are sinuses, which can be the root of much low-level aggravation.

The ear

Ears enable us to hear, but are also instrumental in our sense of balance. As the illustration opposite shows, the ear's structure divides into three parts:

- **The outer ear**: This consists of the pinna, which is the term for the shaped cartilage that forms the visible part of the ear, and the meatus or ear canal, which leads to the ear drum.
- **The middle ear**: Situated beyond the ear drum, the middle ear contains three tiny bones or ossicles, each named after their shape: the malleus (hammer), incus (anvil) and stapes (stirrup). The Eustachian tube, which runs from the middle ear to open into the back of the throat, keeps the middle ear pressure the same as that outside the body.
- **The cochlea**: A fluid-filled tube, the cochlea is found in the inner ear. It is coiled round like a snail shell, from which it gets the name. In the part of the cochlea nearest the middle ear are an 'oval window' and a 'round window', through which the sound vibrations travel. Within the cochlea lies the sensory tissue of the organ of Corti, in which minute hair cells translate sounds into nerve impulses.

Also in the inner ear are three fluid-filled U-shaped tubes, called the semicircular canals. These contain hairs sensitive to movement and cells able to sense bodily positioning, allowing us to keep our balance.

How hearing works

Sound travels in the form of sound waves or vibrations in the air. The folds of the pinna funnel these waves through the ear canal, where they vibrate the ear drum. The ossicles amplify this vibration and transmit it via the oval window to the fluid in the cochlea. Here, cells in the organ of Corti interpret vibrations as nerve impulses, which are carried by the auditory nerve to the brain. Meanwhile, vibrations leave the cochlea through the round window.

The distance between the ears helps the brain to locate the direction of the sound and its source. Sound waves have pitch and volume or intensity. Pitch is determined by the frequency of sound waves. The volume depends on the amplitude of the sound waves, which are measured in decibels.

HEARING SENSITIVITY

Although human beings do not possess very acute hearing in comparison with the auditory powers of some animals, the human ear remains a powerful tool capable of registering an amazing range of noises. The human ear is sensitive to sounds ranging in loudness from 10 to 140 decibels (10 million times as loud as 10) and ranging in pitch from 20 to a high of 20,000 hertz (cycles per second). However, exposure to loud sounds can, over a period of time, reduce the ear's sensitivity and is one cause of partial deafness.

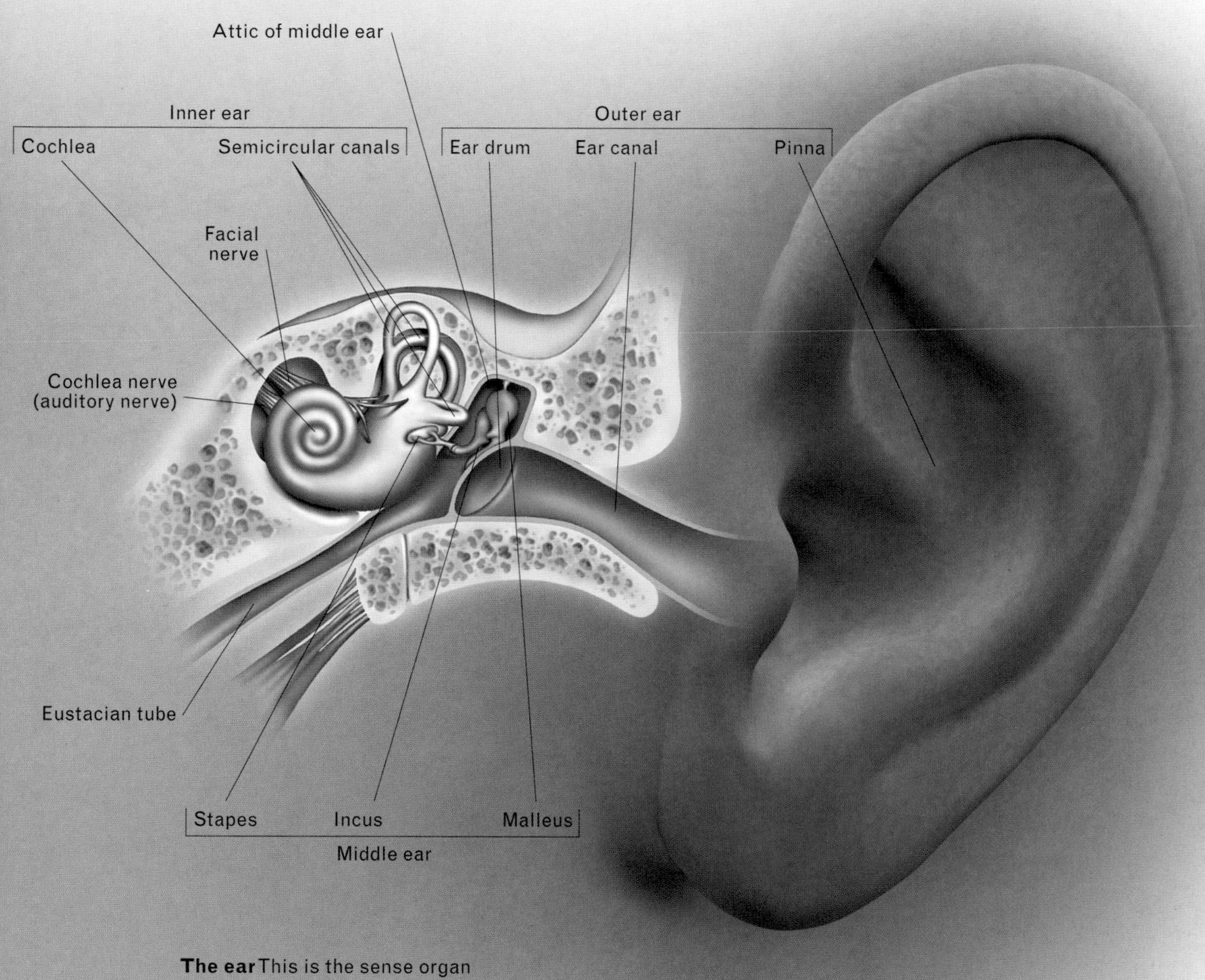

The ear This is the sense organ concerned with hearing and balance. Sound waves transmitted into the external auditory meatus cause the tympanic membrane (eardrum) to vibrate. The semicircular canals in the inner ear are all concerned with balance.

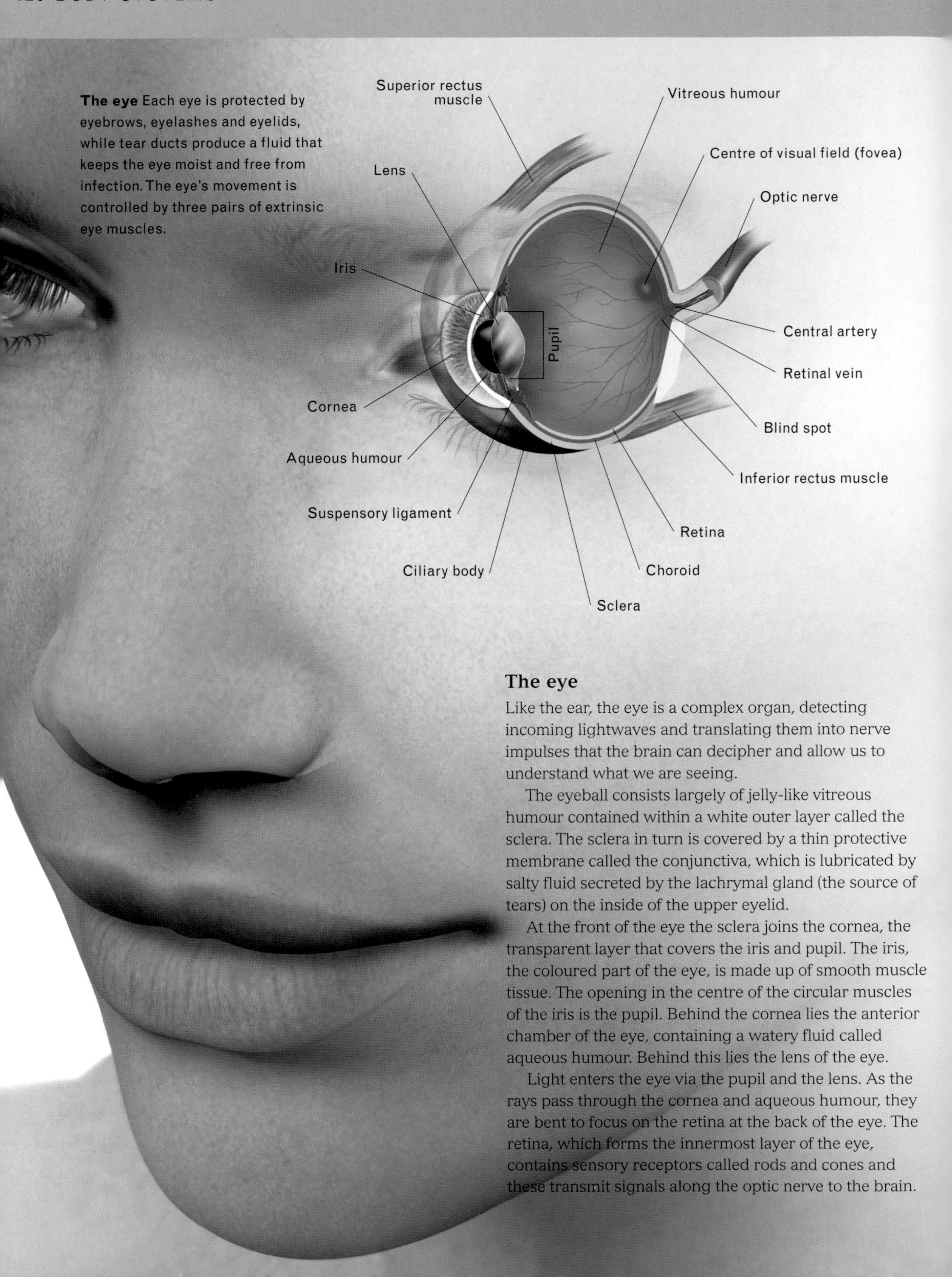

The eye Each eye is protected by eyebrows, eyelashes and eyelids, while tear ducts produce a fluid that keeps the eye moist and free from infection. The eye's movement is controlled by three pairs of extrinsic eye muscles.

The eye

Like the ear, the eye is a complex organ, detecting incoming lightwaves and translating them into nerve impulses that the brain can decipher and allow us to understand what we are seeing.

The eyeball consists largely of jelly-like vitreous humour contained within a white outer layer called the sclera. The sclera in turn is covered by a thin protective membrane called the conjunctiva, which is lubricated by salty fluid secreted by the lachrymal gland (the source of tears) on the inside of the upper eyelid.

At the front of the eye the sclera joins the cornea, the transparent layer that covers the iris and pupil. The iris, the coloured part of the eye, is made up of smooth muscle tissue. The opening in the centre of the circular muscles of the iris is the pupil. Behind the cornea lies the anterior chamber of the eye, containing a watery fluid called aqueous humour. Behind this lies the lens of the eye.

Light enters the eye via the pupil and the lens. As the rays pass through the cornea and aqueous humour, they are bent to focus on the retina at the back of the eye. The retina, which forms the innermost layer of the eye, contains sensory receptors called rods and cones and these transmit signals along the optic nerve to the brain.

The face, nose and sinuses

A blocked nose can affect our hearing and sense of taste, while some smells can bring on a headache and toothache can make the whole face super-sensitive. The nerves in the facial area are so dense and closely linked that it can be difficult to determine the exact source of facial pain.

A common cause of facial discomfort, even severe pain, is blocked sinuses. The sinuses are cavities in bones above and between the eyes and across the cheeks. They give resonance to our voice and lighten the weight of the head on our shoulders (if all the facial bones were solid, the neck would not be able to support the skull).

The sinuses are lined with mucous membrane and if this becomes inflamed, or if, because of excess mucus, one or more of the sinus areas cannot drain, pressure builds up that can be painful. Infection of the sinuses (sinusitis) often follows a heavy cold, leaving you with catarrh. This can also be brought on by hayfever, which irritates the linings of the nose and throat.

The same mucous membrane that lines the sinuses also lines the nasal passages. Inflammation and over-production of mucus here (the most usual reason being the common cold) prevents smells from reaching the olfactory area of the nose, causing a temporary loss of the sense of smell (see box).

The sinuses Hollow porous bones, the sinuses give resonance to the voice and act as drainage for mucus. The hollowness of the bones lightens the weight of the skull on the neck.

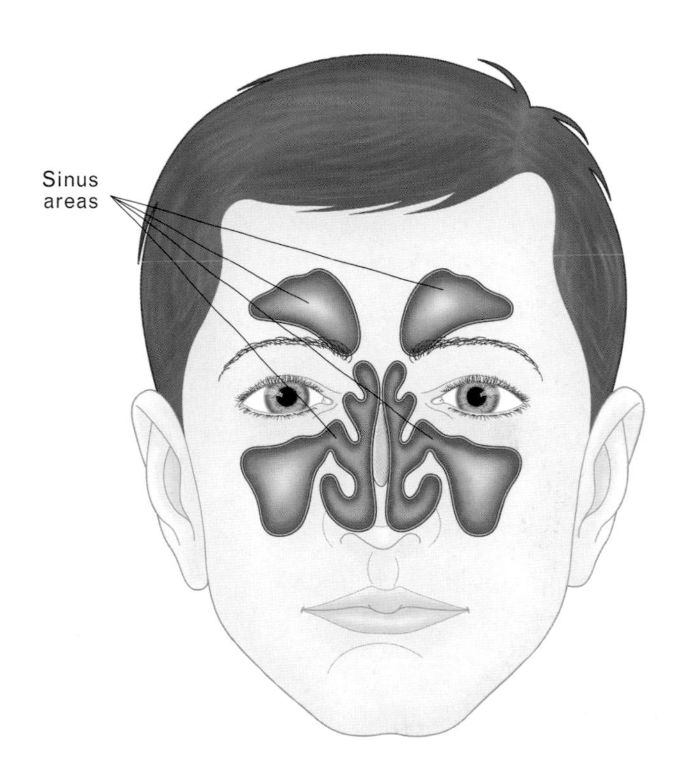

Ear, eye and sinus disorders helped by reflexology

Reflexologists are able to help relieve a number of ear and eye conditions, particularly tinnitus (ringing in the ears), tired or strained eyes, conjunctivitis and constant ear, nose and throat conditions in children.

Many people going through an extremely stressful situation in their lives find that their eyesight deteriorates rapidly. This is caused by tension, and when both stress and tension are relieved with reflexology, their eyesight quickly returns to its normal state.

Sinusitis can be relieved by reflexology, helping neuralgia or any other form of facial pain.

Reflexology can also bring relief from acute pain due to problems with teeth. Search around the fronts of the three toes and you will find an acutely sensitive spot (the right foot if the problem is on the right side of the jaw; the left foot if the problem is on the left side of the jaw). Applying pressure to this sensitive spot will help to alleviate the pain until the sufferer is able to see a dentist. I must stress that this will only relieve the condition temporarily and professional dental help must be sought.

THE SENSE OF SMELL

On each side of the nasal septum, the cartilage that divides the two nostrils, are nerve fibres that have their origins in the roof of the nose. Olfactory receptor cells in these nerves make them sensitive to smell.

Air entering the nose is heated and convection currents carry eddies of air to the roof of the nose. Sniffing sends up more particles more quickly. This increases the number of special cells stimulated and thus the perception of the smell. Continuous exposure to a particular odour quickly decreases perception of that odour, until it is not sensed at all.

The sense of smell is closely associated with the appetite. The smell of good food can make you salivate in anticipation, whereas losing your sense of smell dulls your sense of taste and so your appreciation of food.

Working the associated reflex points

The sinus, ear, eye and other facial reflex points are all found in the toes. In the pictures on pages 123–124, the sinus areas are pinpointed by cross marks.

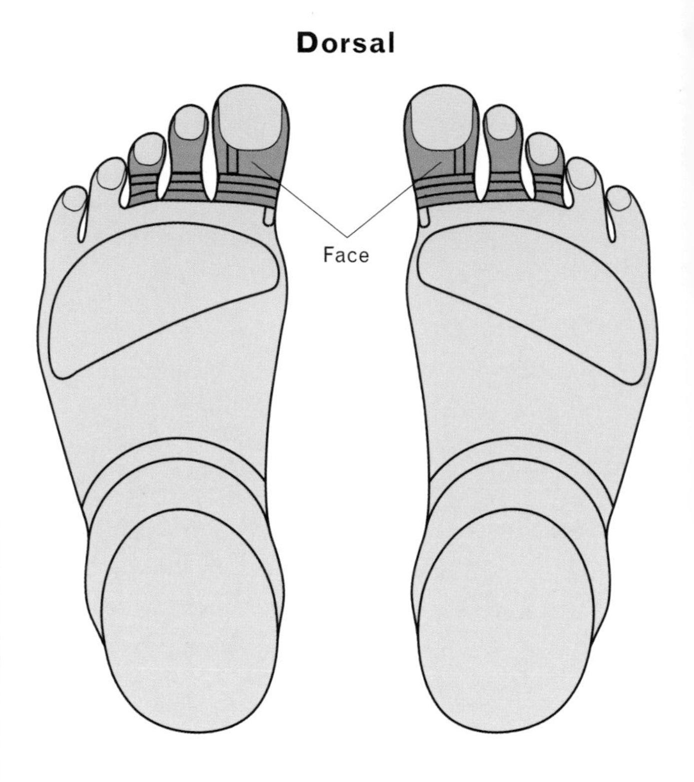

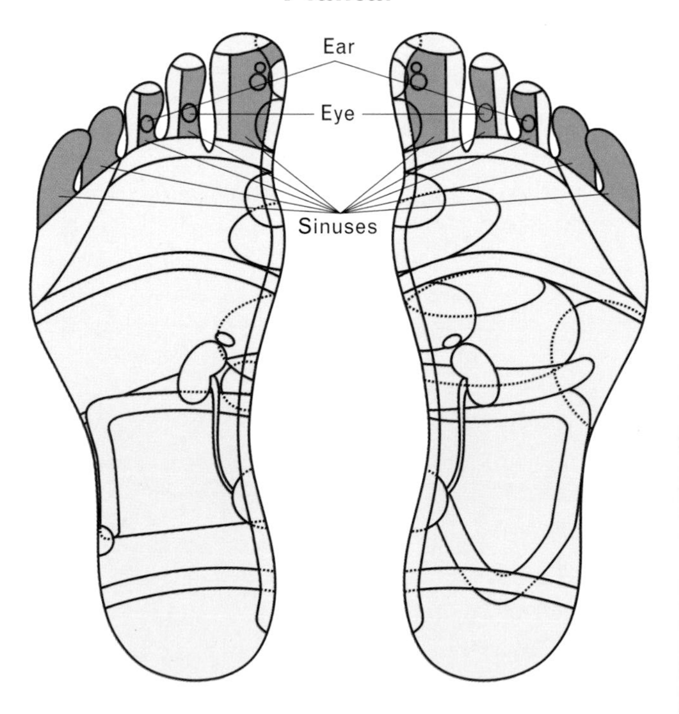

CASE STUDY **SINUSITIS**

CLIENT PROFILE

David had been troubled with sinus problems since his teens and now at the age of 30 he had suffered from three very painful episodes of sinusitis in six months. They had been treated with antibiotics, but although the treatment seemed to clear the infection, it soon returned. David also suffered from hayfever during the summer months when, he said, he always seemed to have a streaming nose.

REGULARITY OF REFLEXOLOGY TREATMENT

Weekly for eight weeks.

REFLEXES

Main reflexes	Assistance
Sinuses, ear, nose and throat	To alleviate inflammation and sensitivity

TREATMENT OUTCOMES

David's sinus reflexes were so sensitive that he could hardly bear any pressure on the toe areas at all, so a very light touch was needed at his first appointment. He telephoned shortly after the appointment to say that he had a severe headache that persisted for 24 hours, and that his nose streamed for hours. This is not an uncommon reaction in these inflammatory states of the sinuses. His sinus problem improved week by week and by the end of the two months was much improved.

The sinus areas

Right foot – plantar
Medial to lateral – top support

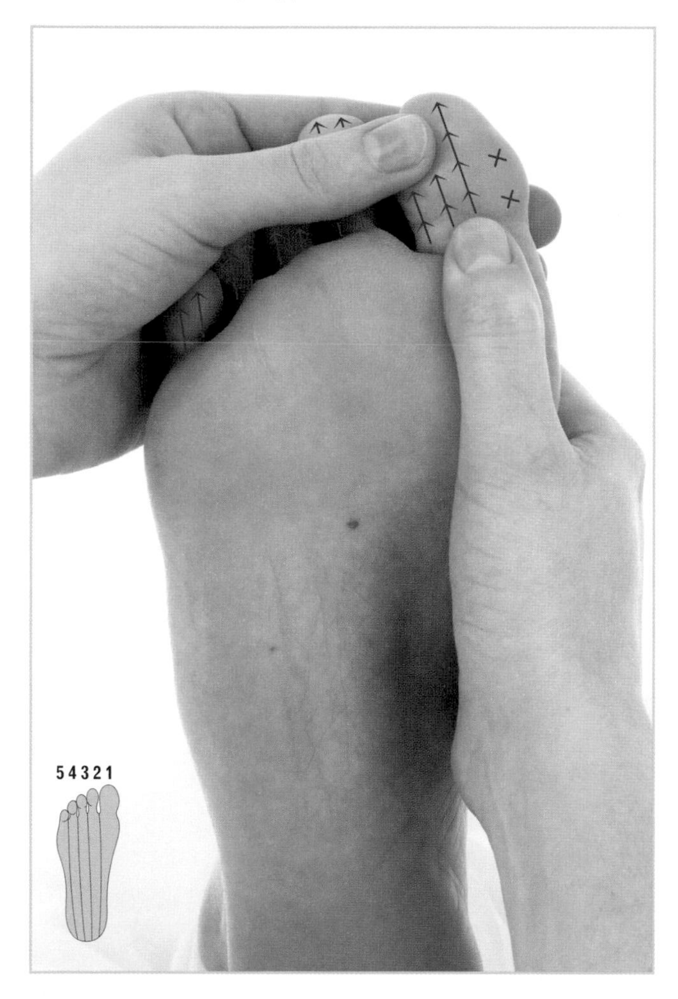

1 Support the right foot with your left hand at the top and, using the right thumb, work upwards in straight lines, from medial to lateral. The crosses indicate the precise reflex areas for the nose and throat.

Right foot – plantar
Lateral to medial – top support

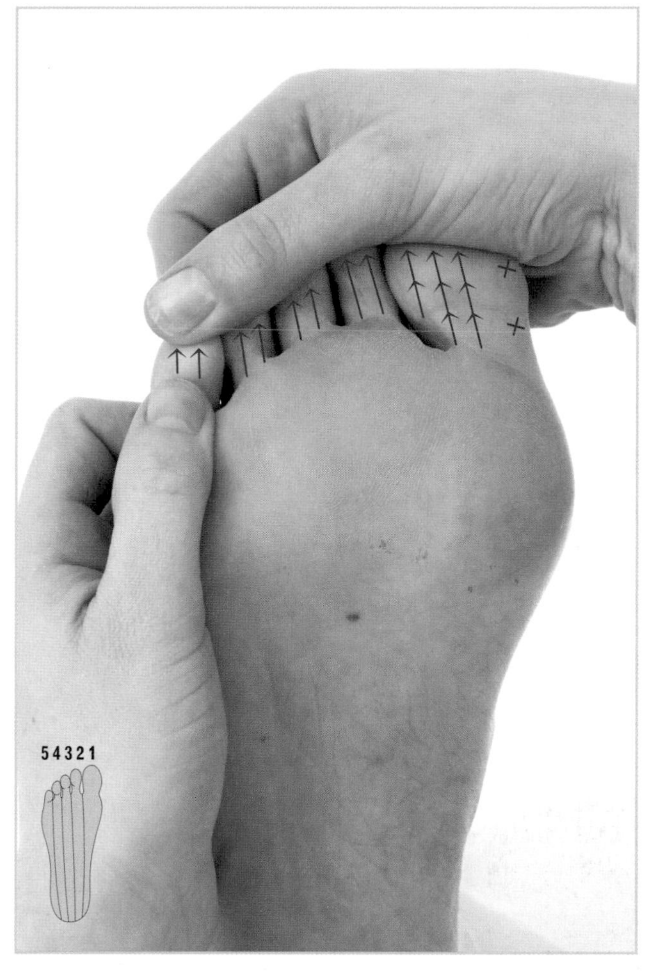

2 Support the right foot with your right hand at the top and, using the left thumb, work upwards in straight lines, from lateral to medial.

The sinus areas

Left foot – plantar
Medial to lateral – top support

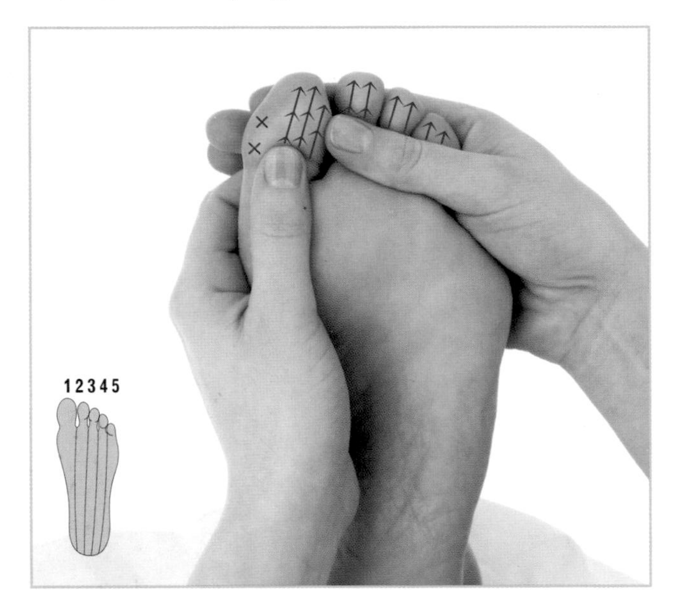

1 Support the left foot with your right hand at the top and, using the left thumb, work upwards in straight lines, from medial to lateral. The crosses indicate the precise reflex areas for the nose and throat.

Left foot – plantar
Lateral to medial – top support

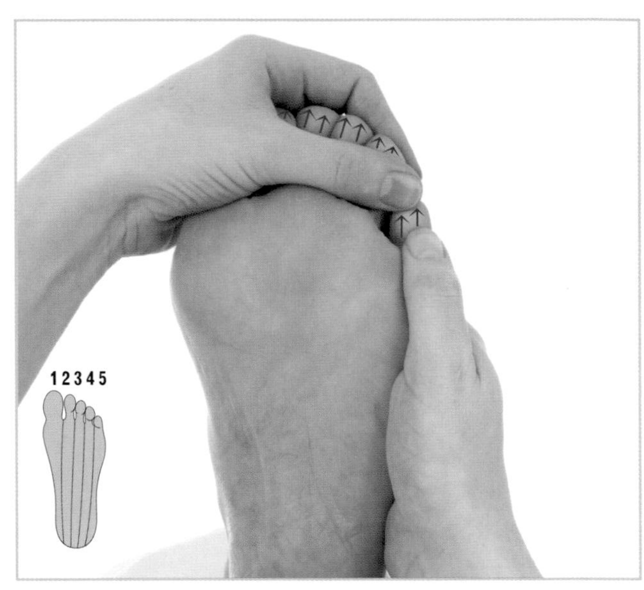

2 Support the left foot with your left hand at the top and, using the right thumb, work upwards in straight lines, from lateral to medial.

The eye and ear

Right foot – plantar
Top support

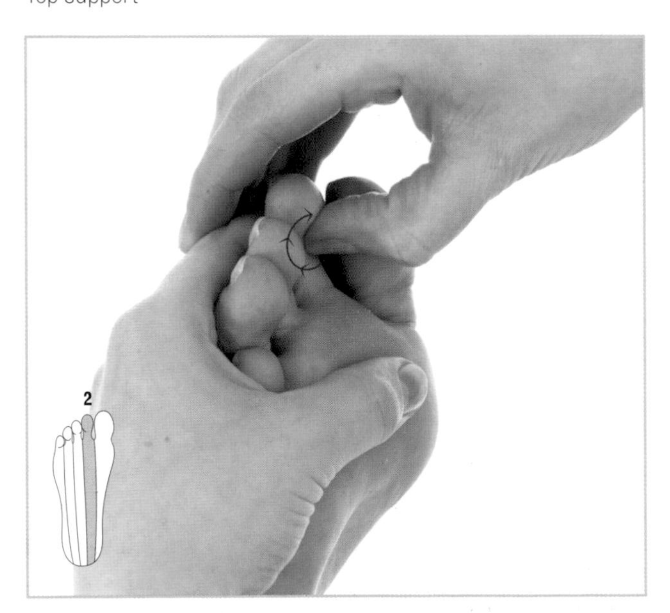

1 Support the right foot with your left hand at the top and, using the right thumb, use a gentle, rotating movement to work the eye area.

Right foot – plantar
Top support

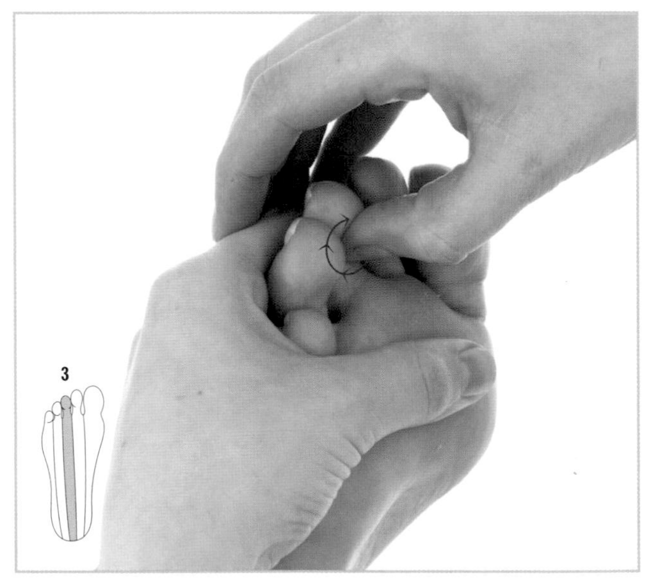

2 Support the right foot with your left hand at the top and, using the right thumb, use a gentle, rotating movement to work the ear area.

The eye and ear

Left foot – plantar
Top support

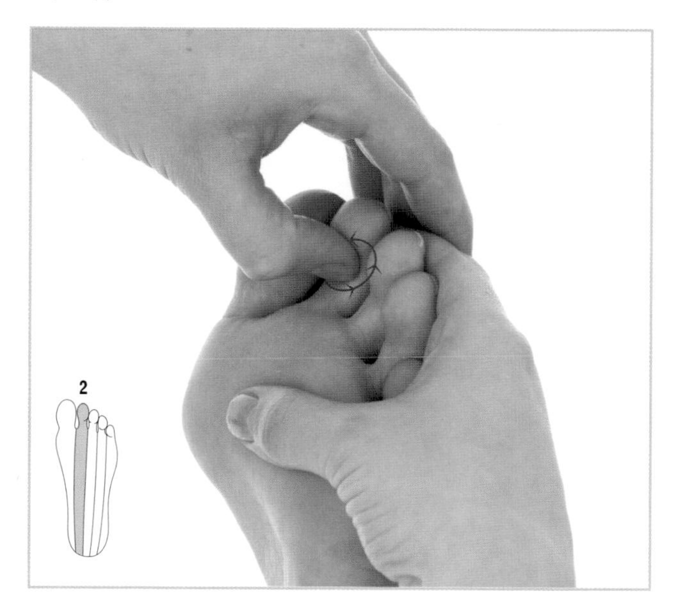

1 Support the left foot with your right hand at the top and, using the left thumb, use a gentle, rotating movement to work the eye area.

Left foot – plantar
Top support

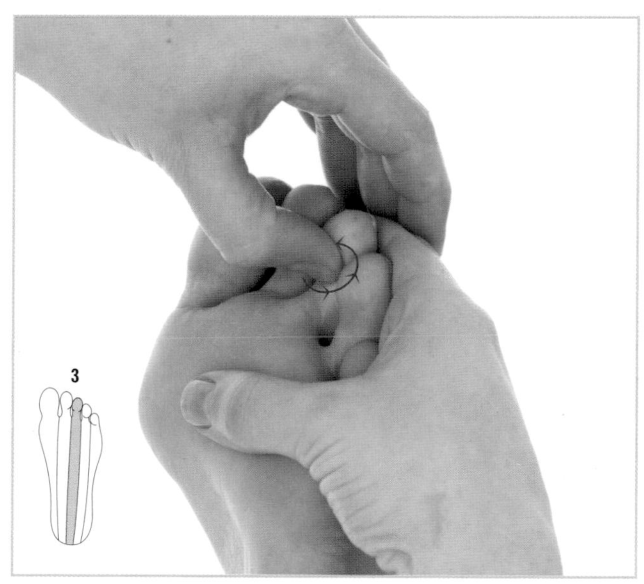

2 Support the left foot with your right hand at the top and, using the left thumb, use a gentle, rotating movement to work the ear area.

The facial area

Right foot – dorsal
Medial to lateral – top support

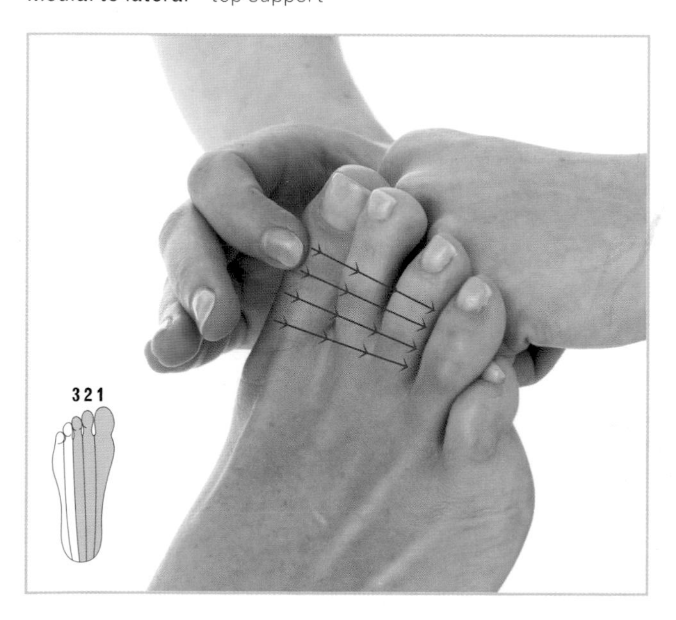

1 Support the right foot with your left hand and, using the right index finger, work across the first three toes, two or three times, from medial to lateral.

Left foot – dorsal
Medial to lateral – top support

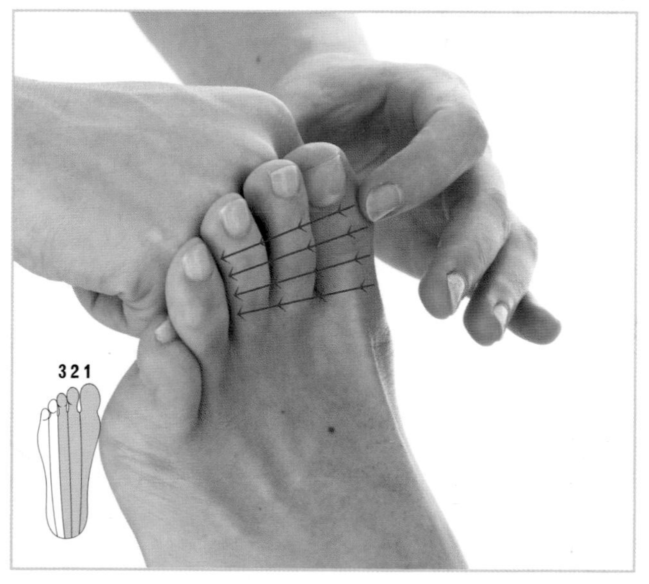

2 Support the left foot with your right hand and, using the left index finger, work across the first three toes, two or three times, from medial to lateral.

The musculoskeletal system

The living skeleton is a strong but flexible structure, articulated with joints that enable it to move, stretch, bend and rotate. As well as controlling movement, from the flicker of an eyelid to a gymnastic backflip, the muscular system is vital to digestion and blood and lymph circulation.

The skeletal system

Bone is more 'alive' than we tend to think, and because of the great age to which people are surviving today, there is obviously more wear and tear in our bones and joints. Operations to replace hips, knees and joints in our spine have become common.

JOINTS

A joint is any meeting point of bones. Some joints are very strong, while others are very mobile. A joint has a strong fibrous capsule surrounding the bone ends and has stabilizing ligaments that bind and strengthen it.

Fibrous joints, such as those in the skull, hold certain bones together with fibrous tissue. In cartilaginous joints, bones are separated by a disc of fibrocartilage, as found between the vertebrae of the spine.

In synovial joints, the most common type of joint, the space between the bones is filled with synovial fluid. This fluid allows frictionless movement between articulating bones. Synovial joints are often capable of a wide range of movement and are classified according to their type of movement:

- Ball and socket joints, such as hip and shoulder joints
- Gliding joints, such as the carpal (wrist) and tarsal (foot) joints
- Pivot joints, such as the atlas–axis joint in the cervical (neck) vertebrae
- Hinge joints, such as elbow and ankle joints
- Condyloid joints, such as knee joints and knuckles
- Saddle joints, such as the base of the thumb.

Bones have five main functions. They provide support, protect the internal organs, give movement by using specialized muscles, produce blood cells and store and release minerals such as calcium and phosphorus.

The skeleton consists of 206 bones, and may be divided into two broad groups: the axial skeleton and the appendicular skeleton.

The axial skeleton consists of the skull, spine, rib cage and sternum. This supplies the basic structure on to which the appendicular skeleton, the limbs, are joined via the pelvic and shoulder girdles. The pelvic girdle is much stronger than the shoulder girdle as it has to support the full weight of the body.

The bones from hip to knee, knee to ankle, shoulder to elbow and from elbow to wrist are referred to as the long bones; the fingers and toes are the short bones; flat bones are those making up the cranium, and the scapula and sternum area. The vertebrae of the spine, the pelvic area and stapes in the middle ear are the irregular bones.

Formation of bones

During fetal development bones form in two ways. Long bones develop from cartilage. The flat bones of the skull, the vertebrae and some other bones develop from a non-cartilaginous connective tissue. Growth takes place in all bones, but is more apparent in the long bones.

Bone is made of specialized cells and protein fibres, interwoven into a gel-like substance that is composed of water, salts and carbohydrates. All bones have an outer, compact layer and an inner, spongy centre. This makes them strong yet light. There is no nerve supply to the bone, but blood vessels enter through the nutrient canal to reach the spongy centre, which contains bone marrow, a soft tissue that produces blood cells.

Each bone is covered by a layer of specialized connective tissue called the periosteum, and the articulating surfaces are covered with hyaline cartilage to supply a smooth surface for the joints.

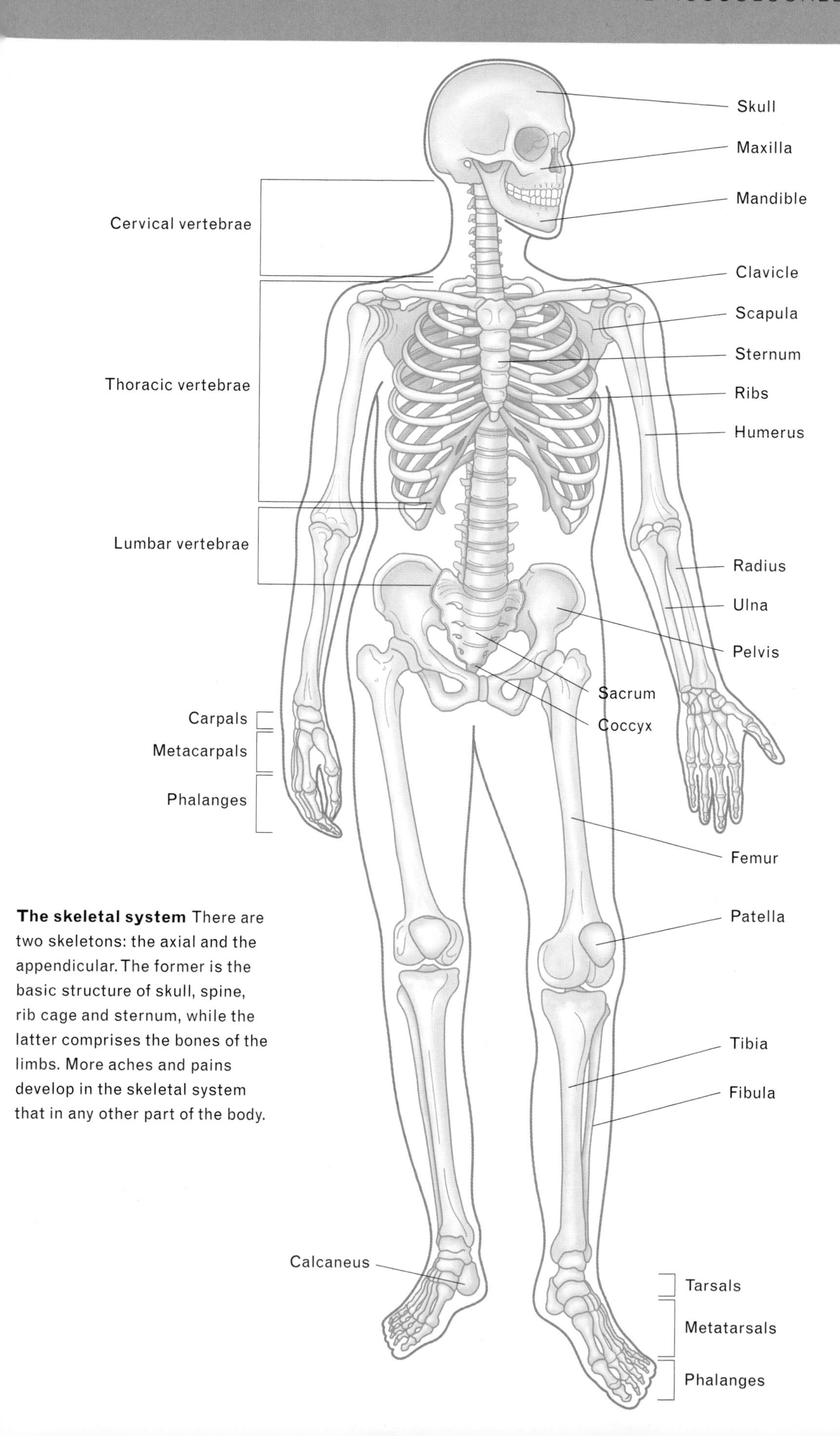

The skeletal system There are two skeletons: the axial and the appendicular. The former is the basic structure of skull, spine, rib cage and sternum, while the latter comprises the bones of the limbs. More aches and pains develop in the skeletal system that in any other part of the body.

The vertebral column

The spine is, literally and metaphorically, the backbone of the skeleton: it is the core of the whole framework, and all other bones relate directly or indirectly to it. The vertebrae that make up the spinal column are very much like cotton reels on a rope, with the central nervous system running as far as the lumbar region inside (see 'The nervous system', page 112).

The spine consists of 33 vertebrae:

- **Seven cervical vertebrae**: Situated in the neck, these are finer and less dense than those lower down as they only have to support the weight of the skull.
- **Twelve thoracic vertebrae**: The main function of these vertebrae is the support of the rib cage structure.
- **Five lumbar vertebrae**: These vertebrae are much denser and stronger than the thoracic vertebrae because the whole weight of the body is supported from this section.
- **Five sacral vertebrae**: These are fused to form the sacrum.
- **Four fused coccygeal vertebrae**: These form a non-protruding 'tail' articulating with the sacrum.

In addition, the atlas and axis are two special vertebrae at the very top of the spine. They allow rotation of the head.

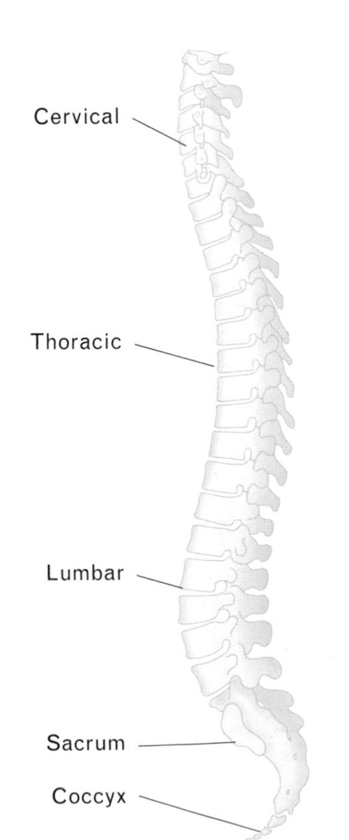

Curves of the spine We have three gentle curves in the spine. The cervical and lumbar sections curve slightly forwards, while the thoracic section curves backwards. Deformation of the spinal column, as in the conditions scoliosis, lordosis and kyphosis, can create exaggerated abnormal curves.

Movement of the spine

Each vertebra is covered with hyaline cartilage and the space between each bone is filled with a thick ring of fibrocartilage with a centre of soft, almost gelatinous tissue. These intervertebral discs act as shock absorbers.

The joints between the vertebrae are held together by anterior and posterior longitudinal ligaments and muscles. As we lie in bed our muscles and ligaments are able to stretch out, but during the course of the day, as we stand, sit and walk, our spines compress, so we are all just a little taller in the morning and become shorter as the day proceeds.

The movement between one individual vertebra and the next is small, but the combined effect down the whole spine is considerable. It can bend forwards, backwards, to the right and left. Most of the flexion and extension is in the cervical and lumbar regions, and bending to the side is principally in the lumbar area.

The joints between the atlas and occiput and between the atlas and axis in the neck are different. Instead of being cartilaginous, they are synovial and surrounded by ligaments (see box on page 126). This permits a much greater degree of movement, allowing the head to turn up to the ceiling and down to the floor as well as rotate on the neck to the left and right.

Attached to each of the 12 thoracic vertebrae is a pair of ribs. The top seven pairs are attached directly to the sternum (breastbone) by costal cartilage; the next three pairs (known as false ribs) are attached to the sternum by a common bar of cartilage to the rib above and the final two pairs, called floating ribs, are not connected to the sternum at all.

The joints between the ribs and their vertebrae are also of the synovial type and are surrounded by ligaments, which allows freer movement.

The muscular system

There are three types of muscle in the body: skeletal, cardiac and smooth muscle. The differences between these types of muscle are outlined on page 70, but here we are concerned with skeletal muscles, which are under voluntary control.

Muscle tissue is composed of cells specialized to contract. These are normally referred to as muscle fibres rather than cells and they are arranged in layers surrounded by connective tissue. Skeletal muscle fibres have a striated appearance.

There are approximately 600 skeletal muscles in the body, each attached to the skeleton by tendons. When a muscle contracts, it pulls on the tendons, which in turn pull on the associated bone, creating movement.

How the body moves

Most movement is the result of carefully controlled coordination of groups of muscles working together. For each movement, the muscles that produce a particular action are called the agonists, and the muscles that cause the opposite action are the antagonists. A simple example of this is to put your hand palm down on a table and lift one finger. Muscles in the back of your hand contract to raise your finger up, then muscles in your palm contract to bring the hand back down again.

Many muscle groups work in opposition to each other in this way. For example, the quadriceps in the front of the thighs straighten the legs and lift them forwards, while the hamstrings in the back of the thighs bend the knees and pull them back. It is important to keep opposing groups of muscles balanced in strength or the skeleton can be pulled out of alignment. Football players, for example, are prone to hamstring injuries because they frequently have very strong quadriceps from running and kicking.

There are often several muscle groups around joints, each stabilizing them from a slightly different angle. If one group becomes stronger than the others, the joints can be pulled out of alignment, causing a knock-on effect throughout the skeleton. For example, shoulder and neck problems often result from a bunching up of the big trapezius muscle in the upper back, while other muscles in the area, such as the latissimus dorsi and serratus anterior, are not functioning effectively.

Injuries, such as a sprained ankle that causes you to favour the other leg when walking, can quickly lead to a tightening of the hip muscles on the underused side, which can pull the spine out of alignment if not corrected.

Each muscle contraction is controlled by motor nerves. Muscle contraction requires energy and the immediate source comes from the energy storage molecule ATP (adenosine triphosphate). Muscle tone is a state of partial contraction of a skeletal muscle. Even when we are not moving, muscle tone keeps our muscles in a slightly contracted state, ready for action.

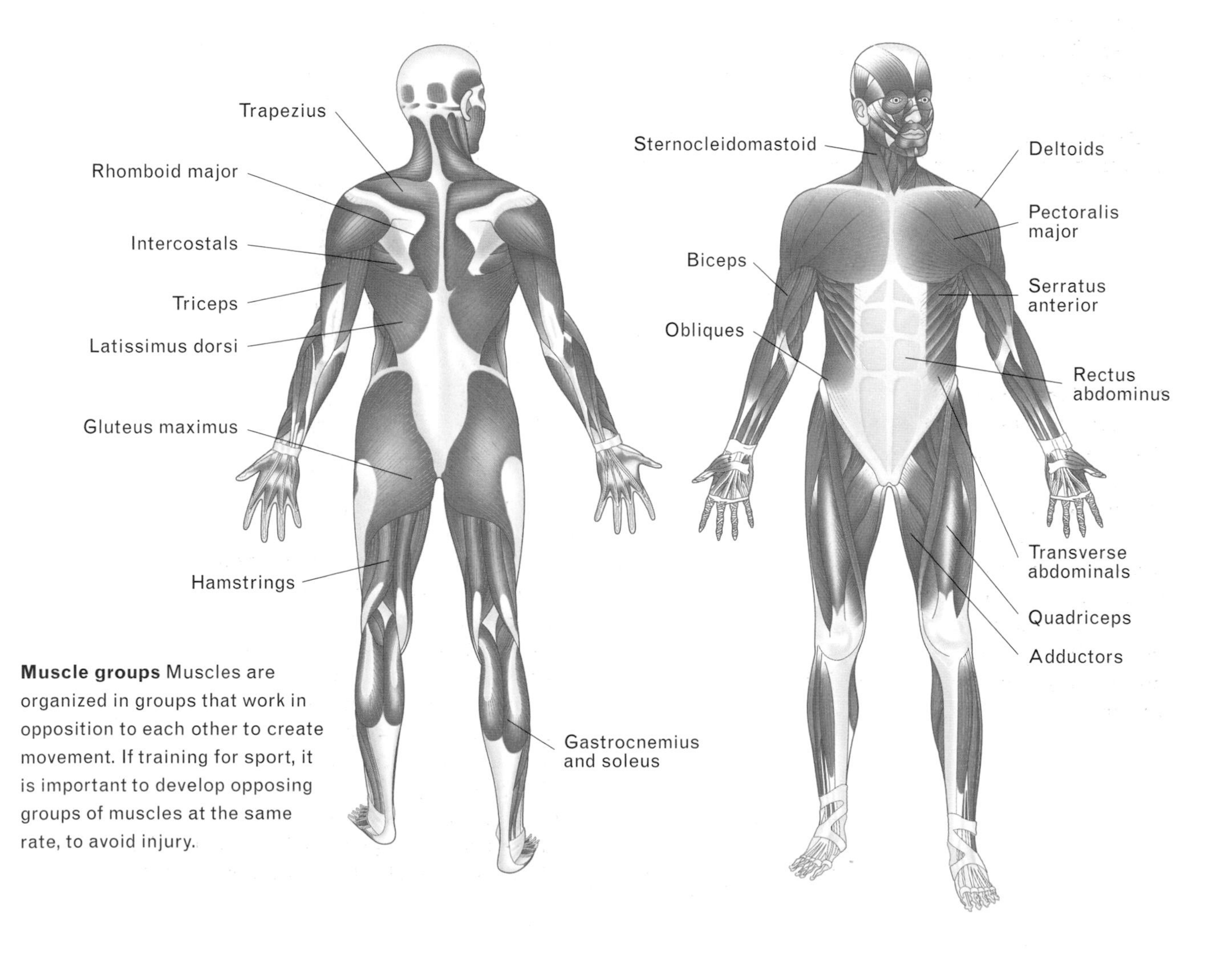

Muscle groups Muscles are organized in groups that work in opposition to each other to create movement. If training for sport, it is important to develop opposing groups of muscles at the same rate, to avoid injury.

Musculoskeletal disorders helped by reflexology

Most skeletal problems that are not due to broken bones stem either from a weak point in the system putting undue strain on other points or from the effect of the wear and tear of age.

Back pain

A great many of the skeletal problems we experience originate in the spine. A back problem hampers every activity and soon makes us begin to feel very aged. More than any other condition, back pain is the most common cause of people taking time off work.

Back conditions are on the increase and this is mainly due to the fact that the human race has grown so much in what is, in evolutionary terms, a very short period of time. Bone-deforming illnesses such as rickets and rheumatic fever are, thankfully, a thing of the past in the Western world, and this, coupled with a great improvement in nutrition and the care and welfare of infants, has meant that people are now taller than they were even a couple of generations ago.

Generally speaking, the taller you are the more likely you will be to suffer from back problems, simply because the spine has more to support. A shorter person is likely to be less prone to postural back trouble.

Extra body fat gives some additional protection against bone and joint problems, such as the higher levels of oestrogen (stored in body fat) that help mobility of joints and retention of a good calcium level in bone. However, being seriously overweight brings its own health problems (high oestrogen levels can increase the likelihood of cancer), and obesity will also naturally put a strain on the joints, because of the extra weight they have to bear.

Another cause of back problems among those living in the Western world is lack of exercise. Always using cars and elevators instead of walking leads to a weakening of the abdominal muscles. If these are not able to give enough support to the upper back, pain will result. Our increasingly sedentary lifestyles can also lead to back problems in other ways: pain can result from poor posture caused by spending the working day hunched over a computer.

Spinal problems often show up as pains or stresses experienced in other areas of the body. Lower back problems can cause pains in the knees, calf muscles and feet. The reverse is also true, as, for instance, when pregnancy or a broken leg cause a patient to adopt a stance that puts strain on the spine and back muscles. Neck conditions can affect the shoulders and arms, with pain and tingling radiating right down to the tips of your fingers.

STRUCTURE GOVERNS FUNCTION

The concept that 'structure governs function' is a guiding principle among many forms of holistic therapy. It means that if a structure (in this case the skeleton and musculature) is sound, it will function efficiently, each element working in coordination without strain. If, on the other hand, there is an imbalance in the structure, such as a weak muscle or a misalignment from bad posture, malfunctions will manifest themselves, and not just in the immediate area of the problem but as a knock-on effect all through the body.

Disc damage

Intervertebral discs tend to wear through the years and can eventually become very thin. This process is called 'narrowing of the disc space' and explains why people become shorter as they get older and deterioration of the joints occurs.

Pressure or injury to a disc may rupture the outer layer, causing pressure on spinal root nerves. This is the main cause for intense back pain and disability and is often referred to as a 'slipped disc'.

Osteoporosis

As we get older, our bones gradually become more porous and thinner. This weakening of the bones is called osteoporosis and can lead to an increased risk of fractures. Osteoporosis is more common in women after the menopause because of reduced oestrogen levels, but men also become prone to calcium loss in bones as testosterone levels decline in later years.

How reflexology can help

The usual medical approach to back pain is to prescribe a range of painkilling and anti-inflammatory medications, and in many instances to advise complete bed rest. Physiotherapy is often recommended, and sometimes helps. However, reflexology can give immense relief to spinal conditions, without the need for confining the

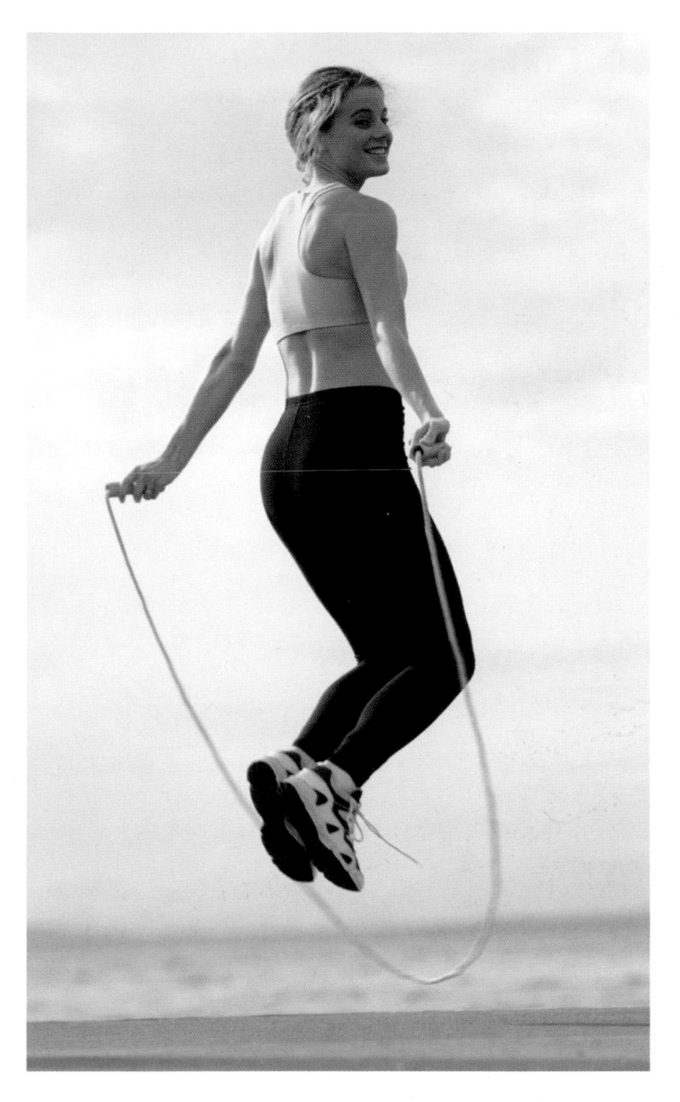

Skipping is good for you Weight-bearing exercise, such as skipping and jogging, increases bone and muscle density.

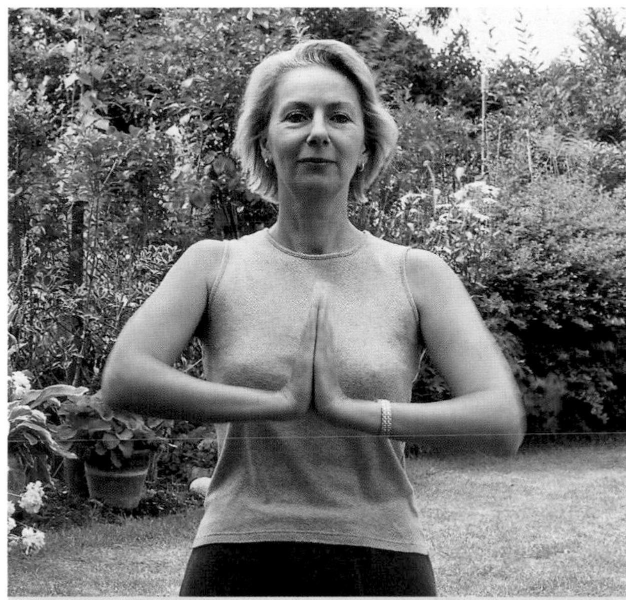

KEEPING YOUR BONES STRONG

We lose bone and muscle density when inactive, so taking suitable exercise is key to protecting your body:

- Jogging is a great weight-bearing exercise that can keep your bones and muscles really fit, but take care to wear appropriate running shoes and avoid running on very hard surfaces such as concrete.
- Daily arm circles and knee bends are gentle exercises that older people can do to keep their joints supple and preserve bone density.
- Even a stroll will help. Sunlight produces vitamin D, which is needed to transport calcium (crucial in bone growth and maintenance) to the bones.

patient to bed. In fact, I would say that reflexologists treat more patients with back conditions than any other health problem. Spinal conditions that respond admirably to reflexology include:

- Lumbago
- Arthritis of the cervical spine
- Chronic neck inflammations
- Sciatica (although sciatic pain does need treatment for many weeks)
- Whiplash injuries, which affect both the neck and lumbar regions.

Reflexology can help in reducing discomfort, settling inflammation and normalizing joint function in the case of many musculoskeletal complaints. It can treat frozen shoulders most successfully, free tension and pain in cases of arthritis and alleviate painful conditions in other joints, such as tennis elbow.

There are obviously limitations to what reflexology can achieve in the degenerative bone and joint conditions suffered by the elderly, but treatment can almost always offer some reduction in pain and stiffness, help reduce inflammation, and provide the patient with an improved quality of life.

Working the associated reflex points

Stimulation of these reflexes helps to relax tense muscles and ligaments, restoring lightness and mobility to the skeleton. The central nervous system and the spinal areas share exactly the same reflex points within the foot, as the spinal cord actually extends from the foramen magnum, a hole in the base of the skull, to the second lumbar vertebra (see page 112).

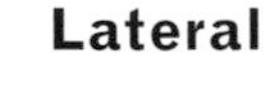

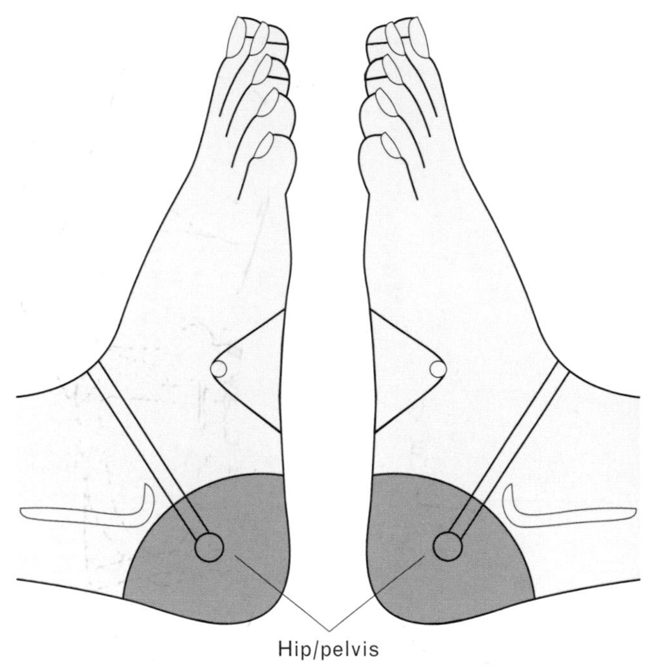

Medial

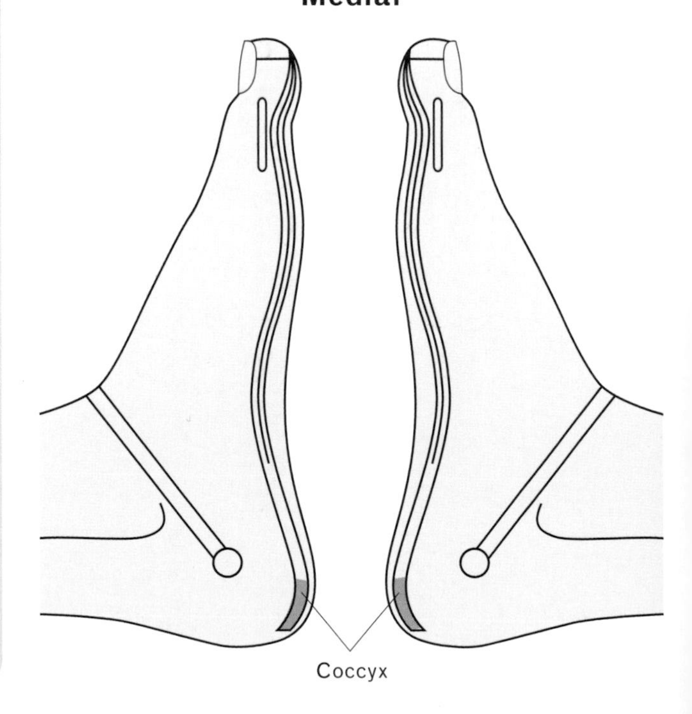

CASE STUDY **LUMBAR PAIN**

CLIENT PROFILE

Gerald had a sudden onset of disabling back pain when he was planting shrubs in his garden. Gardening had been one of Gerald's hobbies since his retirement from a sedentary job two years previously. He had suffered a few episodes of back trouble in the past, which had usually cleared up within a week or two, but this time pain continued into the fourth week.

REGULARITY OF REFLEXOLOGY TREATMENTS

Twice a week for the first two weeks then weekly for a following month.

REFLEXES

Main reflexes	Assistance
Entire spine, coccyx, hips, sciatic areas on both feet	To improve nerve and blood supply to painful areas and reduce pain levels

TREATMENT OUTCOMES

Gerald responded very well to his treatment sessions. Following the first appointment he said that he felt more pain than before in his spine and hip areas, but thereafter every treatment brought about more improvement until at the end of the six weeks he was pain-free and mobile once again.

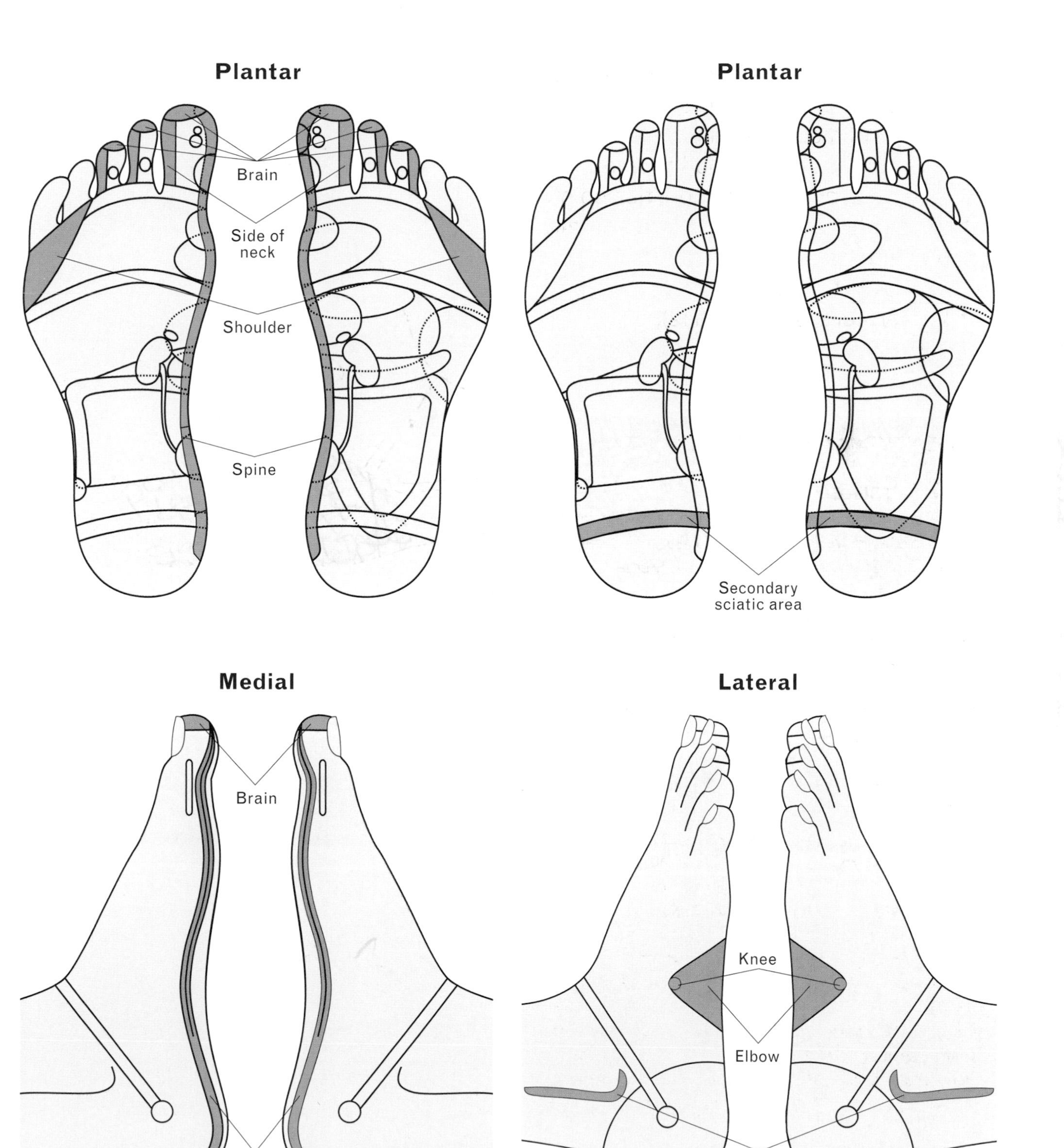
Plantar
Brain
Side of neck
Shoulder
Spine
Plantar
Secondary sciatic area
Medial
Brain
Spine
Lateral
Knee
Elbow
Sciatic nerve

The coccyx and hip/pelvis

Right foot – medial
Medial support

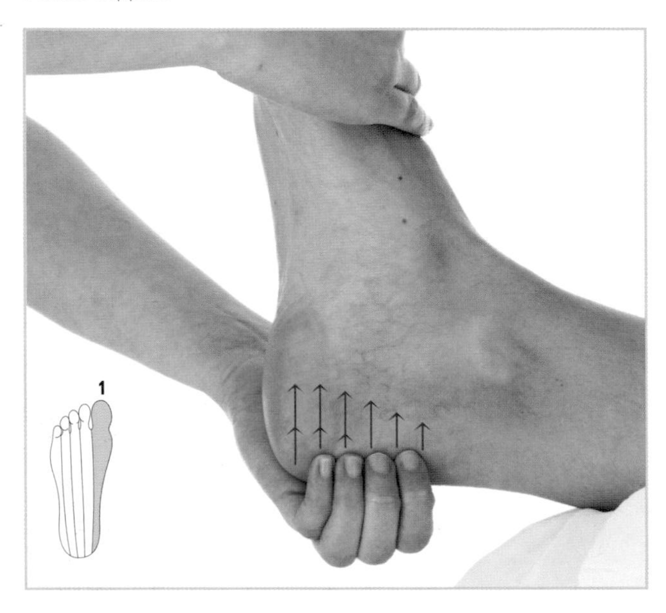

1 Holding the medial side of the right foot with your right hand, use the four fingers of your left hand to work over the coccyx area. Repeat two or three times.

Right foot – lateral
Lateral support

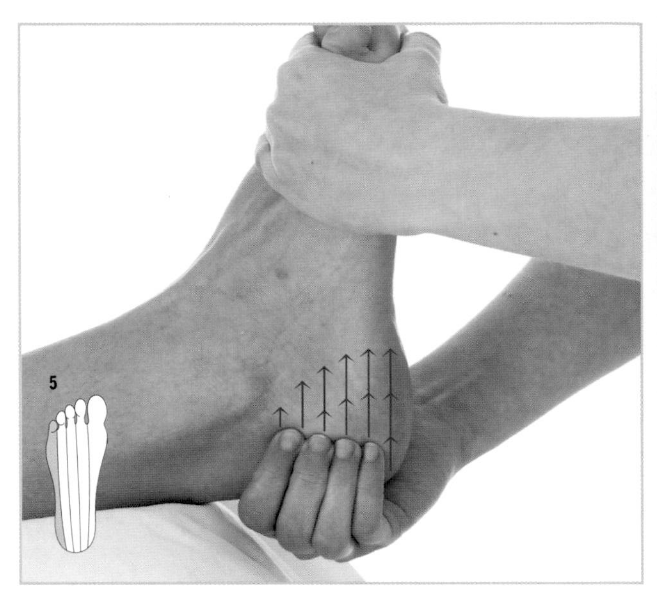

2 Supporting the right foot with your left hand, use the four fingers of your right hand to work over the hip/pelvis area. Repeat this movement two or three times.

The spine

Right foot – medial
Top support

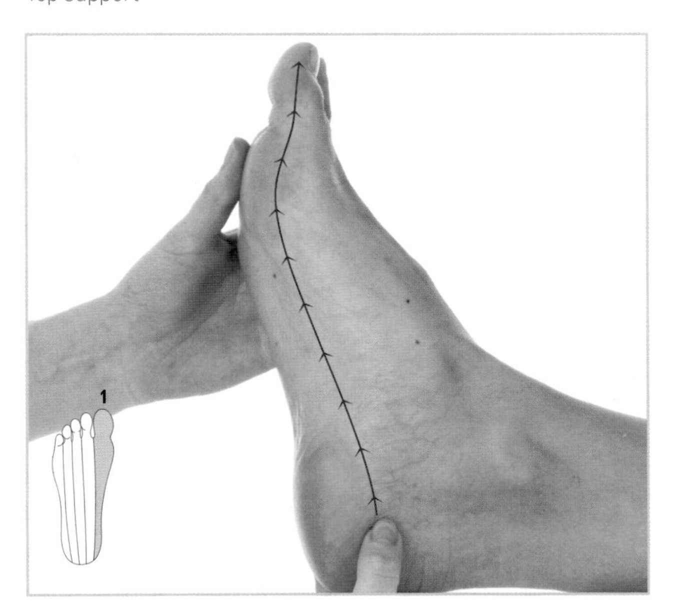

1 Support the right foot with your left hand and, using the right thumb, proceed to work up the vertebral column.

Right foot – medial
Top support

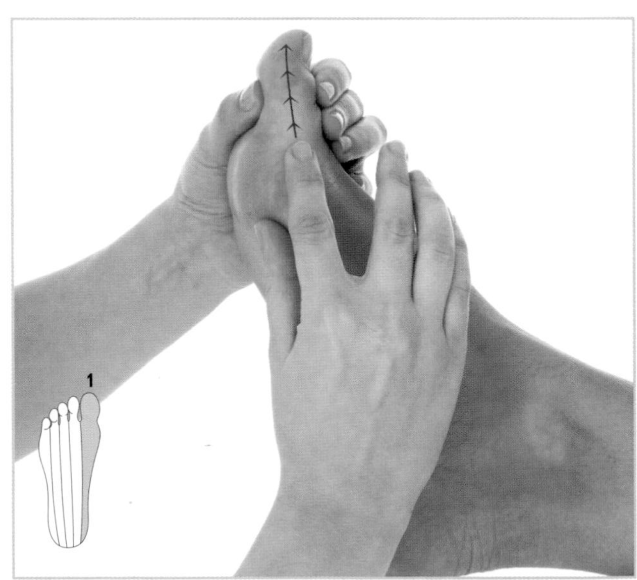

2 Support the right foot with your left hand and, using the right index finger (which will give a better result than the thumb), work up the fine area of the cervical spine.

Side of neck and spine

Right foot – plantar
Top support

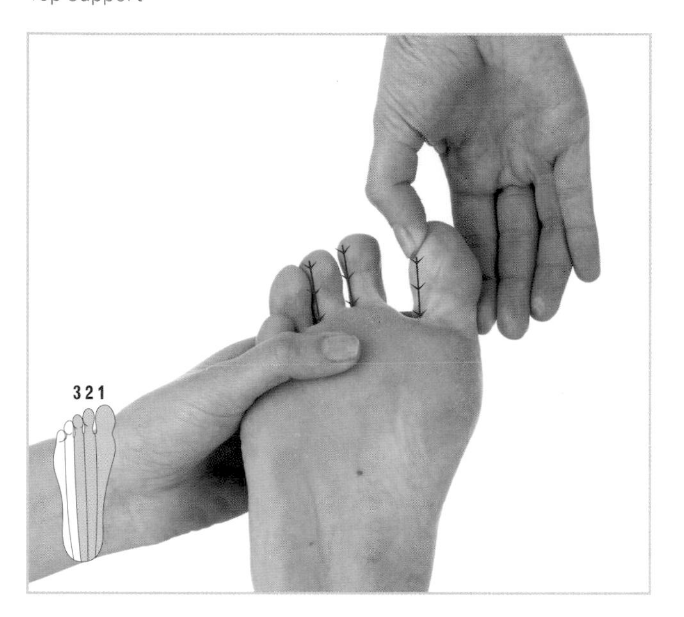

1 Support the right foot with your left hand and proceed to work down the side of neck area on the lateral sides of the first three toes with your right thumb.

Right foot – medial
Top support

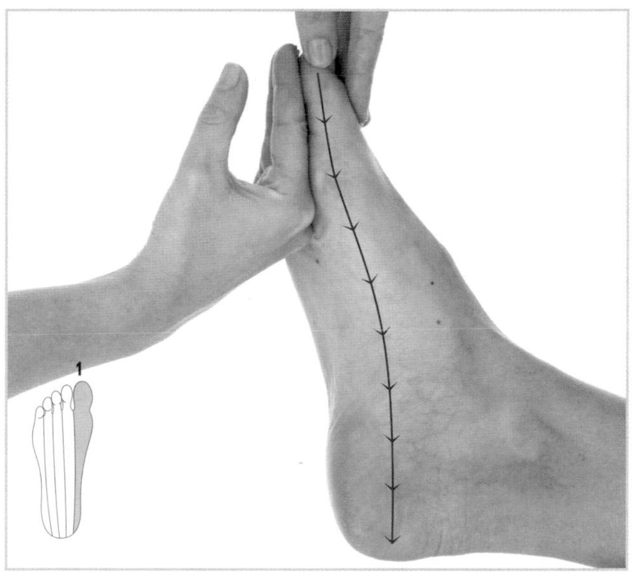

2 Support the right foot with the flat of your right hand and work down the vertebral column using the thumb of the left hand.

The shoulder area

Right foot – plantar
Medial to lateral – top support

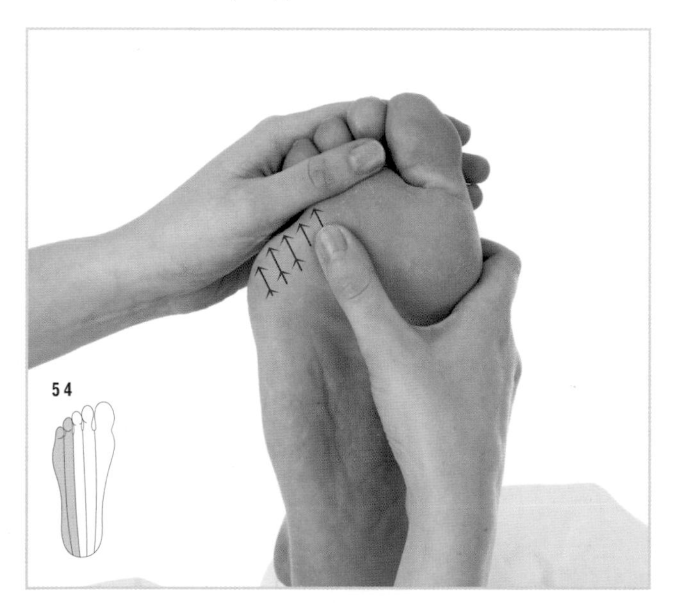

1 Support the right foot with your left hand and work out the area from medial to lateral with your right thumb.

Right foot – plantar
Lateral to medial – top support

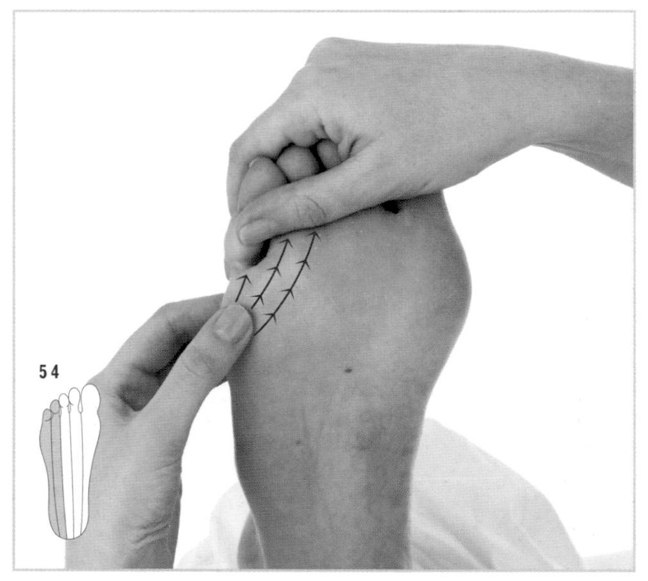

2 Support the right foot with your right hand and work out the area from lateral to medial with your left thumb.

The knee/elbow area

Right foot – lateral
Top support

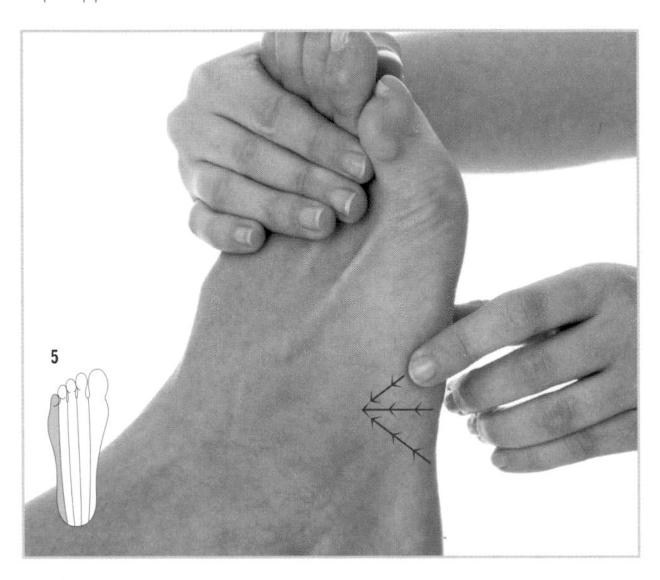

REFERRED PAIN

Always bear in mind that the area where a patient experiences pain or discomfort may not be a true indication of the source of the problem. It is interesting to find on x-ray, for example, that nothing is wrong with a patient's apparently problematic knee joint but that the problem is arising from compression or wear and tear in the lumbar spine.

Support the right foot with your right hand and, using your left index finger, work out the entire triangular area. The knee is at the apex of the triangle. The elbow is found within the triangular area.

The primary and secondary sciatic areas

Right foot – lateral
Top support

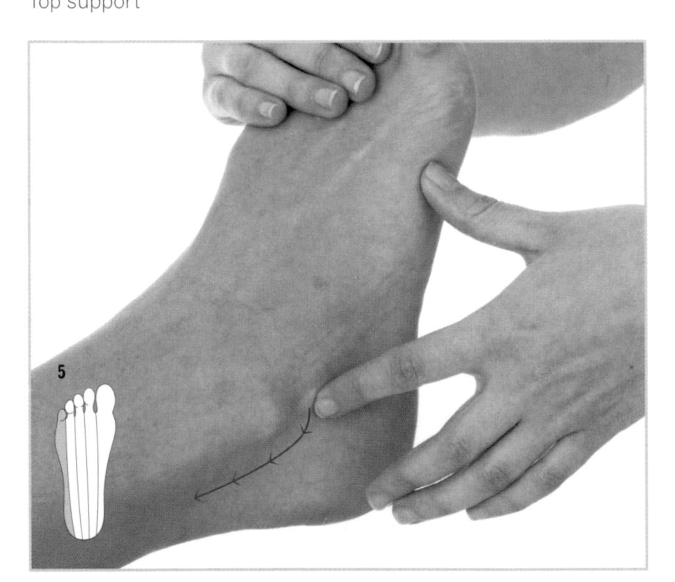

1 Support the right foot with your right hand and, using pressure from the index finger of your left hand, work up the primary sciatic area just behind the ankle bone. Proceed for about 8 cm (3 in).

Right foot – plantar
Medial to lateral – heel support

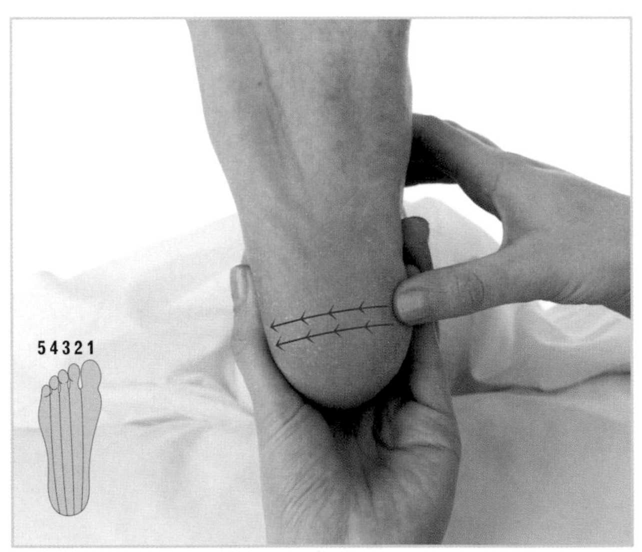

2 Support the right foot in the palm of your left hand and, using the right thumb, work out the secondary sciatic area two or three times.

The coccyx and hip/pelvis

Left foot – medial
Medial support

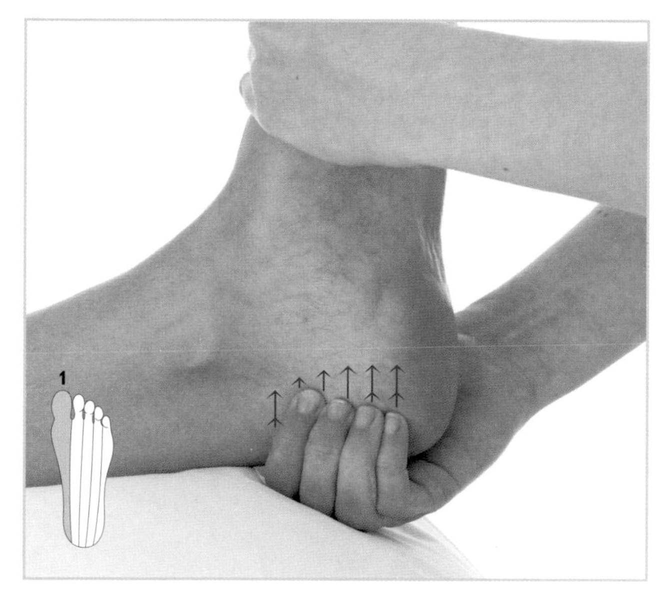

1 Holding the medial side of the left foot with your left hand, use the four fingers of your right hand to work over the coccyx area. Repeat two or three times.

Left foot – lateral
Lateral support

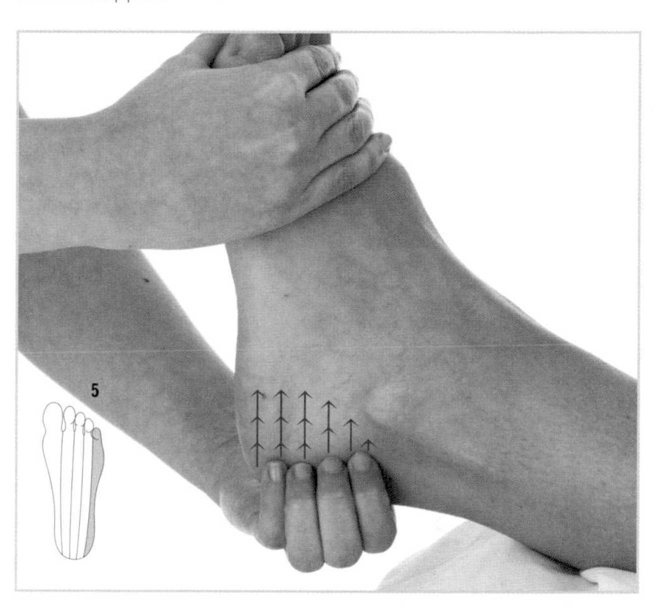

2 Supporting the left foot with your right hand, use the four fingers of your left hand to work over the hip/pelvis area. Repeat this movement two or three times.

The spine

Left foot – medial
Top support

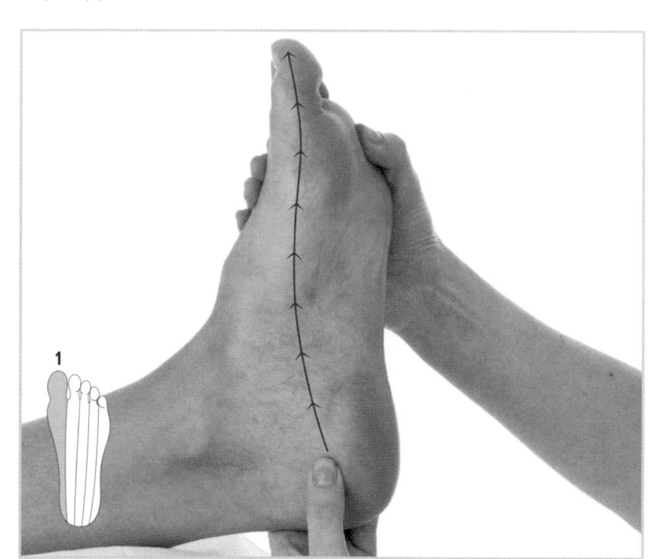

1 Support the left foot with your right hand and, using the left thumb, proceed to work up the vertebral column.

Left foot – medial
Top support

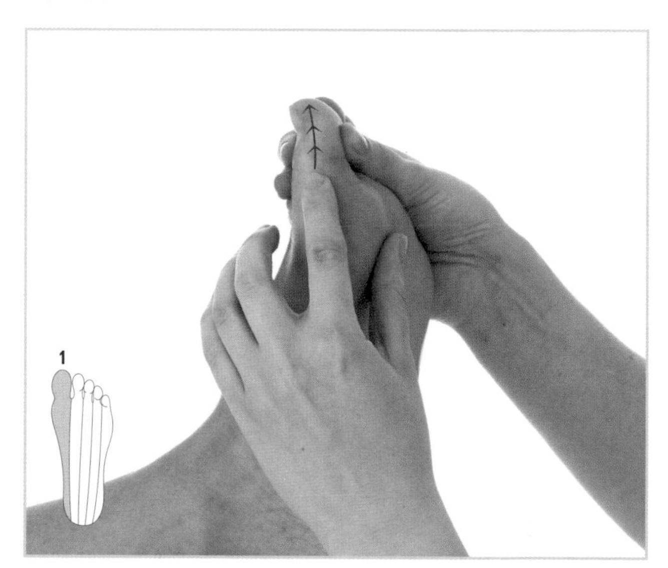

2 Support the left foot with your right hand and, using the left index finger (which will give a better result than the thumb), proceed to work up the fine area of the cervical spine.

Side of neck and spine

Left foot – plantar
Top support

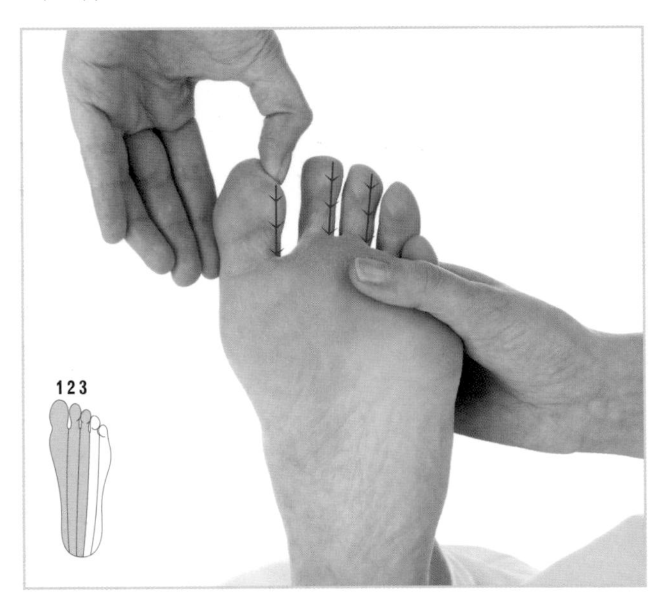

1 Supporting the left foot with your right hand proceed to work down the side of neck area on the lateral sides of the first three toes with your left thumb.

Left foot – medial
Top support

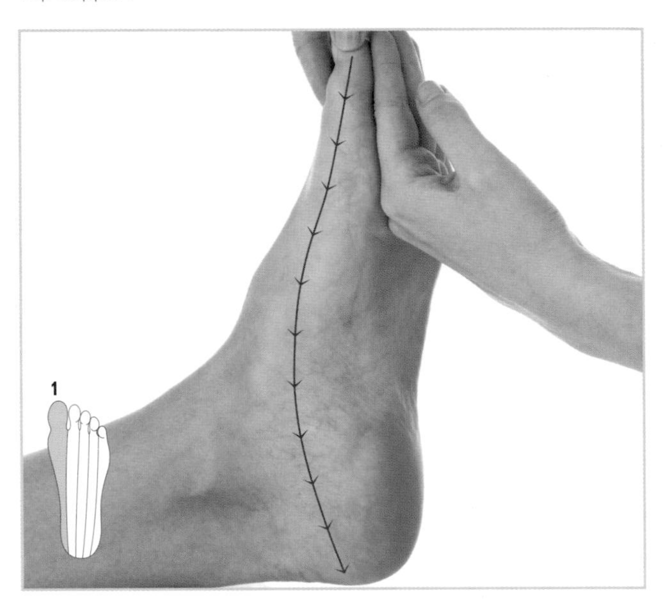

2 Supporting the left foot with the flat of your left hand, work down the vertebral column using the thumb of the right hand.

The shoulder area

Left foot – plantar
Medial to lateral – top support

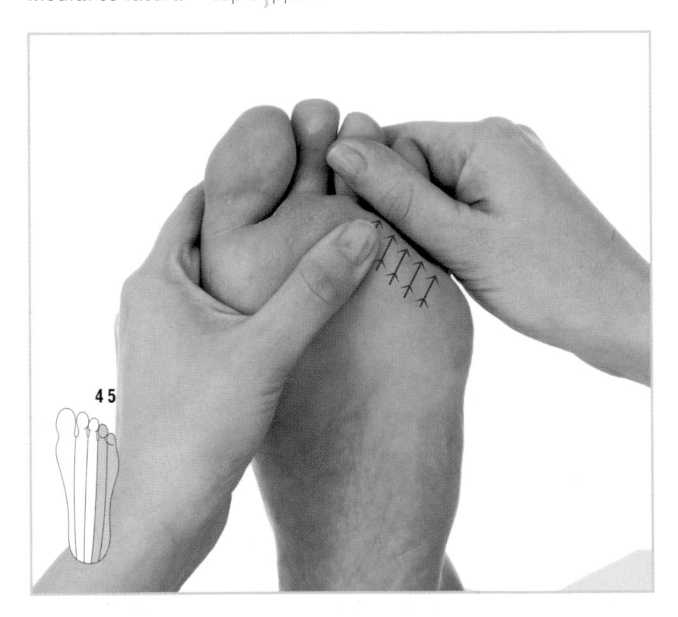

1 Supporting the left foot with your right hand, work out the area from medial to lateral with your left thumb.

Left foot – plantar
Lateral to medial – top support

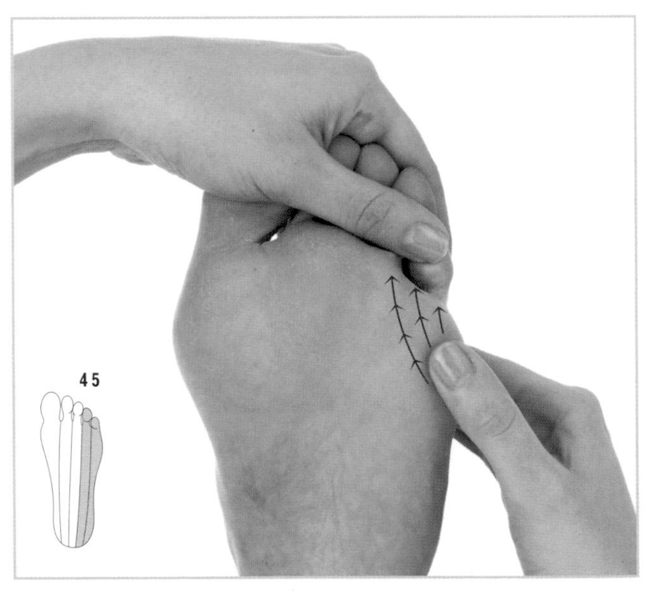

2 Supporting the left foot with your left hand, work out the area from lateral to medial with your right thumb.

The knee/elbow area

Left foot – lateral

Top support

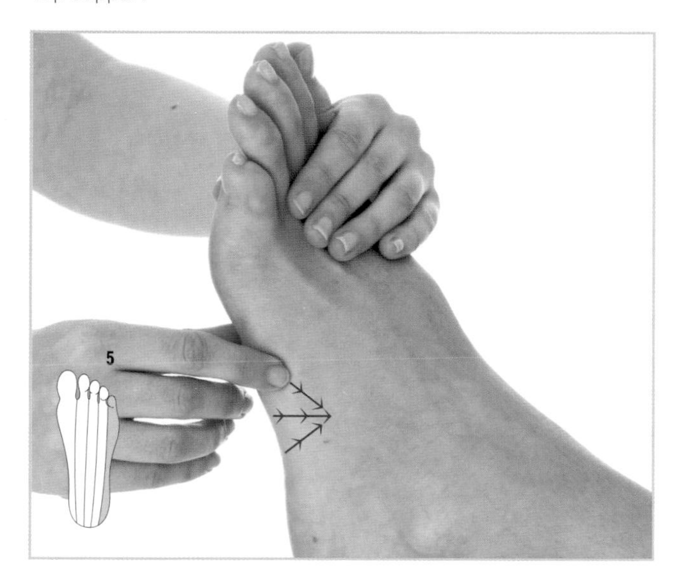

Support the left foot with your left hand and, using your right index finger, work out the entire triangular area. The knee is at the apex of the triangle. The elbow is found within the triangular area.

SCIATICA

Sciatica occurs when a disc is compressed in the spine (usually L5 or S1), causing irritation to the sciatic nerve. This is the largest single nerve in the human body, running from each side of the lower spine and radiating deep into the back of the thigh and down to the lower leg and foot. In a bout of sciatica, pain will be felt in the buttock, back of thigh and calf, occasionally extending as far as the foot. Reflexology can bring great relief and treatment should be given on a daily basis until the symptoms subside.

The primary and secondary sciatic areas

Left foot – lateral

Top support

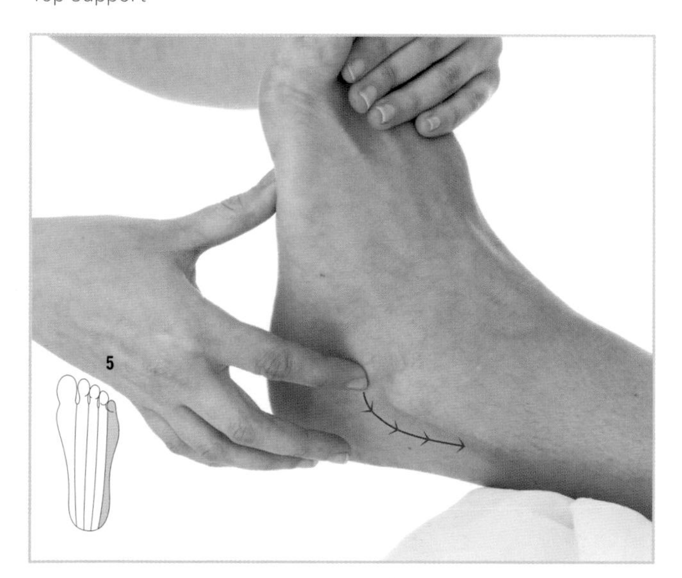

1 Support the left foot with your left hand and, using pressure from the index finger of your right hand, work up the primary sciatic area just behind the ankle bone. Proceed for about 8 cm (3 in).

Left foot – plantar

Medial to lateral – heel support

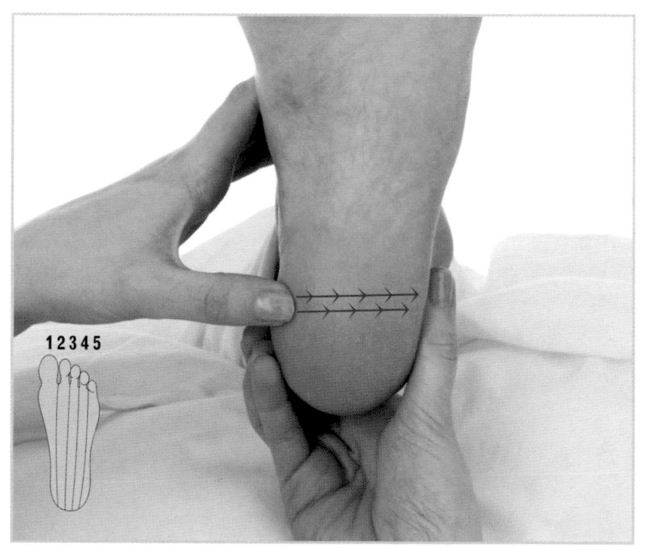

2 Support the left foot in the palm of your right hand and, using the left thumb, work out the secondary sciatic area two or three times.

The urinary system

The urinary system comprises two kidneys, two ureter tubes and a bladder. The kidneys act as a waste-processing system, filtering out unwanted matter from the blood. If permitted to accumulate, these wastes could reach toxic concentrations, so how well the kidneys function becomes reflected in our general health.

The kidneys

The kidneys are a pair of bean-shaped organs. They are encapsulated in fat and lie behind the stomach, facing inwards towards the spine. Together, the kidneys are the same size as their owner's heart.

Each kidney consists of a central medulla and the surrounding cortex. Blood carrying waste products flows into the kidney in order to be filtered, entering the medulla from the renal artery, which branches directly from the aorta, the main artery in the body. The cortex and medulla both contain tiny blood-filtration units known as nephrons. A single kidney will contain more than a million nephrons.

Inside the medulla, the artery splits into minute coiled blood vessels called glomeruli that spread throughout the medulla and cortex. Almost completely surrounding each glomerulus is a sac the size of a pinhead called a Bowman's capsule in which fluids from the blood in the glomerulus are collected. The filtered liquid then continues through a tubule surrounded by capillaries. These tiny blood vessels reabsorb into the blood most of the water and useful chemicals such as amino acids and glucose. One pair of kidneys can process 180 litres (45 gallons) of blood a day.

The treated, purified blood then leaves the kidney via the renal vein and re-enters the blood circulatory system. The extracted waste material flows on via a collecting tube to an area known as the kidney's pelvis. These wastes now form urine.

THE NATURE OF URINE

Urine is largely made of water, nitrogen wastes (mainly urea), inorganic salts and other substances of which the body has no need. Our urine output, naturally, is linked to how much fluid we drink, but it drops while we are asleep and also when we perspire a lot. Sweating is just ridding the body of excess fluid by another means.

The consistency and smell of urine varies according to what we eat and drink. When we drink a large amount of water, our kidneys produce well-diluted urine which is a light straw colour; too few fluids and not only will the amount drop, it will also be much more concentrated, darker in colour and stronger smelling.

Medical tests conducted on urine can pick up on various infections or malfunctions in the body, from cystitis to diabetes to toxaemia in pregnancy.

The ureters, the bladder and the urethra

From the pelvis in each kidney, the collected urine passes through a tube called the ureter. The two ureters lead in turn to the bladder.

The bladder is situated in the pelvis, behind the pubic bone, and functions as a temporary storage sac for the urine. An empty bladder is flat, but its lining is constructed in folds that permit it to expand. As urine drips into the bladder through the ureter tubes, the bladder walls relax and stretch. When it is full, a bladder can hold about 600 ml (1 pint) of urine.

When the bladder is full, urine is released via a broader tube, called the urethra, which opens from the base of the bladder and leads to the body's exterior. A ring of muscles known as the urethral sphincter normally keeps this outlet closed, but when the bladder holds about a cupful of urine, nerves start sending signals to the brain to urinate. When urination takes place, the external urethral sphincter muscle relaxes and the bladder wall contracts, forcing urine through the urethra and out of the body.

The urinary system Including the kidneys, ureter, bladder and urethra, the urinary system conducts urine from the kidneys to the exterior of the body. The female urethra is much shorter than that of the male.

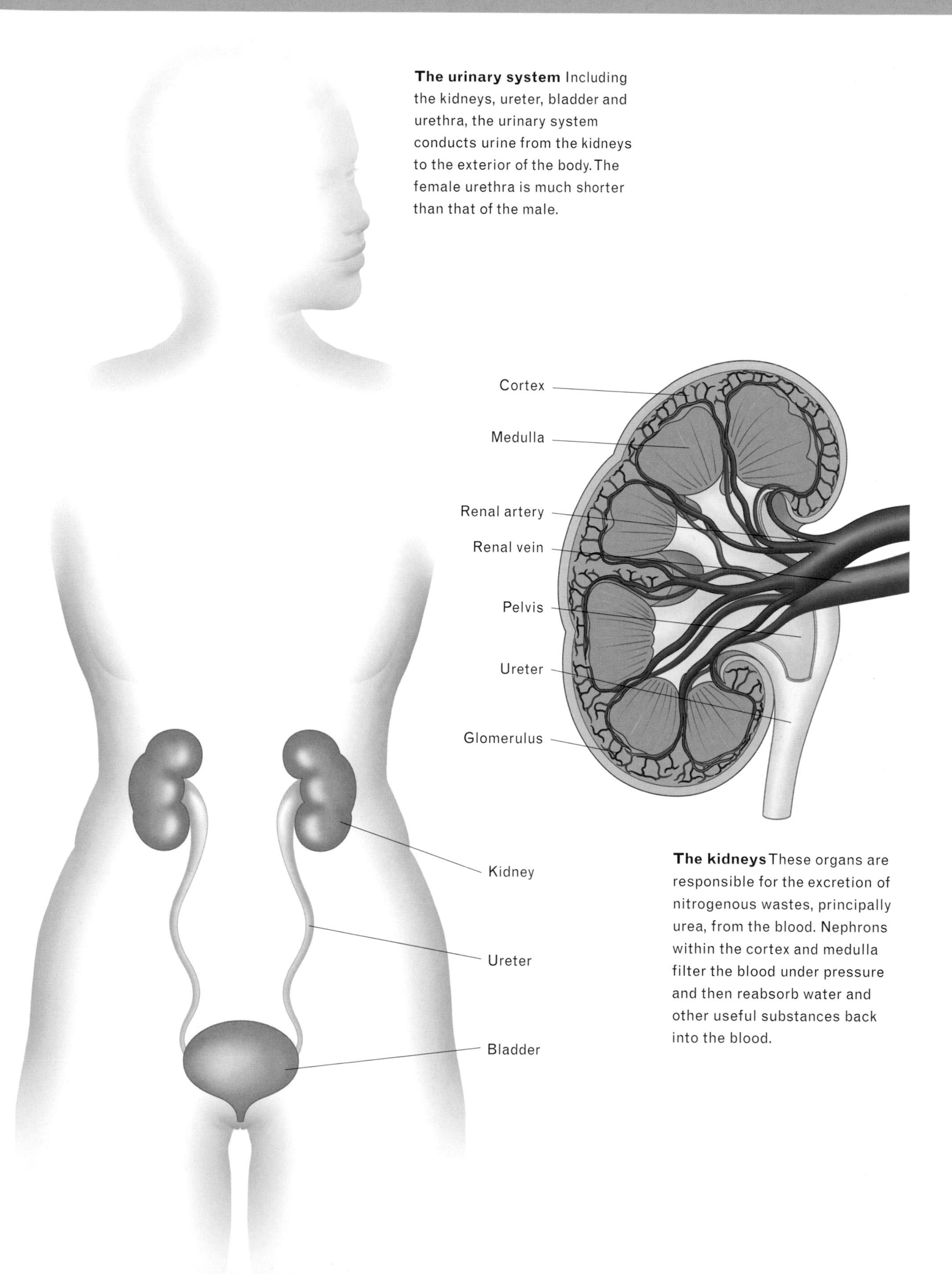

The kidneys These organs are responsible for the excretion of nitrogenous wastes, principally urea, from the blood. Nephrons within the cortex and medulla filter the blood under pressure and then reabsorb water and other useful substances back into the blood.

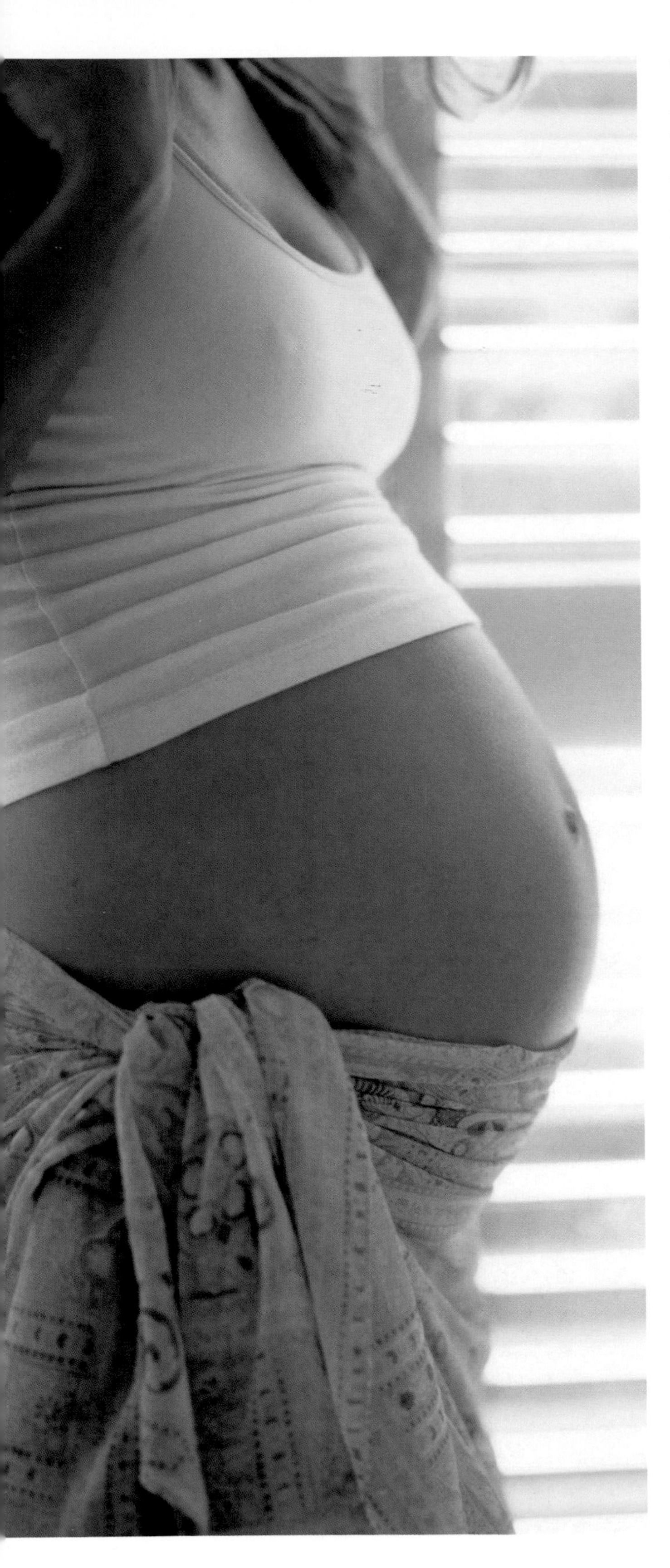

Urinary conditions helped by reflexology

The female urethra is short, emerging just above the vagina, but the male urethra, which runs the length of the penis, is about 20 cm (8 in) long and passes through a small gland called the prostate. Both of these different configurations can bring their own problems.

Bladder infections

These are more common in women than men because the long male urethra acts as a barrier to bacterial invasion. The most common bladder infection is cystitis, which is caused by bacteria invading the delicate membranes of the bladder. It results in pain, frequent urination and a feeling of being generally unwell.

The prostate gland encircling the base of the male urethra often enlarges as men grow older. This may compress the urethra or distort it, causing problems with frequency of urination and a weakened flow. As the bladder does not always empty completely, a tendency for urine infections becomes more common. Cancer of the prostate is a common disorder in men over 50 years old (see also page 152).

Urinary incontinence

Involuntary leakage of urine is especially common in elderly people and often accompanies senile dementia as brain cells die off and the brain–bladder coordination becomes poor. However, urinary incontinence can occur at any age and for a number of reasons. The leakage can take place after suddenly coughing or sneezing, or on picking up a heavy object. Incontinence occurs more frequently in women than in men, mainly because women often have a weakness in their pelvic floor muscles if they have had children or a difficult delivery that resulted in a forceps birth. Pregnant women also have the frequent desire to urinate and may experience temporary incontinence because of the pressure the swelling uterus is putting on the bladder, which is situated just below the uterus. Damage to the spinal cord as the result of an accident in the lumbar spinal area is yet another cause of incontinence.

Urinary conditions in pregnancy In pregnancy, the bladder can become squashed under the weight of the baby, potentially leading to urinary infections and temporary incontinence.

Kidney problems

More frequent in men than women, kidney stones are a common complaint. Stones form in the urine-collecting part of the kidneys or the ureter tubes when certain concentrated substances in the urine coagulate and create solid deposits. Larger stones (more than about 5 mm (¼ in) across) cannot be flushed out easily with the flow of urine and the pain they cause as they try to pass through the system has been said to be the most excruciating that one can suffer. Stones in the kidneys or ureters may show up on an x-ray or scan.

High blood pressure has close associations with the kidneys. People suffering from chronic hypertension often find that the kidney function can eventually become impaired. The increased pressure of blood being forced through the kidney tubules often causes a collapse of these delicate nephrons and results in less efficient function of the filtering system. Inflammation of the nephrons is called nephritis.

As the kidneys face inwards towards the lumbar region of the spine, kidney pain can often be confused with back pain and is therefore sometimes suffered for a long period of time before a doctor is consulted.

Pregnancy can put extra stress on the kidneys, as they are eliminating waste products for two beings instead of one. Fluid retention, showing as puffy ankles and fingers, is common, but if a urine sample also reveals protein in the urine and there is raised blood pressure, toxaemia may be indicated. Immediate attention from a specialist would be needed to decide whether bed rest can improve the situation, or whether the mother and baby would both benefit from an early birth.

Long-term diabetes can also lead to complications in the kidney function and may progress to kidney failure.

How reflexology can help

Reflexology has proved to be very successful in relieving many of the conditions described above. Stimulating the whole pelvic cavity has the effect of improving the nerve and blood supply to the urinary system and this helps to rid the body of its impurities. Reflexology also breaks down tension that has accumulated in the body, further encouraging the healing process.

Reflexology is safe to use in pregnancy and, by improving urinary function, it will ease the effects of pregnancy-related urinary conditions.

By taking the stress off the kidneys we are able to improve the kidney function, which has an effect on lowering the blood pressure. Patients with high blood pressure will very often have very sensitive reflexes in the kidney areas.

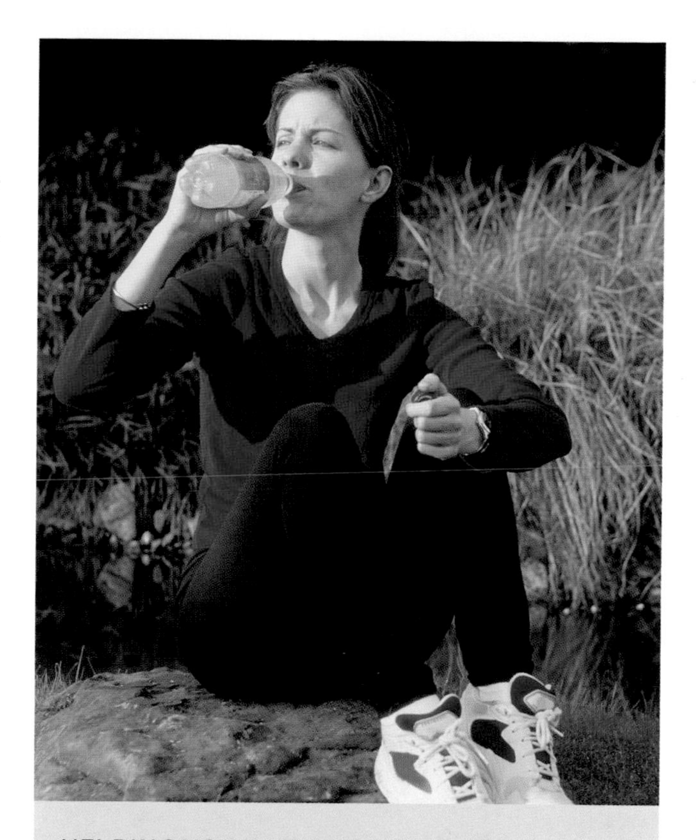

HELPING YOUR URINARY SYSTEM

Every living thing depends on water for its survival. Water transports hormones and nutrients around the body, helps dilute toxic substances and absorbs waste products. It is crucial to replace the fluids lost in exhaled air, perspiration and excreted waste. Without sufficient fluids, the kidneys cannot keep the body's chemistry in perfect balance. Here are some ways in which you can assist your urinary system:

- Drink 2 litres (4 pints) of fluid daily and more if you are exercising or the weather is hot. Remember that water comes in other forms, such as fruit juice.
- Cranberry juice is excellent if you suffer from cystitis as it helps to prevent bacteria sticking to the bladder wall and multiplying.
- Cut out caffeine and any food stuffs that contain caffeine if you have an infection.
- Apple cider vinegar is a great natural antiseptic and anti-inflammatory. If you have a urinary infection, take three teaspoons morning and evening in a large glass of warm water.

Working the associated reflex points

The kidney reflex area sits in the arch of each foot, while the bladder points are found on the medial side of the pelvic (heel) line. As in the body itself, the ureter reflex runs between these two areas. Be sure to work out the areas connected to the pelvic, hip and coccyx areas and also the lumbar spine whenever you are treating bladder and kidney problems.

CASE STUDY **KIDNEY STONES**

CLIENT PROFILE

Tom was 65 and had suffered from kidney stones for many years. As the stones passed through the delicate ureter tubes to the bladder he suffered agonizing pain and bleeding. On most of these occasions he had to be admitted to hospital in order for the pain to be controlled. Although he got over these attacks each time, they left him feeling exhausted and depressed. He decided to try reflexology to see if he could get some relief.

REGULARITY OF REFLEXOLOGY TREATMENTS

Weekly sessions for eight weeks.

REFLEXES

Main reflexes	Assistance
Kidney, ureter tube, bladder	To ease inflammation in these areas due to laceration of stones
Lumbar spine/nerves	To help urinary function

TREATMENT OUTCOMES

Tom responded well to his reflexology sessions and had one quite amazing experience: he actually passed and collected a kidney stone following one appointment. Although he had a dull, aching sensation in his low back, he certainly did not experience the severe pain felt previously. He continued with reflexology treatments for many years and, despite continuing to produce more stones, he never suffered the painful episodes of the past. Reflexology relaxed the painful spasms in his ureter tubes and allowed the stones to pass with ease.

Plantar

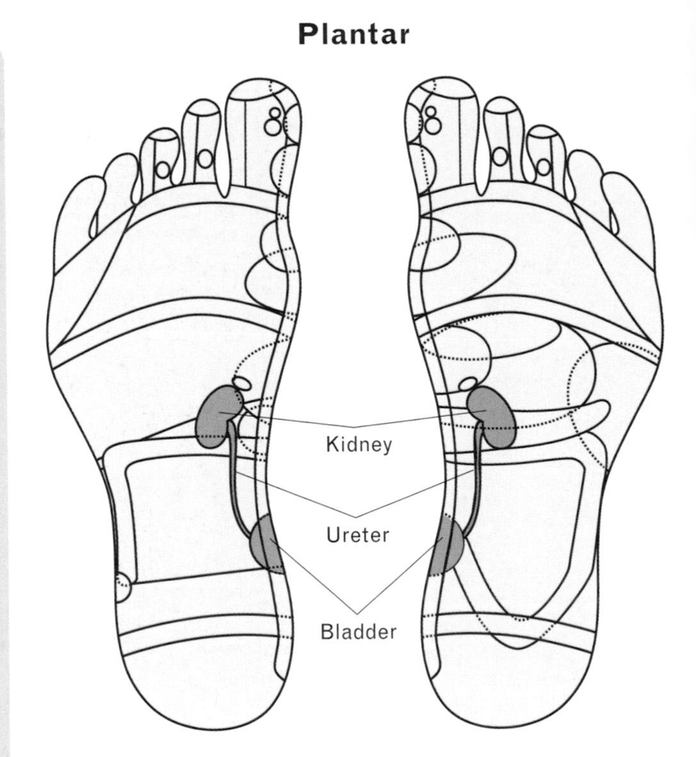

The bladder/ureter tube and kidneys

Right foot – medial
Top support

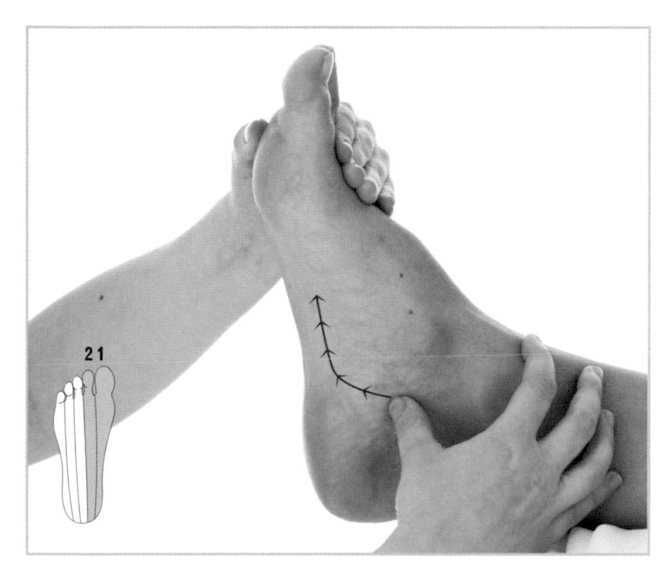

1 Supporting the right foot at the top with your left hand, work on and over the bladder area with the right thumb. Proceed up the medial side of the ligament line to work out the ureter tube.

Right foot – medial
Top support

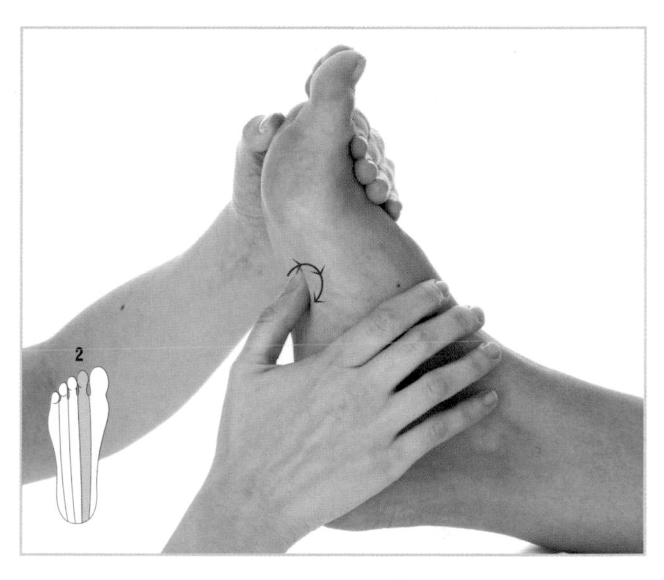

2 Supporting the right foot with your left hand and placing the right thumb on the lateral side of the ligament line, work out the kidney area as shown.

The bladder/ureter tube and kidneys

Left foot – medial
Top support

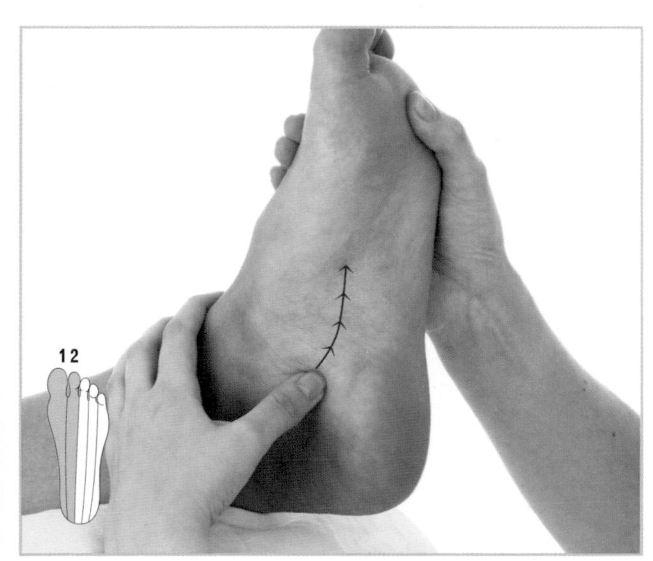

1 Supporting the left foot at the top with your right hand, work on and over the bladder area with the left thumb. Proceed up the medial side of the ligament line to work out the ureter tube.

Left foot – medial
Top support

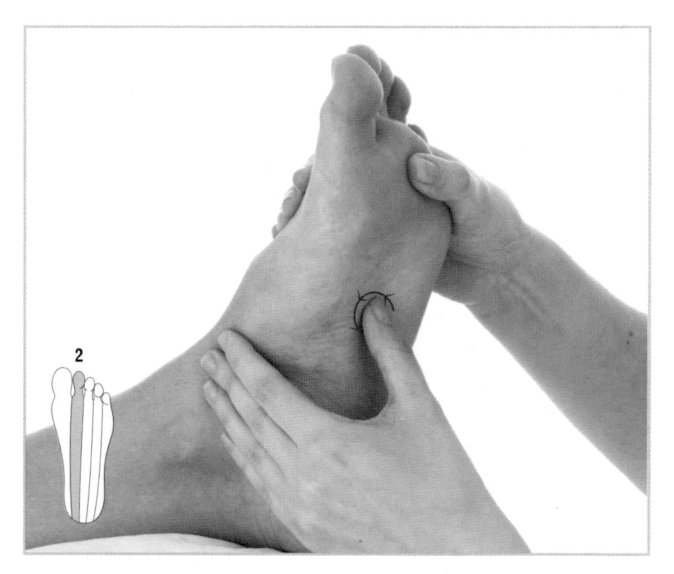

2 Support the left foot with your right hand and, placing the left thumb on the lateral side of the ligament line, work out the kideny area as shown.

The reproductive system

Hormones are responsible for the different ways in which men and women develop through childhood and beyond, and for the separate functions of our reproductive systems. Although these may appear very different, the underlying anatomical structure is similar and this is reflected in the reflex points of the feet.

Hormones at work

The reproductive systems of both men and women are regulated and controlled by hormones. Even before birth, hormones shape an individual's sex and sexuality, and at certain stages in life they become particularly active, triggering physical changes. At puberty, for example, they are responsible for changes such as secondary hair growth, a boy's voice dropping in pitch, a girl's breast development and the onset of menstruation.

Two hormones, orchestrated by the pituitary gland in the brain (see 'The endocrine system', page 98), are the main instigators of a woman's monthly reproductive cycle. Follicle stimulating hormone (FSH) stimulates the development and ripening of the ovarian follicle. During its development, the ovarian follicle secretes its own hormone, oestrogen. As the level of oestrogen increases in the blood, so the secretion of FSH is reduced. Then the luteinizing hormone (LH) promotes a final maturation of the ovarian follicle and ovulation. The main function of LH is to promote the formation of a body called the corpus luteum, which secretes a second ovarian hormone, progesterone.

FSH and LH are also at work in the male body. FSH stimulates the epithelial tissue of the seminiferous tubules in the testes to produce spermatozoa, while LH stimulates the interstitial cells in the testes to secrete testosterone.

The female reproductive system, unlike the male one, is the only system in the body that has a shorter lifespan than any of the others. The average age of the onset of the menopause, and therefore the cessation of ovulation, menstruation and child-bearing, is around 52 years (see page 149).

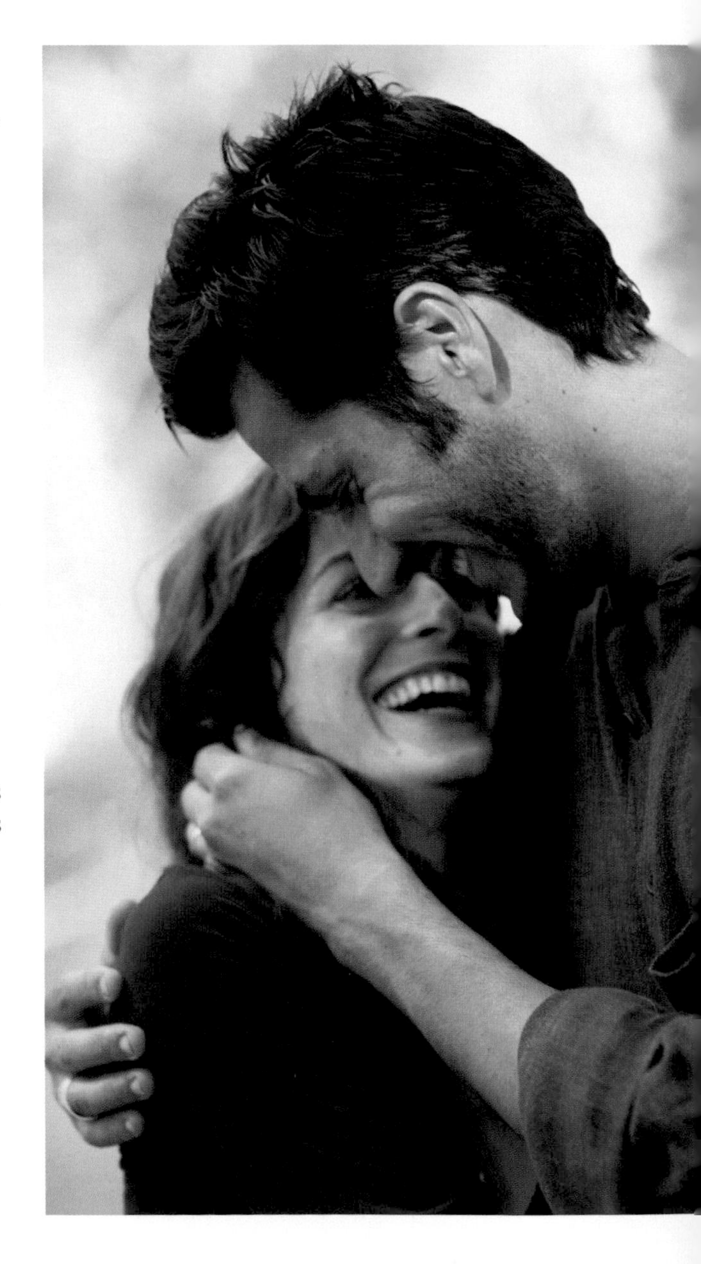

The role of hormones The sex and sexuality of men and women is shaped from before birth by hormones produced by the endocrine system.

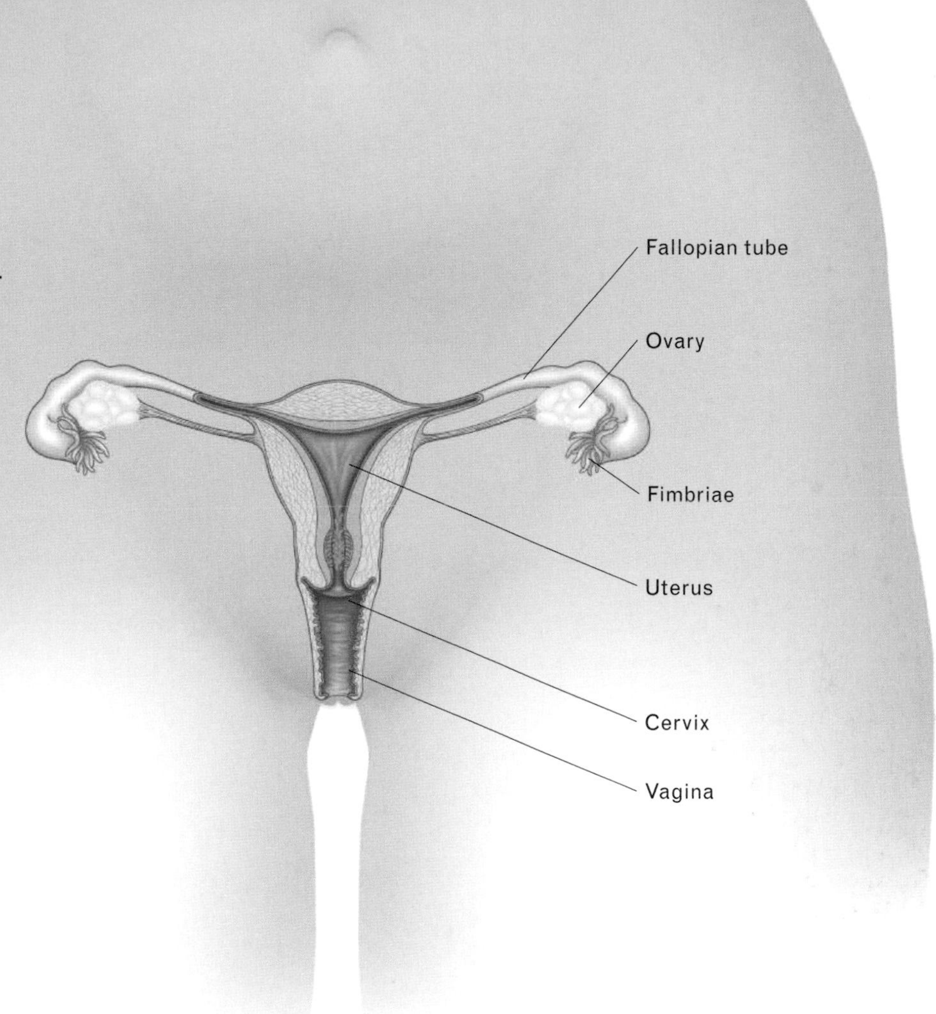

The female reproductive system Once the egg has been released from an ovary, it is drawn into the Fallopian tube. Slight contractions of the tube and the movement of tiny cilia move the egg towards the uterus. It can survive in the Fallopian tube for 24 hours and, if it is not fertilized, it will be reabsorbed by the body.

The female reproductive organs

The ovaries, uterus and vagina all work together in a harmonious cycle to keep a woman's reproductive system in readiness for pregnancy and childbirth.

The vagina

The vagina, an elastic tube 10–15 cm (4–6 in) long, lined with moist epithelial tissue (see page 70), provides both access for the penis during sexual intercourse (vagina comes from the Latin *vaina*, meaning 'sheath for a sword') and the birth canal for a baby.

At the entrance to the vagina are a pair of lip-like folds, the larger and thicker being the labia majora, and the smaller and inner being the labia minora. They lie on either side of the vaginal entrance and blend in the front into the padded area of the mons pubis. At the front they enclose the exit of the urethra, just behind the small projection which is the external portion of the clitoris.

The cervix, uterus and Fallopian tubes

At the top end of the vagina is the uterus, or womb, the entrance to which is guarded by the cervix, also called the 'neck of the womb'. This is a thick, fibrous, muscular structure lined with special cells that form a mucus.

The uterus itself is small and pear-shaped. It lies behind the bladder and in front of the rectum, held in place by muscles and four strong fibrous ligaments of the pelvic floor. To the sides, pairs of round suspensory ligaments also hold it in place, running in folds of peritoneum, the strong lining of the abdominal cavity.

The uterus is covered with peritoneum, a thick wall of interweaving muscle fibres. Uterine muscles are always contracting and relaxing slightly. The inner walls of the uterus are lined with special endometrial cells, which react and change under hormonal influences.

To the left and right of the uterus extend the Fallopian tubes, each 12 cm (5 in) long. On their free ends, close to the ovaries, are finger-like projections called fimbriae.

The ovaries

These two small, oval-shaped, pearl-coloured organs lie just below the Fallopian tubes on each side of the uterus. Within the ovaries are the eggs (ova) that provide the start of a new human life.

A female has the greatest number of ova in her ovaries that she will ever have (about 20 million) when she is a 20-week fetus inside her mother's womb. A woman's biological time clock for reproduction begins ticking before she is even born.

Ovulation, fertilization and menstruation

From about the age of 13 or so for the next 40-odd years, one or other of the ovaries releases an ovum about once a month. (The ovum is the largest single cell in the human body, although it is no larger than the full stop at the end of this sentence.) This 'maturation' of an ovum, decreeing it is ready for release, is controlled by a hormone from the pituitary gland. Cells of the follicles in the ovaries secrete another hormone, oestrogen, causing a small cyst to erupt each month and this eruption releases a watery fluid, known as liquor folliculi, propelling the ovum out of the ovary and towards the Fallopian tubes.

The Fallopian tube adjacent to whichever ovary has ovulated provides the route for the ovum into the uterus. Its fringe-like extremity draws in the released ovum and contractions in the muscular tube wall and hair-like cilia along its length helps move the ovum to the uterus.

To coincide with ovulation, the pituitary gland triggers the release of another hormone, LH, which stimulates the development of a temporary mass of tissue in the ovary follicle known as the corpus luteum. This secretes further hormones, progesterone and oestrogen, which stimulate the uterus to prepare for a possible pregnancy.

Fertilization takes place high in the Fallopian tube. Of the thousands of sperm that have swum up the vagina, only one penetrates the ovum's outer layer. It then sheds its tail and body while the head, which contains all the genetic material, moves to the ovum's nucleus. The nuclei of the sperm and ovum each contain 23 chromosomes, which together provide the genetic data required for life.

When the ovum is fertilized the work of the corpus luteum in producing progesterone will be taken over by the placenta within the uterus. If there is no fertilization, and so no need for the uterus to prepare for pregnancy,

ANCIENT BELIEFS

Not surprisingly, the ability to create new life has long been associated with powerful beliefs and rituals. Menstruation and giving birth have historically been marked by cleansing rituals and in some cultures women's reproductive organs have been endowed with a talismanic quality. In prehistoric societies, vulvas and pubic triangles were frequently drawn or inscribed on cave walls to symbolize a sacred place, a gateway to life. In Taoist cultures, the ovaries are thought to contain the life force that produces sexual energy.

Some traditions regarded the umbilical cord with reverence, not as a waste product to be discarded at birth. It was seen as a powerful link, reflecting the unity and protection of child and mother. Some Native American tribes wrapped the cord around a stone and laid it to dry in the sun, then stored it in a container, keeping a record of the date and time of birth. When the time came for the child to be taught to ride, the cord was braided into the pony's mane in the belief that the mother–child link would offer the child protection.

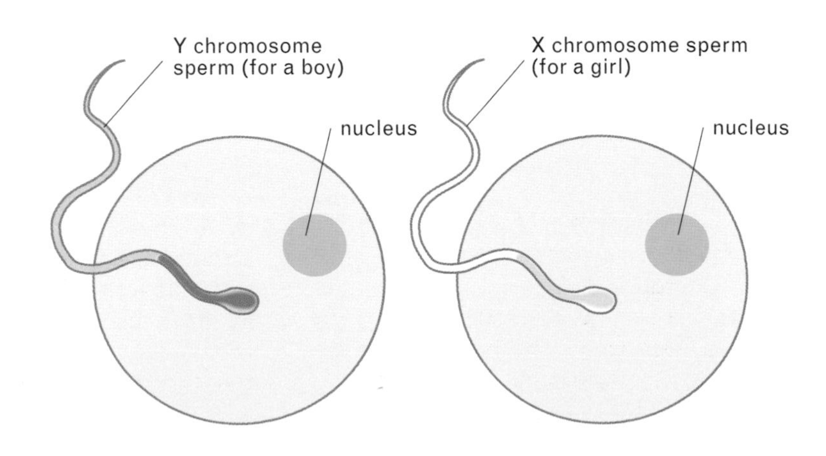

How sex is determined Each egg contains a single X sex chromosome, while each sperm contains either an X or a Y sex chromosome. If the fertilizing sperm contains a Y chromosome, the baby will be a boy; if it contains an X chromosome, the baby will be a girl.

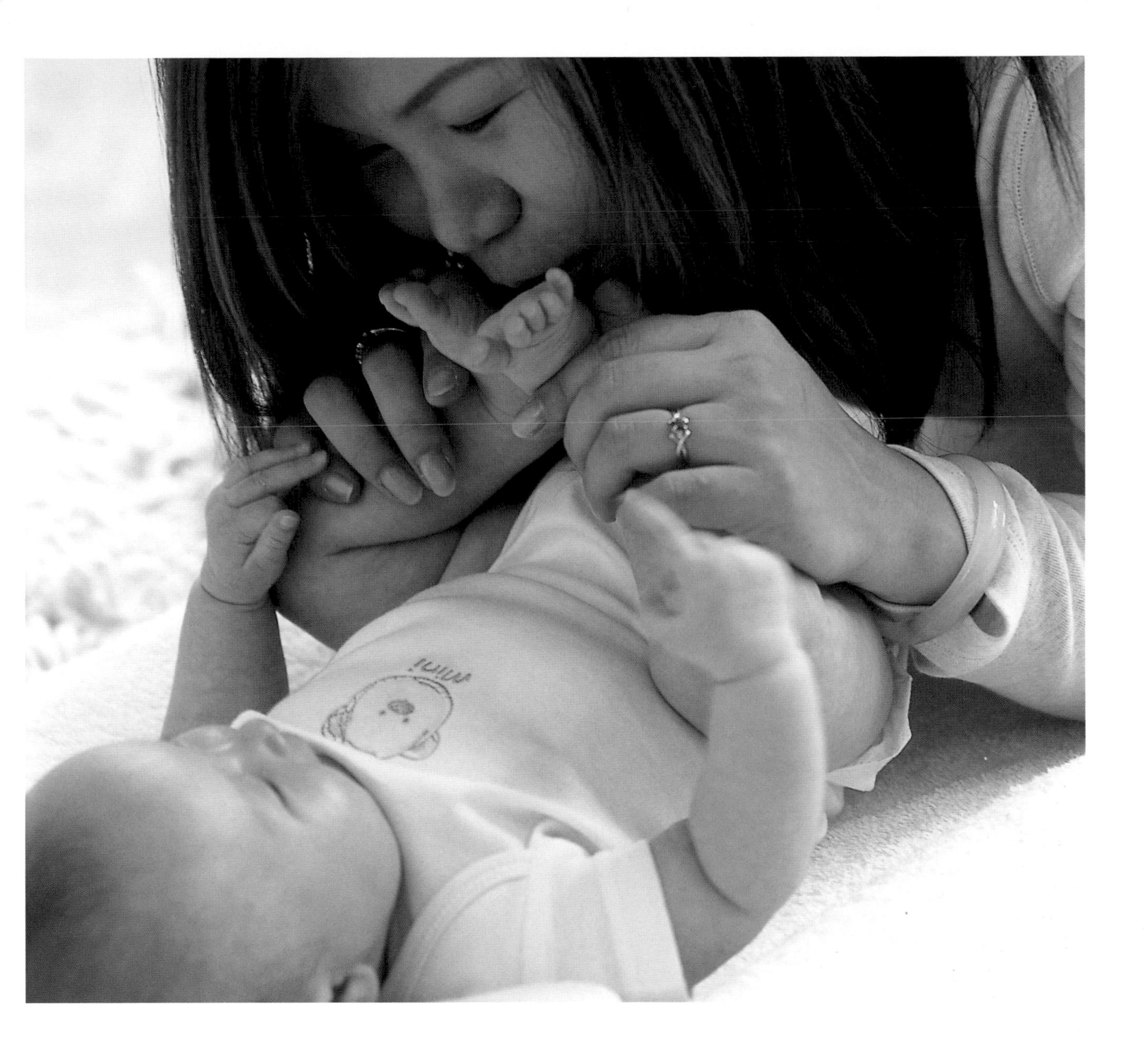

the corpus luteum will 'switch off' and die back. The thickened, blood-engorged lining that had been formed in the uterus is then shed as menstrual blood, about 14 days after ovulation.

The umbilical link This is one of the most powerful protective energies of the body, persisting undiminished after the actual physical connection has been severed.

The menopause

A baby girl is born with thousands of ova, only a few of which will ever become mature enough to develop into a fetus. When a woman runs out of her supply of ova her reproductive years cease and her menstrual cycles come to an end. This is the menopause. The passage into the post-menopausal years can involve uncomfortable symptoms, including hot flushes, migraine headaches and vaginal dryness, as the woman's body adapts to different hormonal levels (see the case study on helping menopausal symptoms on page 153).

The ovaries get smaller when the reproductive years are over, but they still produces hormones that help a woman's general health. For this reason, the ovaries should be respected and considered as valuable organs at every age.

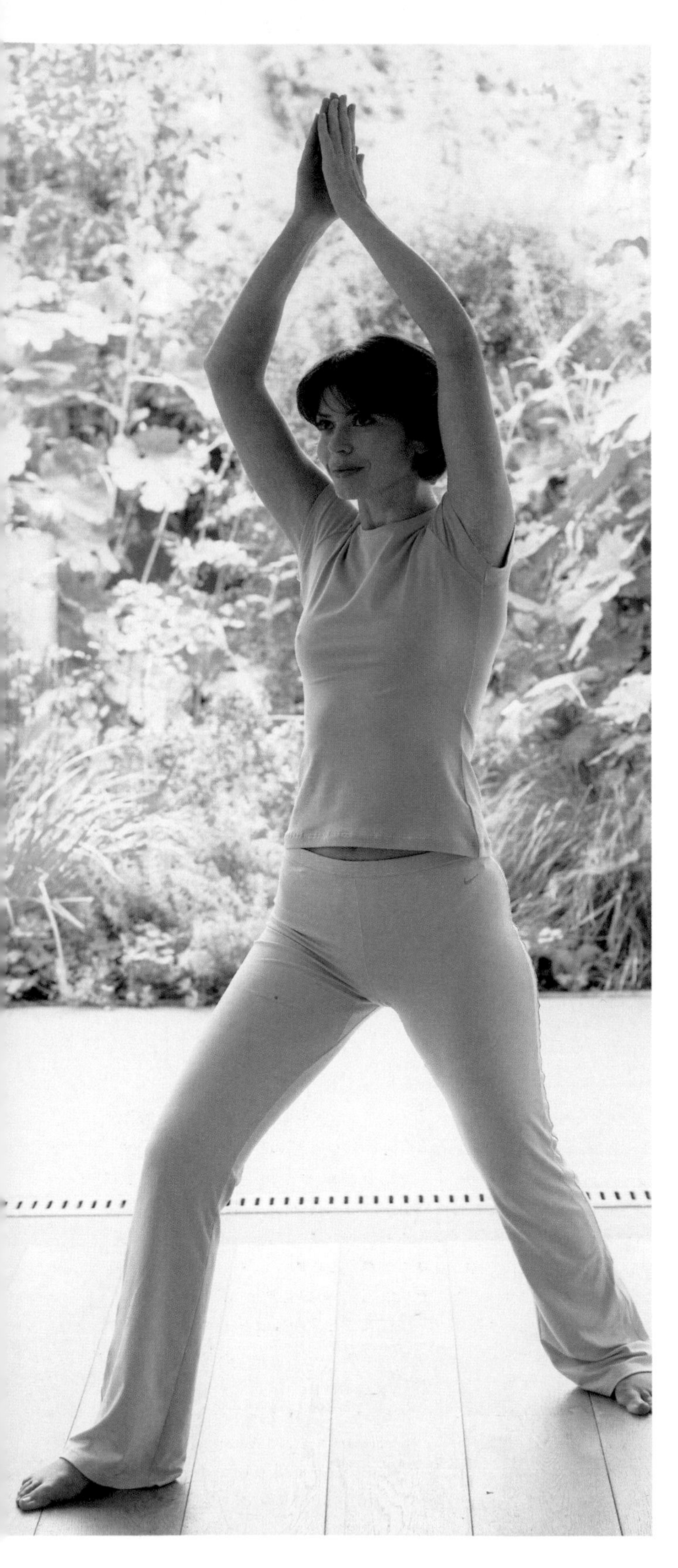

Female reproductive disorders helped by reflexology

It is not surprising that a system that is so dependent on a range of hormones all acting in perfect synchronization should show problems if the fine balancing act is disturbed in any way. Ovarian cysts and polycystic ovaries are usually due to a hormonal dysfunction. Many cysts erupt of their own accord and dissipate. However, some become very large and cause pressure on organs in the pelvic cavity, creating discomfort; these are then treated medicinally or surgically. Ovarian cancer, too, is unfortunately on the increase.

Stress can interrupt the regularity of the menstrual cycle and plays a major part in making conception more difficult. This stress can be of the psychological or physical kind. Athletes who drive their bodies too hard or women, particularly adolescent girls, who overdo the dieting or are anorexic, frequently find their periods stop. Worry can also affect the ovulation/menstrual cycle, which is ironic if the stress stems either from not conceiving or from the fear of becoming pregnant.

How reflexology can help

At the time of ovulation many women get ovulation pain. It is interesting to note that reflexology picks up the sensitivity in the ovary, as it does in any other part of the body that is inflamed, congested or tense. If ovulation is occurring on the right side you will find a sensitive reaction when you apply pressure on the right foot; and if ovulation occurs on the left side a sensitive reaction will be found on the left foot.

Many patients coming for reflexology treatments for ovarian cysts have found that within weeks the discomfort subsides and the cyst disappears, so it is well worth trying reflexology before you resort to other measures. Surgery should always be used as a last resort instead of a first choice.

When treating patients suffering from premenstrual symptoms, the aim will be to normalize the imbalance in the hormonal system that gives rise to the unpleasant side-effects such as irritability, breast pain, food cravings, headaches, and dull, congested pain in the uterus.

Reflexology sessions for infertility or an irregular menstrual cycle should be designed to relax the body. They can be of great benefit in restoring natural rhythm.

Period pain Sitting about will make the pain worse so try some gentle, stress-relieving exercise.

The male reproductive system
Male sperm production begins at puberty and continues until very late in life, although it starts to slow down in late middle age. Of the hundreds of million sperm in any one ejaculation, only a couple of thousand survive the journey into the uterus and on to the Fallopian tube.

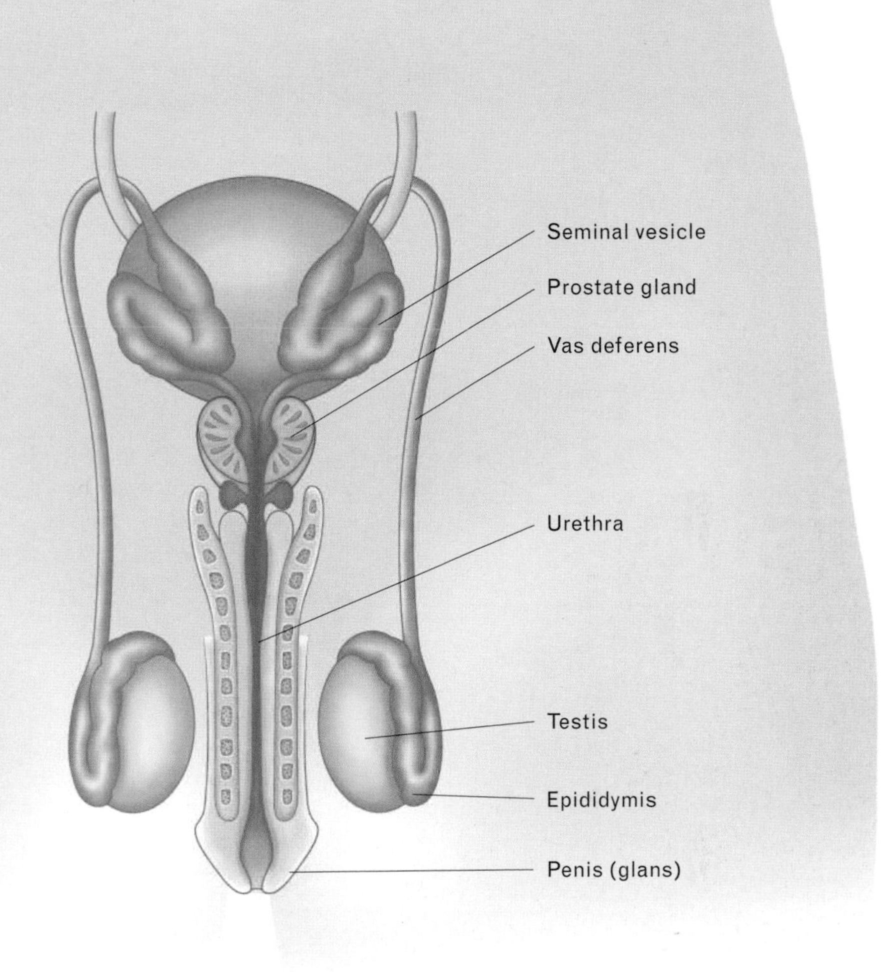

The male reproductive organs

The male reproductive system comprises two testes (testicles) that hang in the scrotal sac, the seminal vesicle, the prostate gland, various ducts and the penis.

Testes have two functions: the production of testosterone and of spermatozoa. Testosterone responds to the gonadotropic hormones from the pituitary gland at various stages in a boy's life (the first while still in the womb), but the best-known effect it has is the development of male secondary sexual characteristics: pubic and facial hair growth, increased aggressiveness, muscle bulk and deepening of the voice.

The tubules inside the testes produce large quantities of sperm every day, which pass into a series of communicating ducts. The first of these, the epididymis, is a coiled tube that empties into the vas deferens. This passes from the scrotum through the inguinal canal to the seminal vesicles, where mature sperm is stored. A duct from the seminal vesicles leads into the ejaculatory duct and then opens into the urethra. Unlike the female reproductive system, where the urinary and reproductive systems are completely separate, the penis has a dual function: the ejaculation of sperm as well as the excretion of urine from the bladder.

The prostate gland lies around the upper part of the urethra, at the base of the bladder, and its secretions help maintain sperm activity. An additional pair of glands, Cowper's, release a few drops of fluid that neutralize the acidity of the urethra and lubricate the urethra and penis.

Common disorders of the male reproductive system

Changes in the prostate gland are commonly found in men aged over 50, and because of the urethra's shared roles of urination and ejaculation, enlargement of the prostate has an effect on erection and sexual performance as well as on urination. Alterations in the prostate may be brought about by cancerous growth, but that is not necessarily the case; a deficiency of zinc in the diet also has this effect (see below).

Swollen testicles are another common complaint relating to the male reproductive system. Swellings may be due to a collection of fluid called a hydrocele. Most swellings are painless but they should be checked out by a doctor. Testicular trauma may also be caused by a sports injury. Even mild injuries can lead to severe pain, bruising or swelling.

Another condition is varicocele. This is a varicose (abnormally swollen) vein in the network of veins that runs from the testicles. It occurs quite frequently in boys going through puberty and can lead to a decrease in sperm production.

Zinc deficiency

Incidents of prostate enlargement are increasing and this is often due to a lack of the mineral zinc in the diet. Zinc used to be found in abundance in our soil and as a result we had sufficient in our diets for the needs of reproduction in both men and women. However, the use of chemicals in modern farming methods has depleted the soil of minerals, including zinc. At the same time, the level of minerals in our diet has been reduced because foods are being picked before they are ripe to enable them to be transported long distances.

The male reproductive system relies on an adequate zinc intake to produce sperm and to create sufficient fluid in the prostate for the sperm to reach the ovum. If the system is deficient in zinc, the prostate becomes enlarged. This leads to pain and difficulties in passing urine and often increased frequency in urination, particularly at night. To counteract this, it is advisable for men (and women) to take a daily allowance of zinc in tablet form.

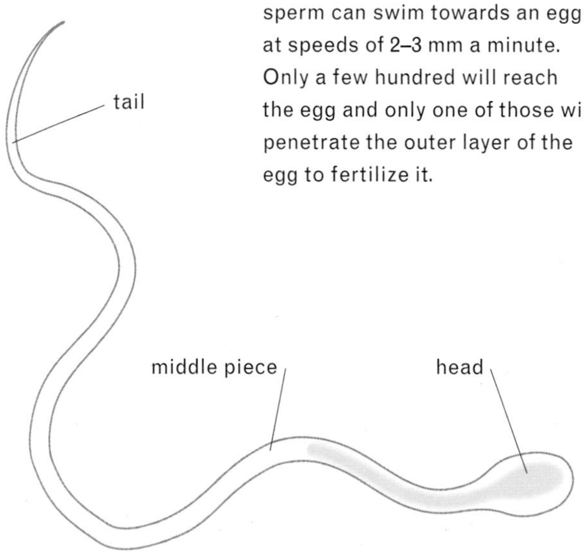

Anatomy of a sperm Healthy sperm can swim towards an egg at speeds of 2–3 mm a minute. Only a few hundred will reach the egg and only one of those will penetrate the outer layer of the egg to fertilize it.

tail

middle piece

head

How reflexology can help

One patient, Paul, suffered from a hernia just a few months after having extensive bowel surgery. The incisions made through the low abdominal walls were thought to be the cause of the hernia. Reflexology helped relieve his pain and swelling, until he was able to have the hernia repaired. He continued his reflexology treatments after the surgery and was sure that it had eased the discomfort and swelling following the operation.

Reflexology can be beneficial in treating many of the male reproductive conditions. Many men consult their doctor with problems relating to impotence. The usual procedure would be to eliminate various possible causes such as diabetes, forms of neurological disease or reactions to medication such as sleeping tables, anti-depressants or drugs for high pressure. Frequently, however, the cause is the stress that is so often a part of modern living. Regular reflexology treatments can come to the rescue in reducing stress and helping to counteract its effects on the body.

Reflexology can also assist with sports injuries such as testicular trauma. These usually heal well with a few treatment sessions.

Working the associated reflex points

The health of the reproductive system is always important, not just in reproductive years. Reflecting fundamental similarities, the reflex points are the same for both sexes, running across the dorsal side of the foot like an ankle strap.

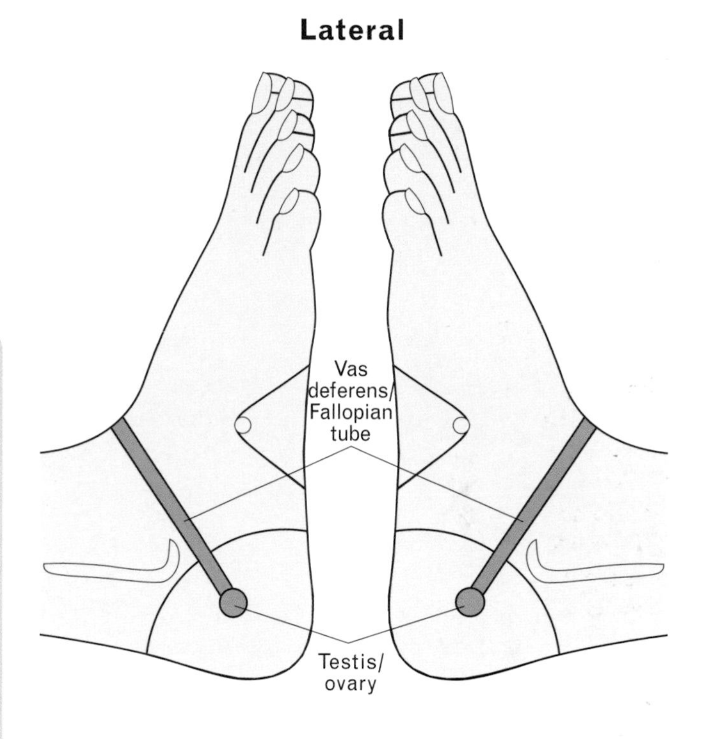

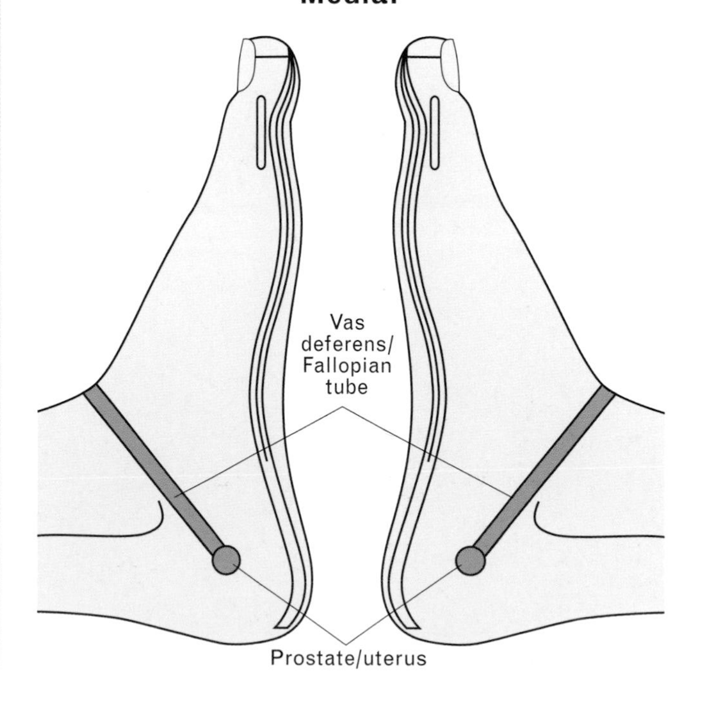

CASE STUDY
MENOPAUSAL SYMPTOMS

CLIENT PROFILE

Gloria had been fit and active all her life and at 52 did not anticipate the symptoms she would suffer when her periods became irregular and eventually ceased. From having lots of energy she became very listless. She suffered from night sweats, which disturbed her sleep, and had a dry, sore vagina, which made intercourse impossible. She was not keen to take hormone replacement therapy and wanted to try reflexology.

REGULARITY OF REFLEXOLOGY TREATMENTS

Weekly for eight weeks and then a monthly appointment for as long as she felt that the treatment was of benefit.

REFLEXES

Main reflexes	Assistance
Entire endocrine system: pituitary, hypothalamus, thyroid, adrenals	To stimulate endocrine system
Reproductive system, especially uterus	To help this system

TREATMENT OUTCOMES

After her first appointment, Gloria's night sweats were worse than ever. (Sometimes reflexology makes symptoms a little worse before they start to get much better, see page 61.) After her second appointment, her night sweats were a little better and she could sleep for longer periods. Her depression lifted and energy improved, and after eight sessions her quality of life was much better. Gloria decided to have a monthly appointment on a regular basis in order to maintain her improved health.

The uterus/prostate area

Right foot – medial
Top support

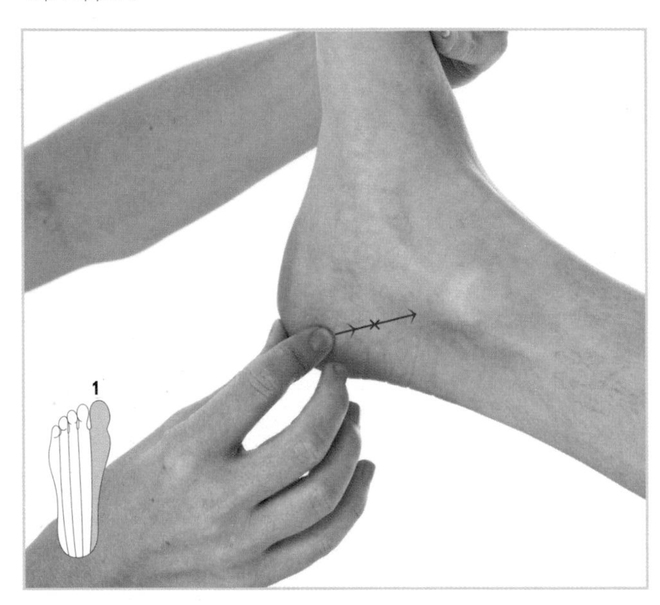

Support the right foot with your left hand and, using the right index finger, work in a straight line over the uterus/ prostate area as marked. Repeat two or three times.

The ovary/testis

Right foot – lateral
Top support

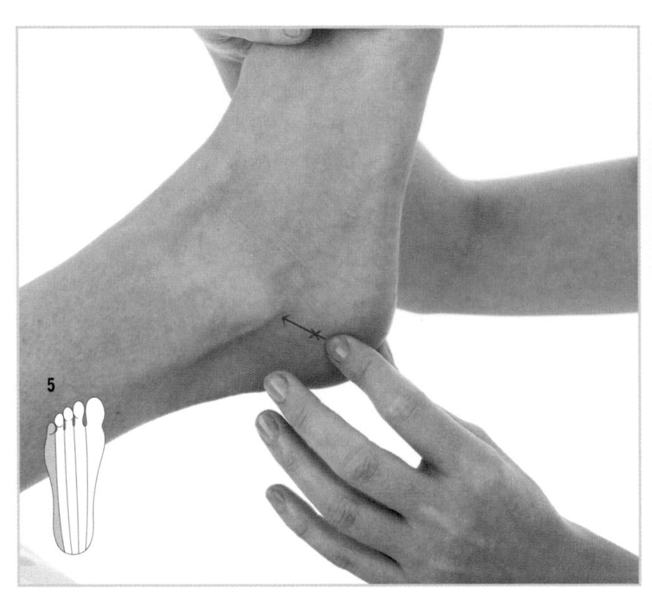

Support the right foot with your right hand and, using the left index finger, work in a straight line over the ovary/ testis area (marked with a cross) two or three times.

Fallopian tubes/vas deferens

Right foot – dorsal
Heel support

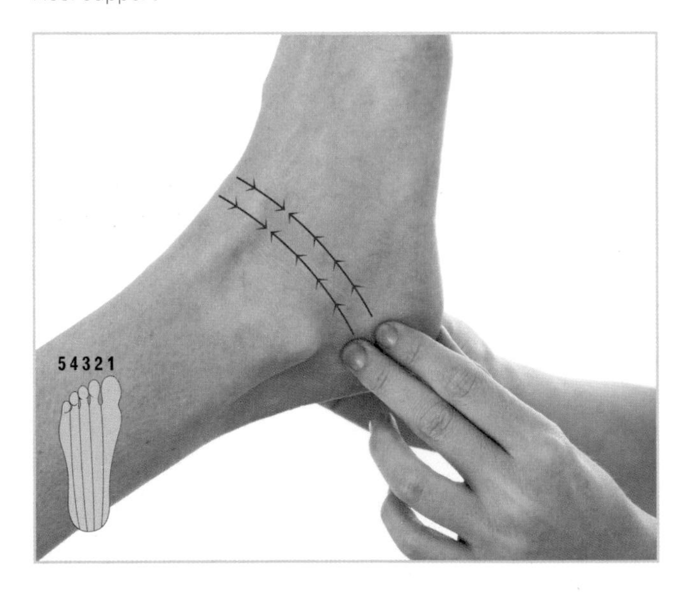

Support the plantar side of the right foot and, pressing in for support with both thumbs, work the Fallopian tubes/vas deferens area around the front of the foot with the index and third finger together. Repeat two or three times.

The uterus/prostate

Left foot – medial
Top support

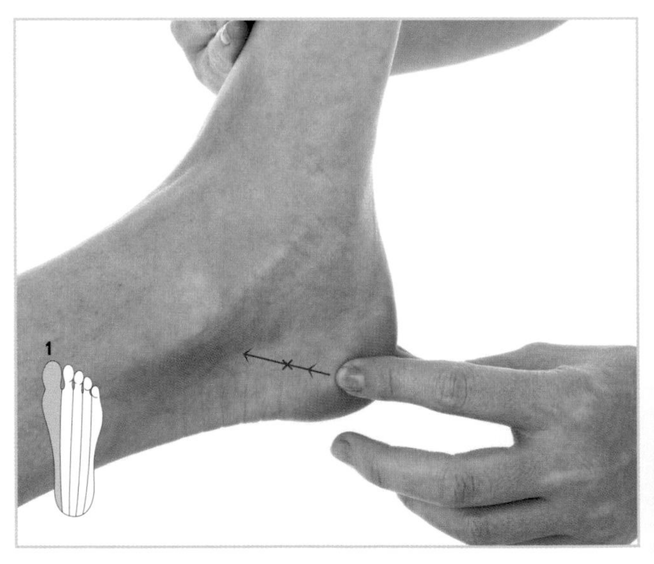

Support the left foot with your right hand and, using the left index finger, work the uterus/prostate area (marked with a cross) in a straight line. Repeat two or three times.

The ovary/testis

Left foot – lateral
Top support

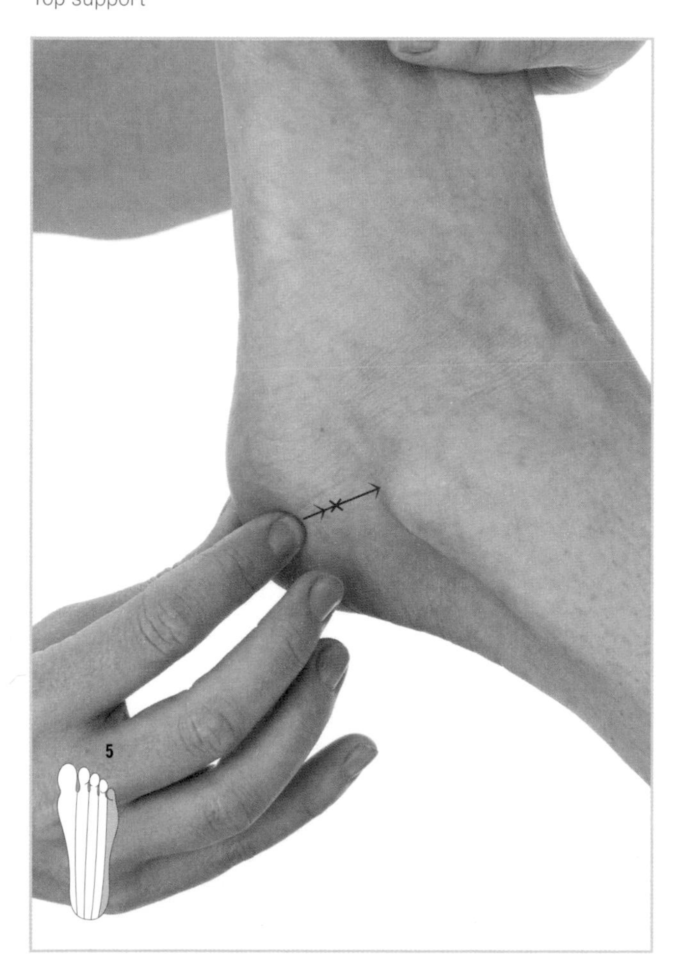

Support the left foot with your left hand and, using the right index finger, work the ovary/testis area (marked with a cross) in a straight line two or three times.

Fallopian tubes/vas deferens

Left foot – dorsal
Heel support

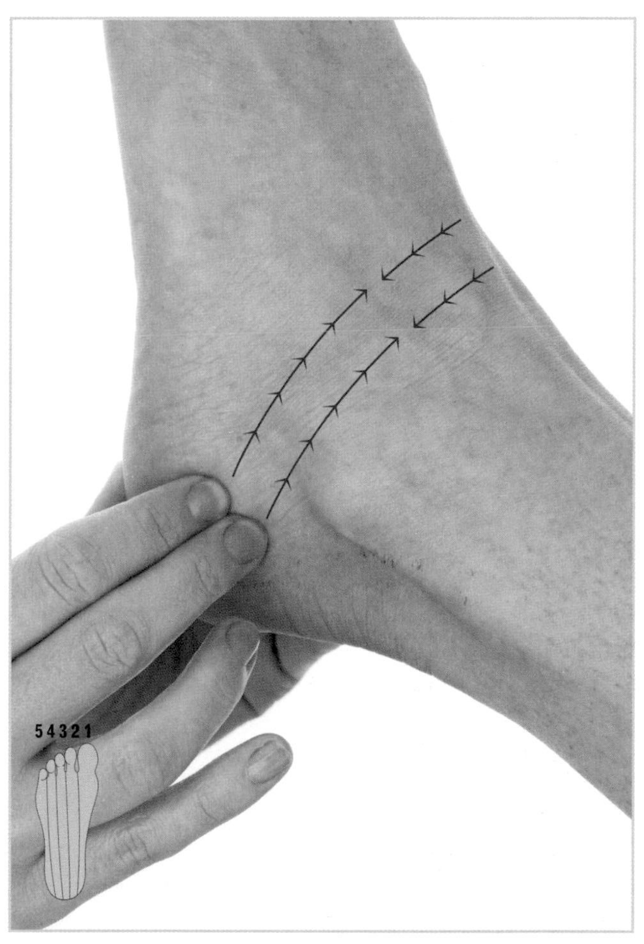

Support the plantar side of the foot and, pressing in for support with both thumbs, work the Fallopian tube/vas deferens area around the front of the foot with the index and third finger together. Repeat two or three times.

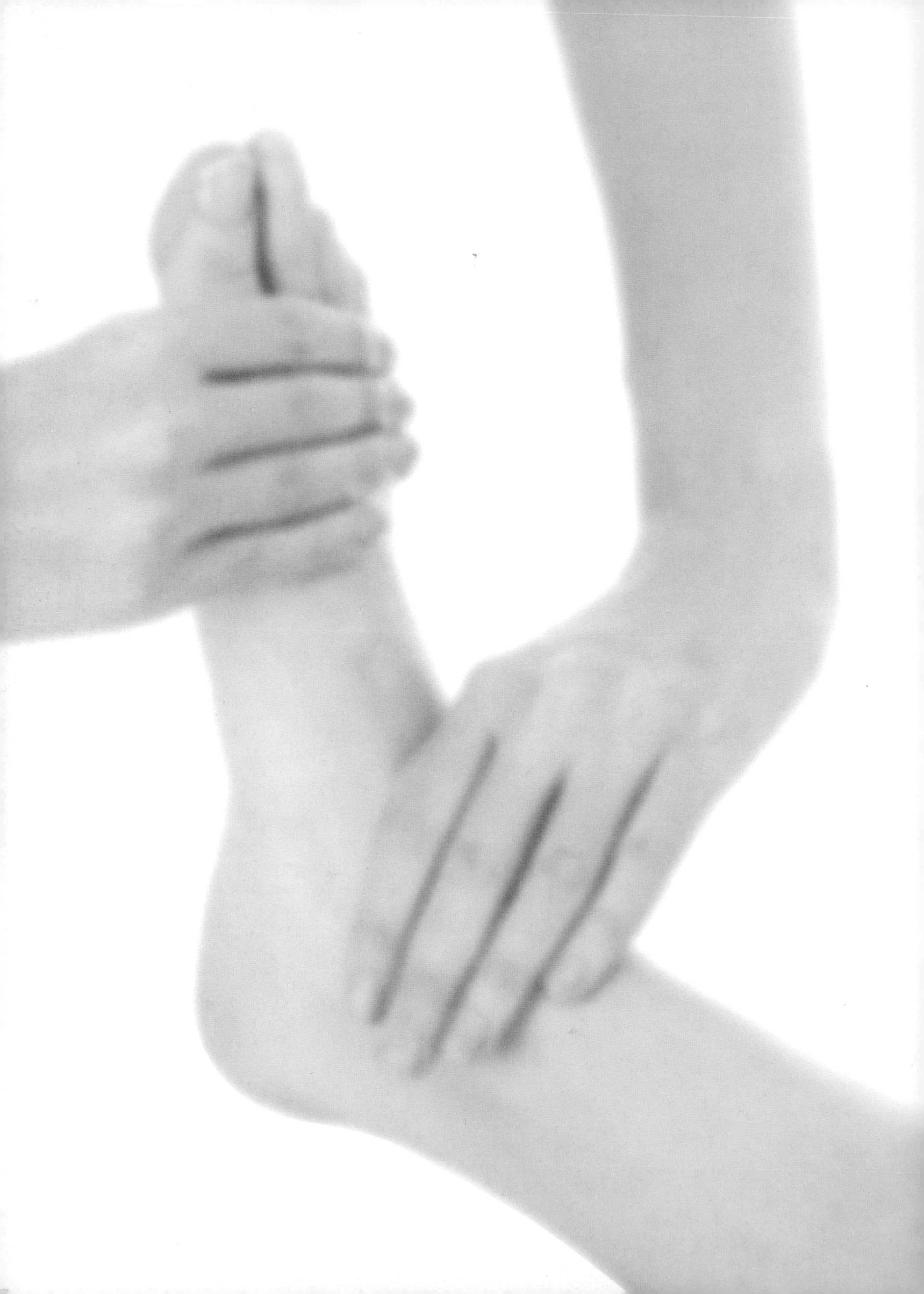

The whole routine

When treating a patient you should run through the whole routine in the order outlined in this chapter, so that you can be sure of picking up any areas of sensitivity and treating every body system. Take care when you are working close to reflexes that relate to organs or systems with which the patient has problems.

Preliminary relaxation exercises

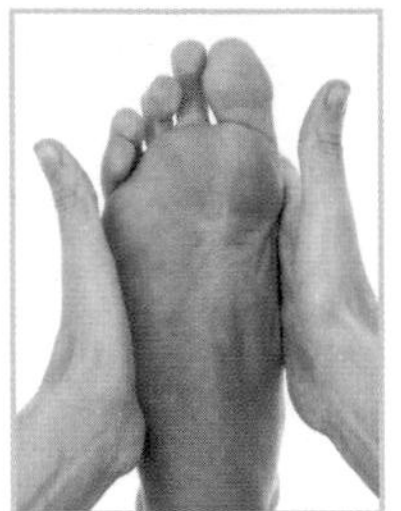
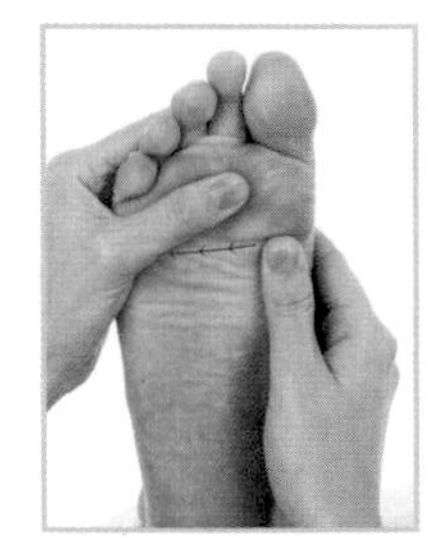
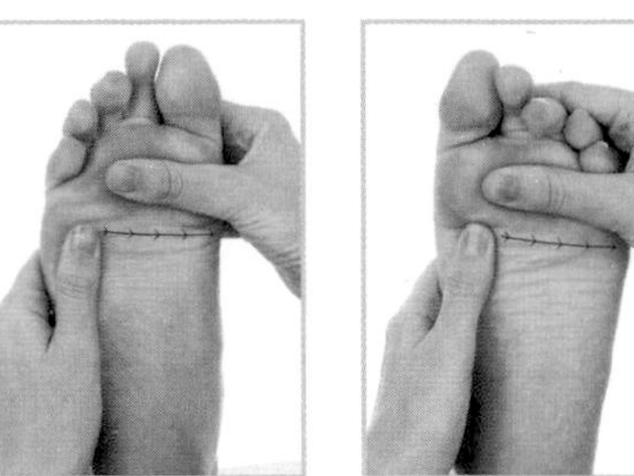
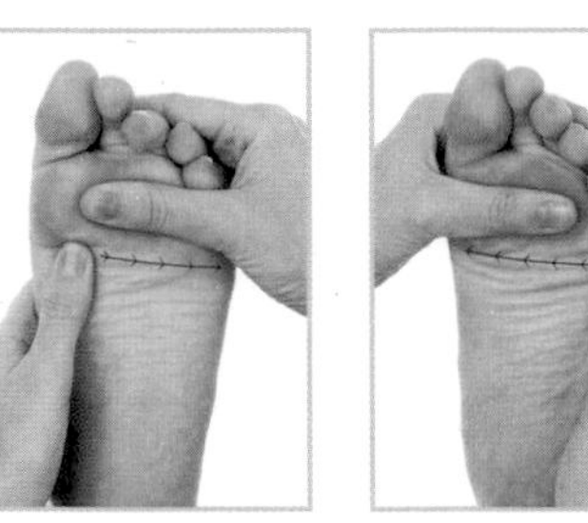

1 Start with the Side-to-side relaxation exercise on the right foot. Then repeat this on the left foot. See page 54.

2 Now use the Diaphragm relaxation exercise. First work on the right foot.

3 Then work the left foot. This helps to slow the patient's respiratory rate. See page 55.

The right foot

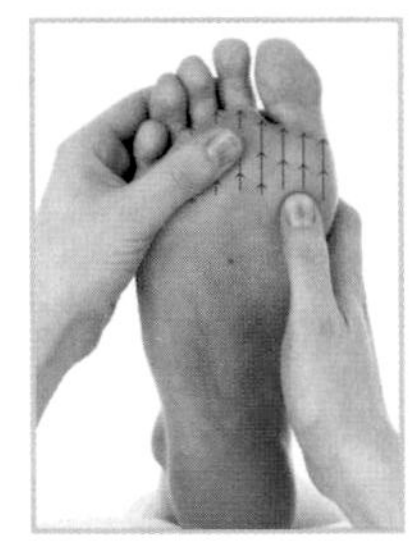
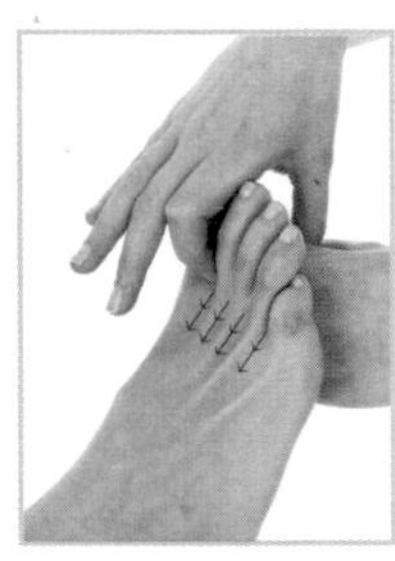
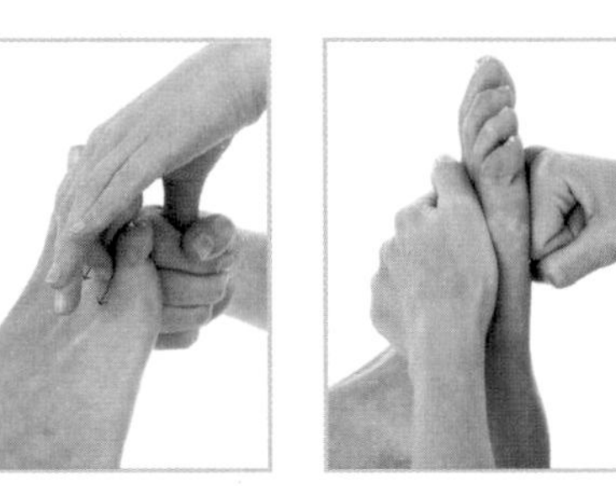

1 Work up the lung area on the plantar side (remember to work from medial to lateral then lateral to medial). See page 86.

2 Work down the lung/breast area on the dorsal side. See page 86.

3 Use the Metatarsal kneading relaxation exercise. See page 56.

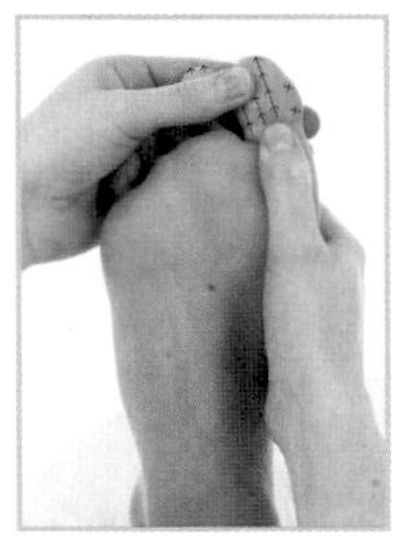
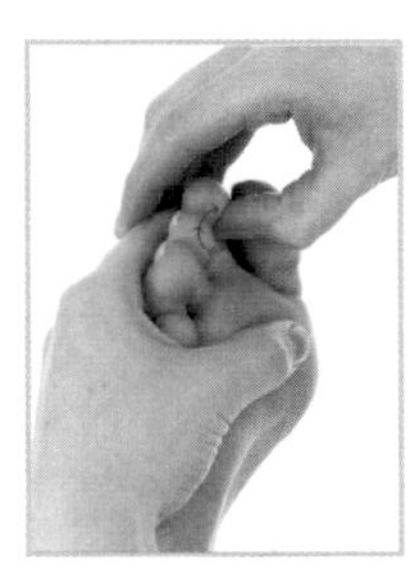
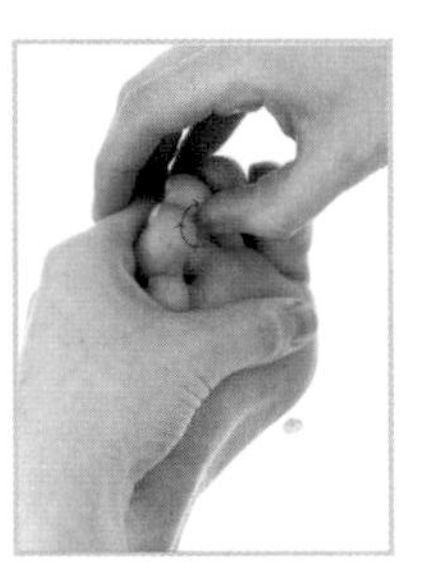
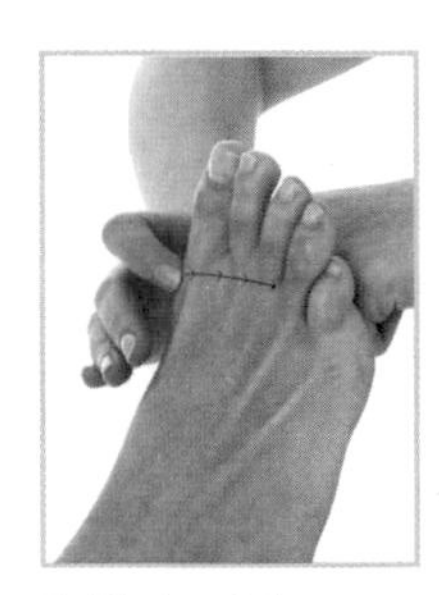

4 Work up all the toe areas. These include the sinus areas as well as the pituitary gland, which is on the medial side of the big toe. See pages 105 and 123.

5 Work out the eye and ear using the rotating method. See page 124.

6 Work out the neck/thyroid (plantar side). See page 105.

7 Work out the neck/thyroid (dorsal side). See page 105.

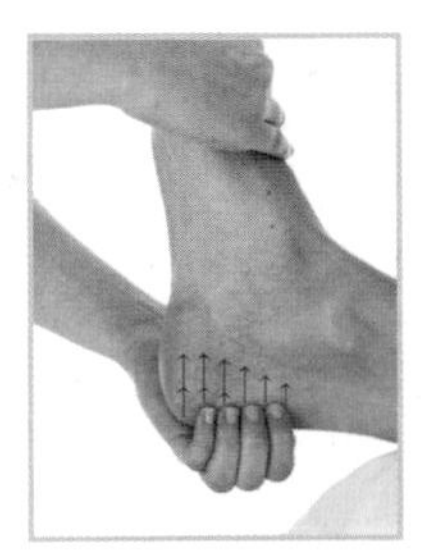
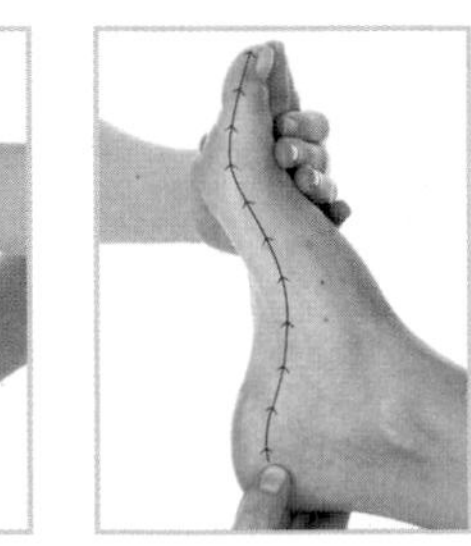
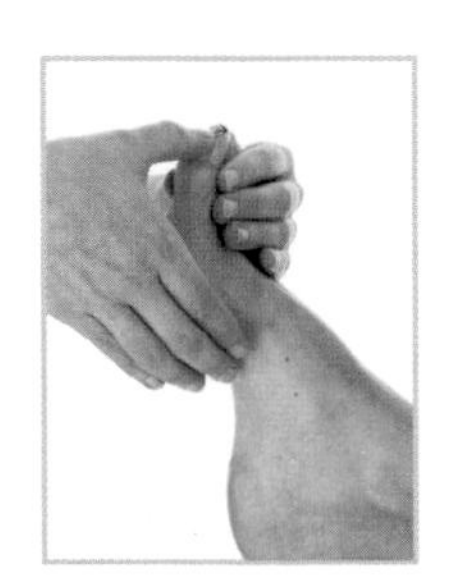

8 Work out the coccyx, pelvis and hip. See page 134.

9 Work up the spine over the brain (which simultaneously works the central nervous system. See page 115.

10 Work the neck side. See page 135.

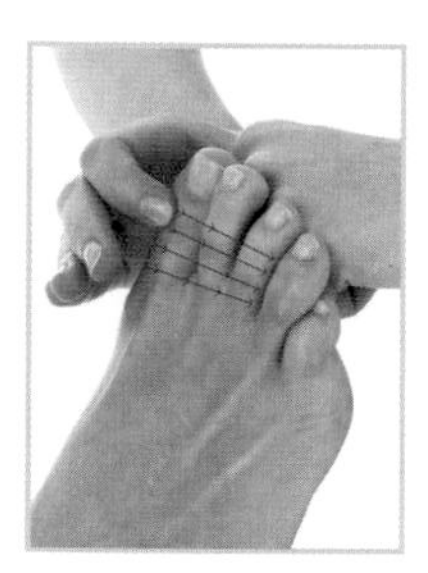

11 Work out the front of the face. See page 125.

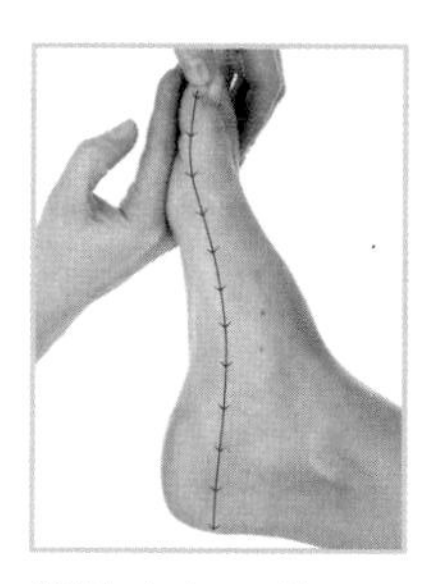

12 Work down the spine. See page 115.

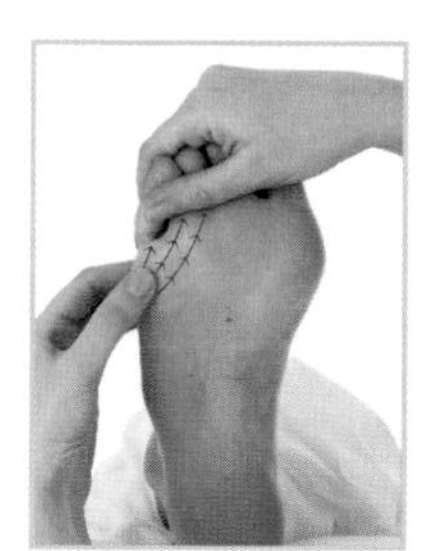

13 Work out the shoulder area. See page 135.

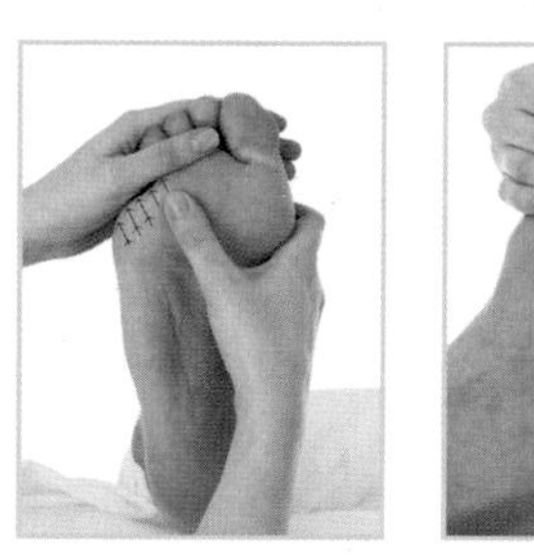

14 Work out the knee/elbow area. See page 136.

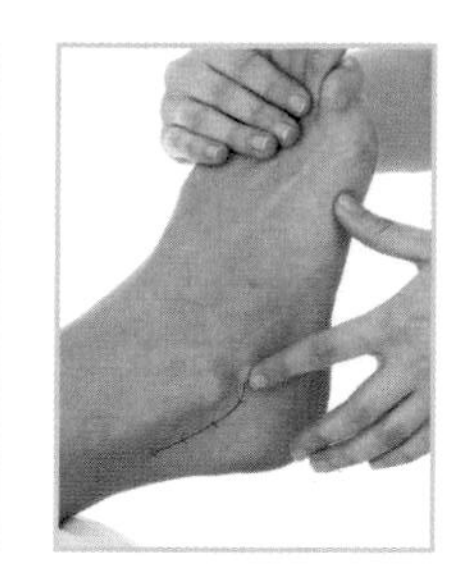

15 Work out the primary sciatic area. See page 136.

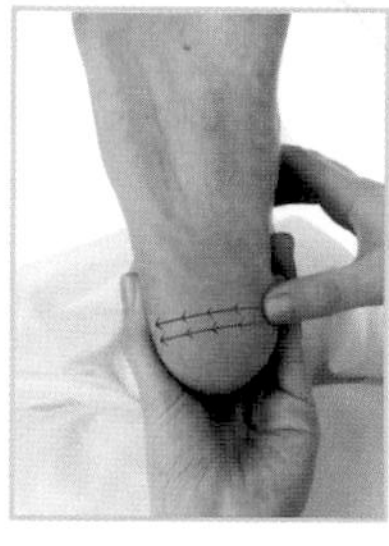

16 Work out the secondary sciatic area. See page 136.

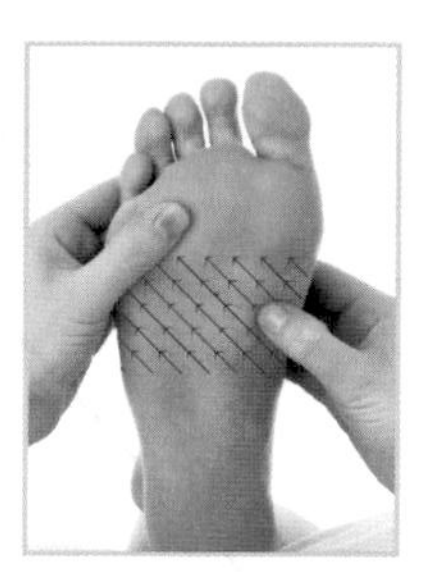

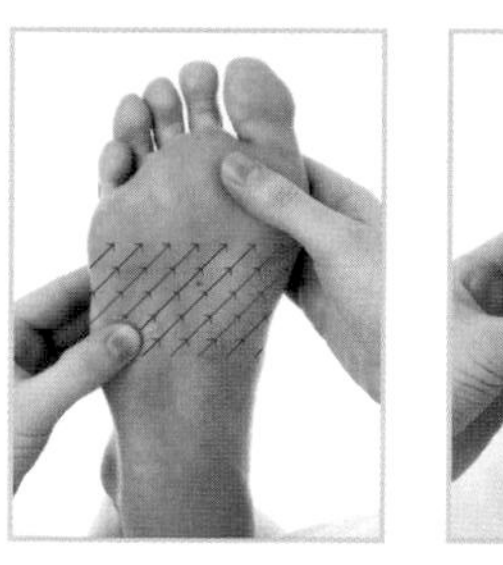

17 Work out the liver area. See page 79.

18 Use the hooking-out technique on the ileocecal valve. See page 80.

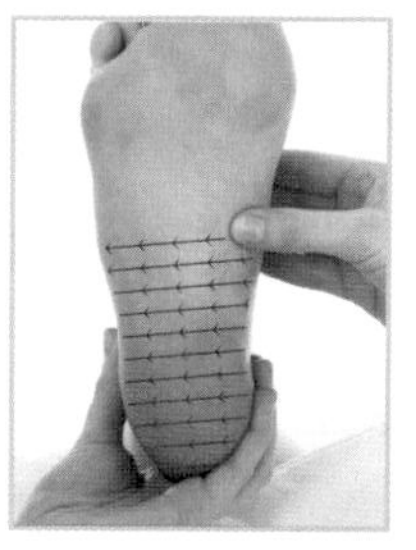

19 Work out the entire intestinal area to the base of the heel. (This includes the buttock and back of the pelvic area.) See page 80.

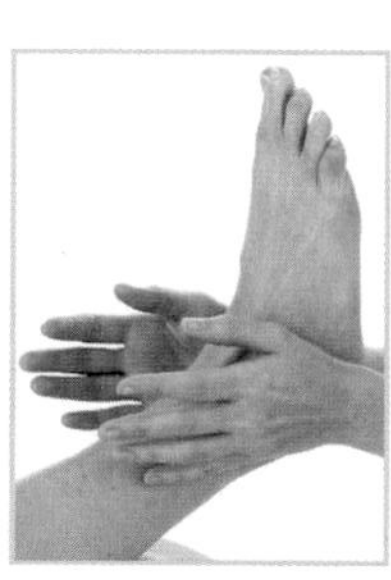

20 Use the Ankle-freeing relaxation exercise. See page 57.

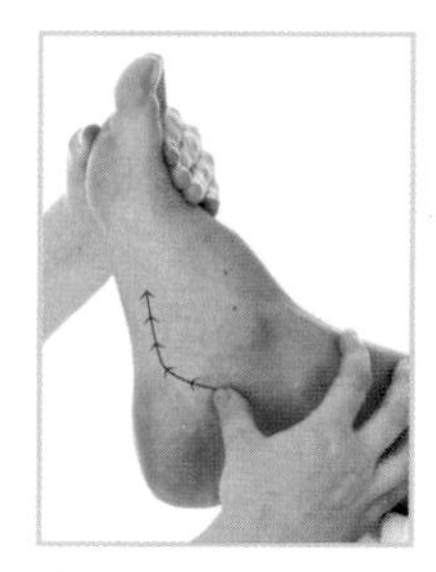

21 Work out the bladder, ureter tube and kidney. See page 145.

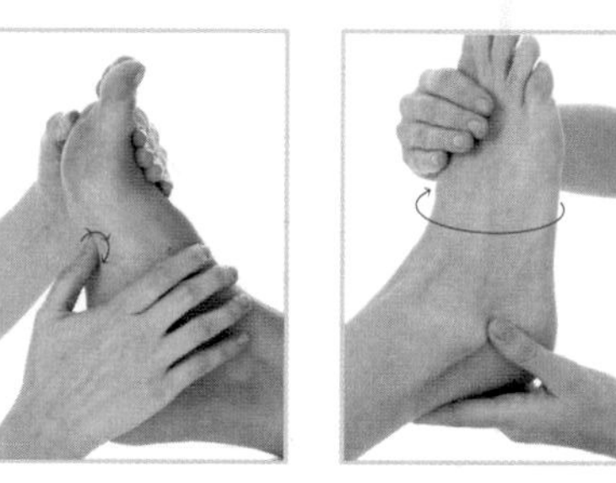

22 Use both the Undergrip and Overgrip relaxation exercises. See page 57 and 58.

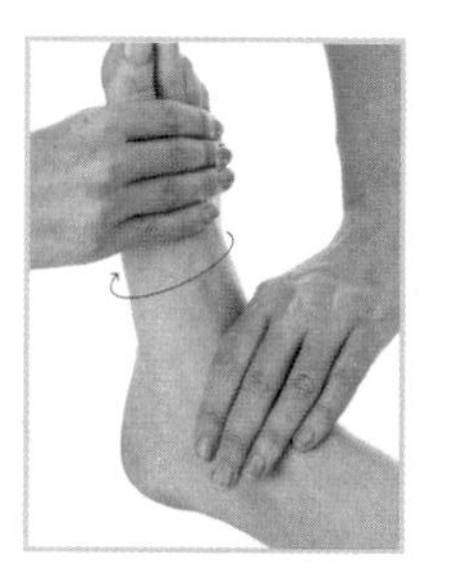

23 Work out the area of the uterus/prostate. See page 154.

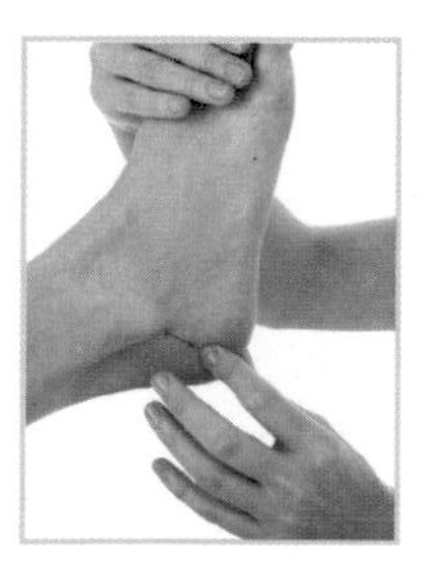

24 Work out the ovary/testis. See page 154.

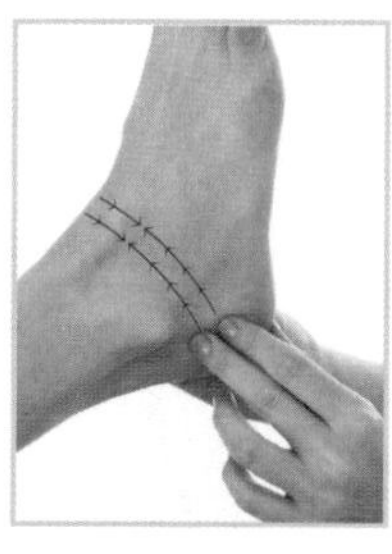

25 Work the Fallopian tube/vas deferens. See page 154.

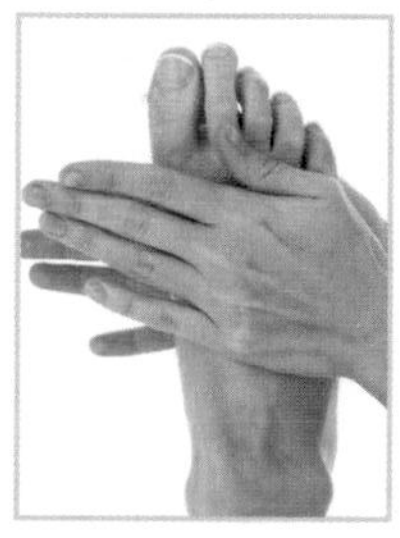

26 Use the Foot-moulding relaxation exercise. See page 59.

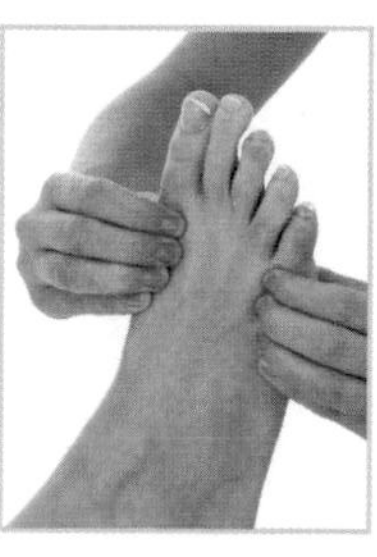

27 Use the Rib cage relaxation exercise. See page 60.

At this stage, highlight the sensitivities you have found on the right foot on your patient's treatment record card (see page 47), using a red pen. This card then acts almost like an x-ray, showing how internal congestions, inflammations and irritations reflect as sensitivities in the reflexes in the feet.

The left foot

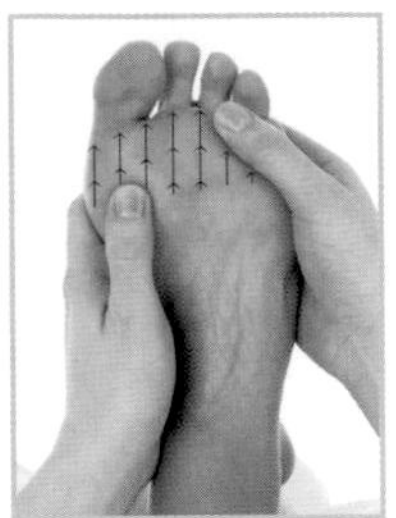

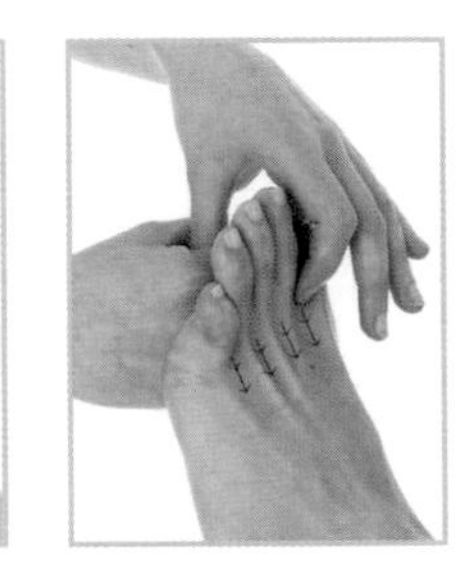

1 Work up the lung area on the plantar side. See page 87.

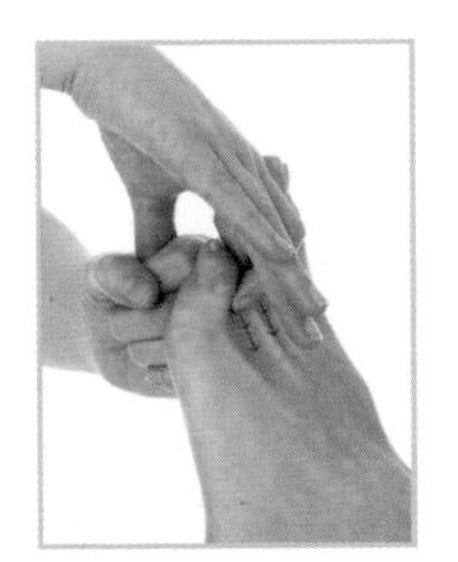

2 Work down the lung/breast area on the dorsal side. See page 87.

3 Work out the heart area. See page 93.

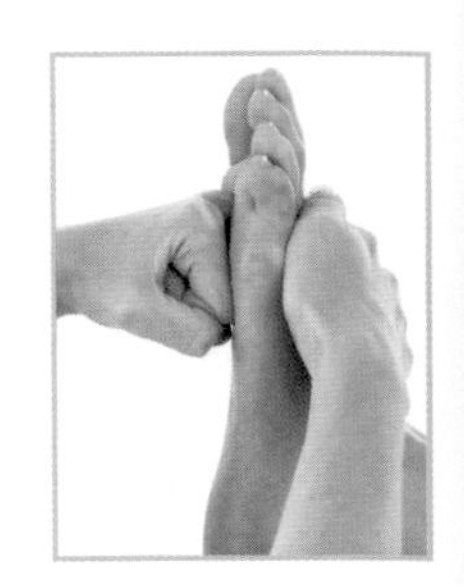

4 Use the Metatarsal kneading relaxation exercise. See page 56.

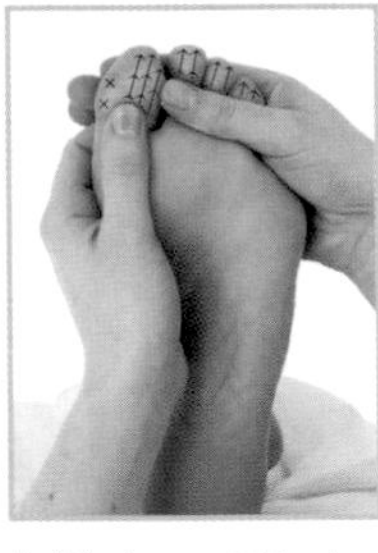

5 Work up all the toe areas. These include the sinus areas as well as the pituitary gland, which is on the medial side of the big toe. See pages 106 and 124.

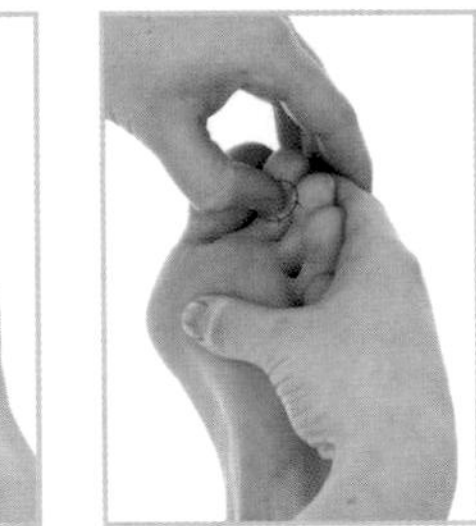

6 Work out the eye and ear using the rotation technique. See page 125.

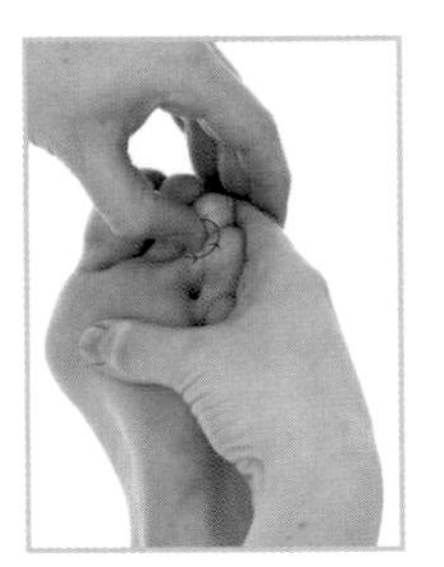

7 Work the neck/ thyroid (plantar side first). See page 106.

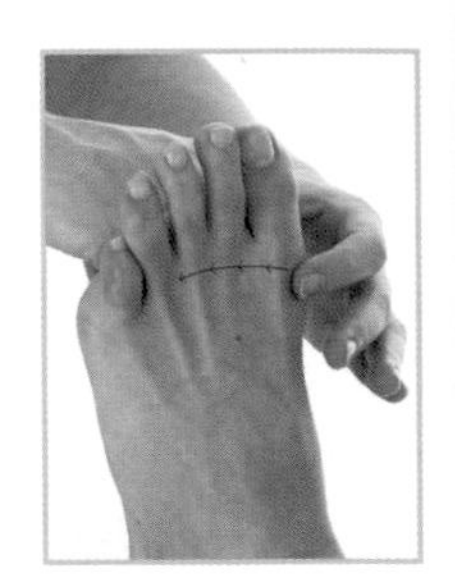

8 Work out the neck/thyroid (dorsal side). See page 106.

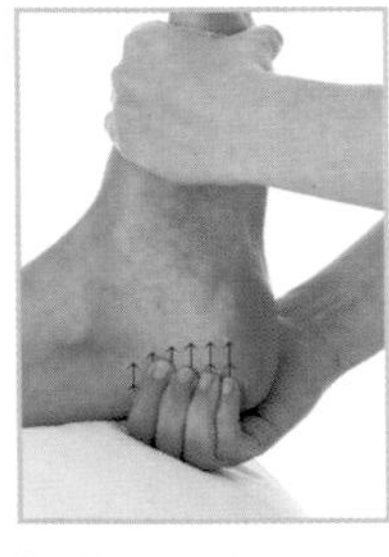

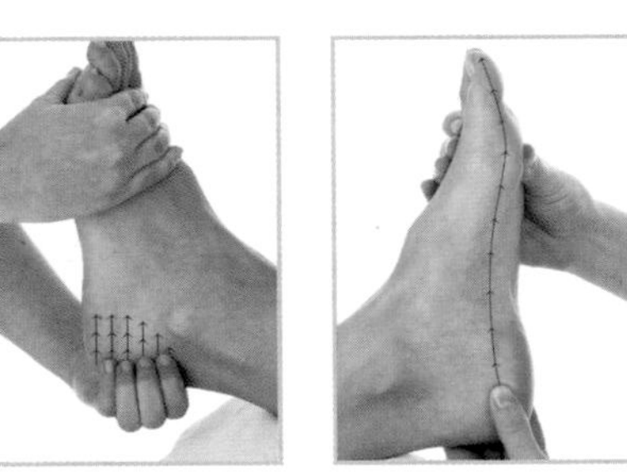

9 Work on the coccyx, then pelvis and hip. See page 137.

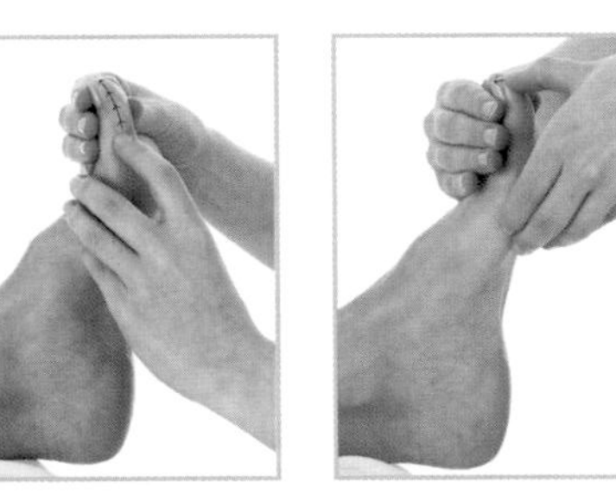

10 Work up the spine over the brain. See pages 116–117.

11 Work out the side of the neck. See page 138.

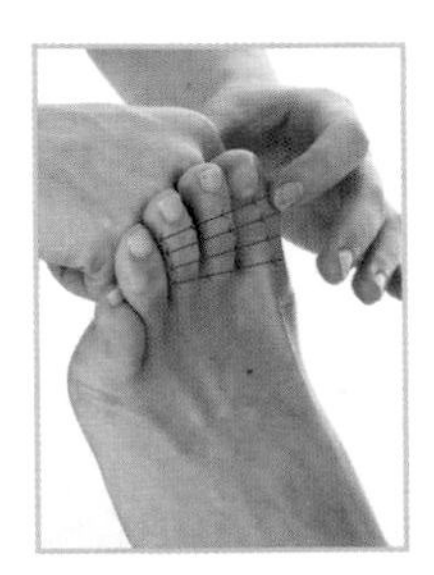

12 Work the front of the face. See page 125.

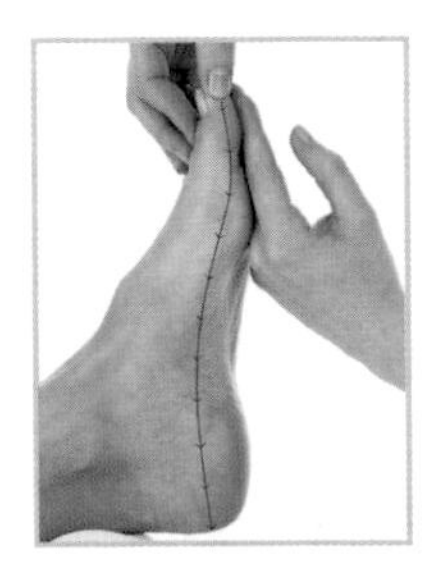

13 Work down the spine. See page 117.

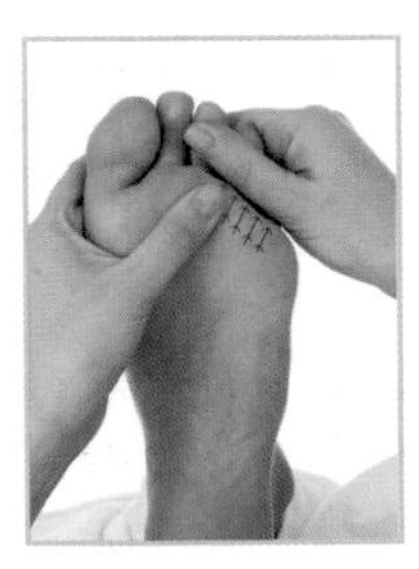

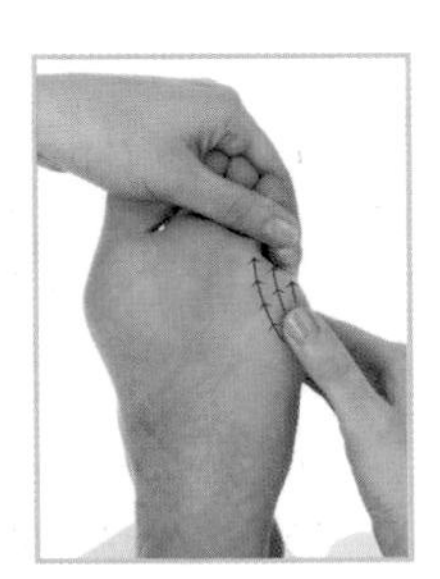

14 Work out the shoulder area. See page 138.

15 Work out the knee/elbow area. See page 139.

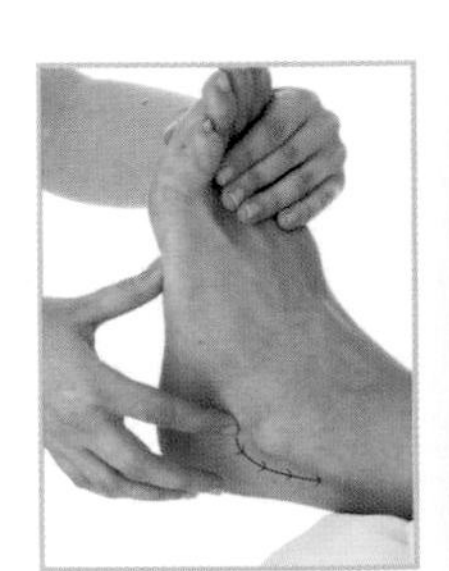

16 Work out the primary sciatic area. See page 139.

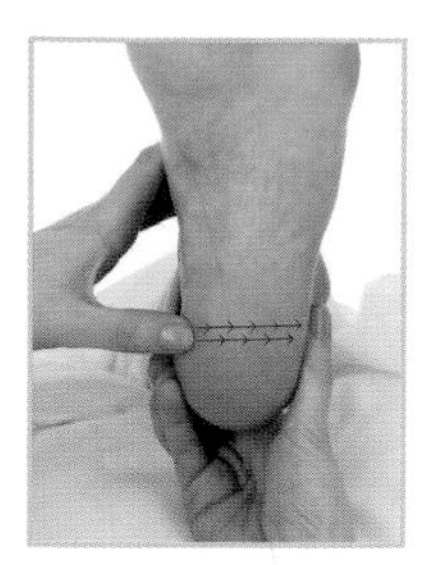

17 Work out the secondary sciatic area. See page 139.

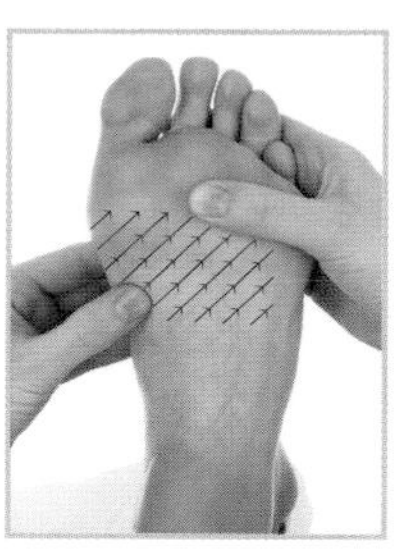

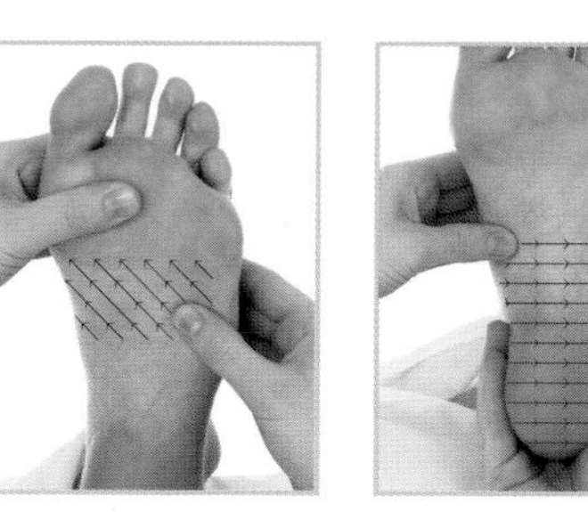

18 Work out the stomach, pancreas and spleen. See page 79.

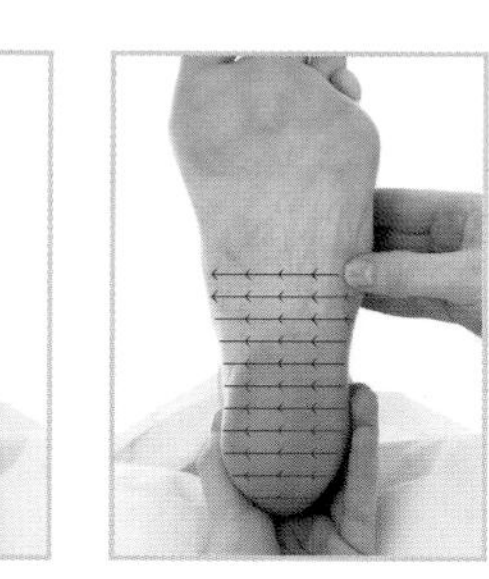

19 Work out the transverse and descending colon. See page 81.

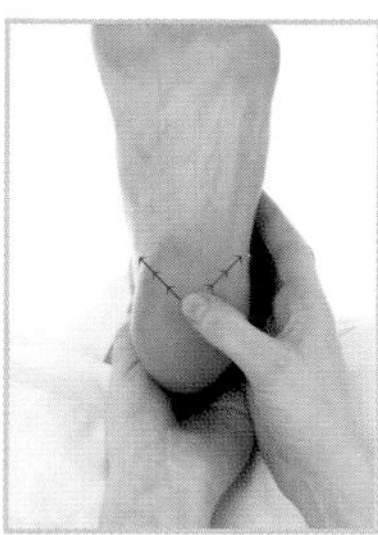

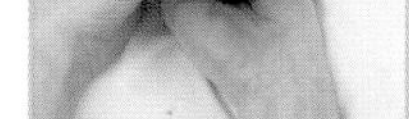

20 Work out the sigmoid colon. See page 81.

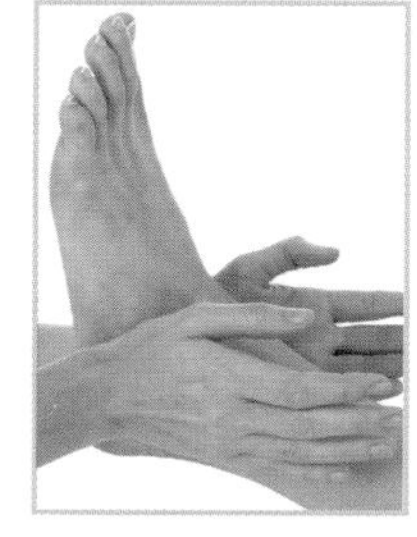

21 Use the Ankle-freeing relaxation. See page 57.

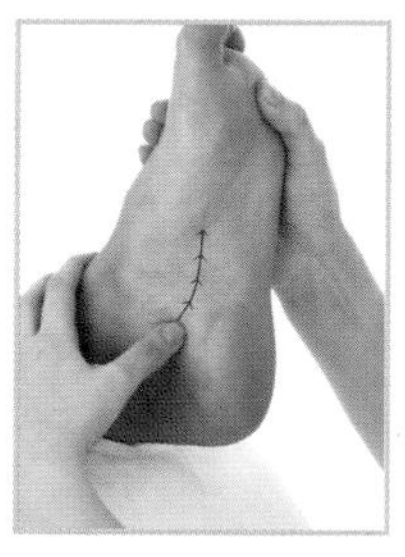

22 Work out the bladder, ureter tube and kidney. See page 145.

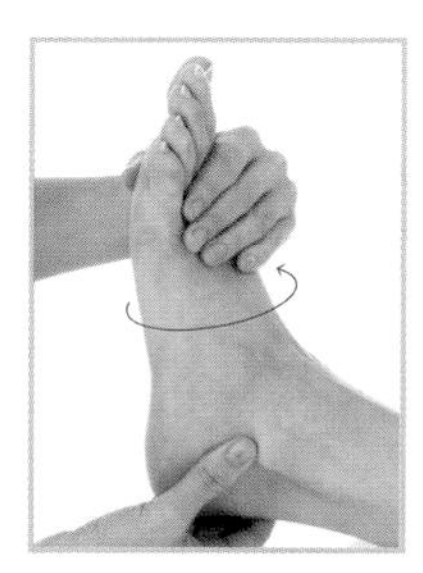

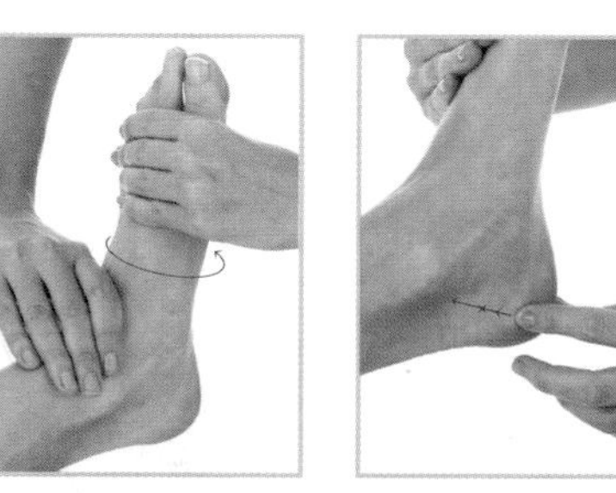

23 Use both the Undergrip and Overgrip relaxation exercises. See page 58.

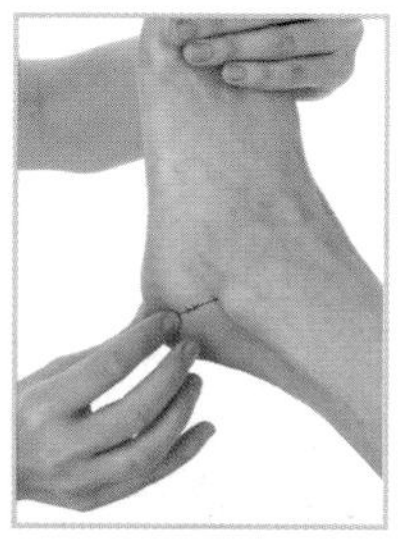

24 Work the area of the uterus/prostate. See page 154.

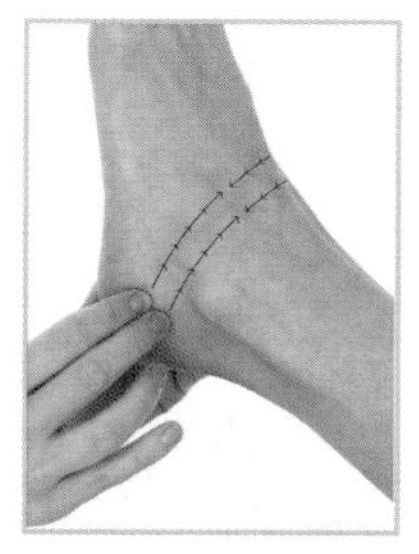

25 Work out the area of the ovary/testis. See page 155.

26 Work out the Fallopian tube/ vas deferens. See page 155.

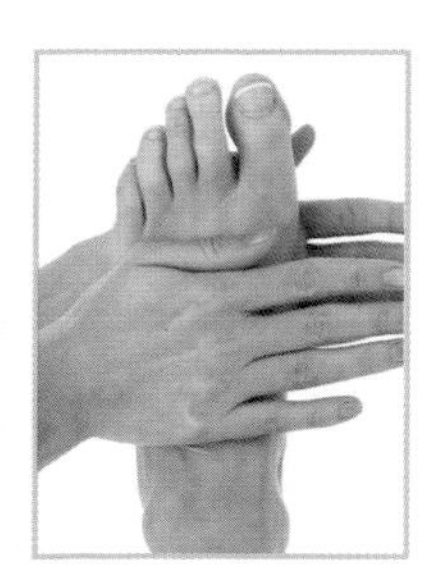

27 Use the Foot-moulding relaxation exercise. See page 59.

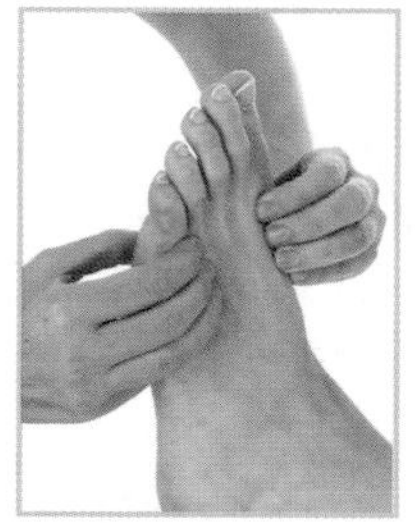

28 Use the Rib cage relaxation exercise. See page 60.

Record the sensitivities found on the left foot. Then return to the right foot and work only the sensitivities in the right foot, two or three times. Repeat the same procedure on the left foot. You should find that the sensitivities have already decreased, which means that you have effected a good treatment session.

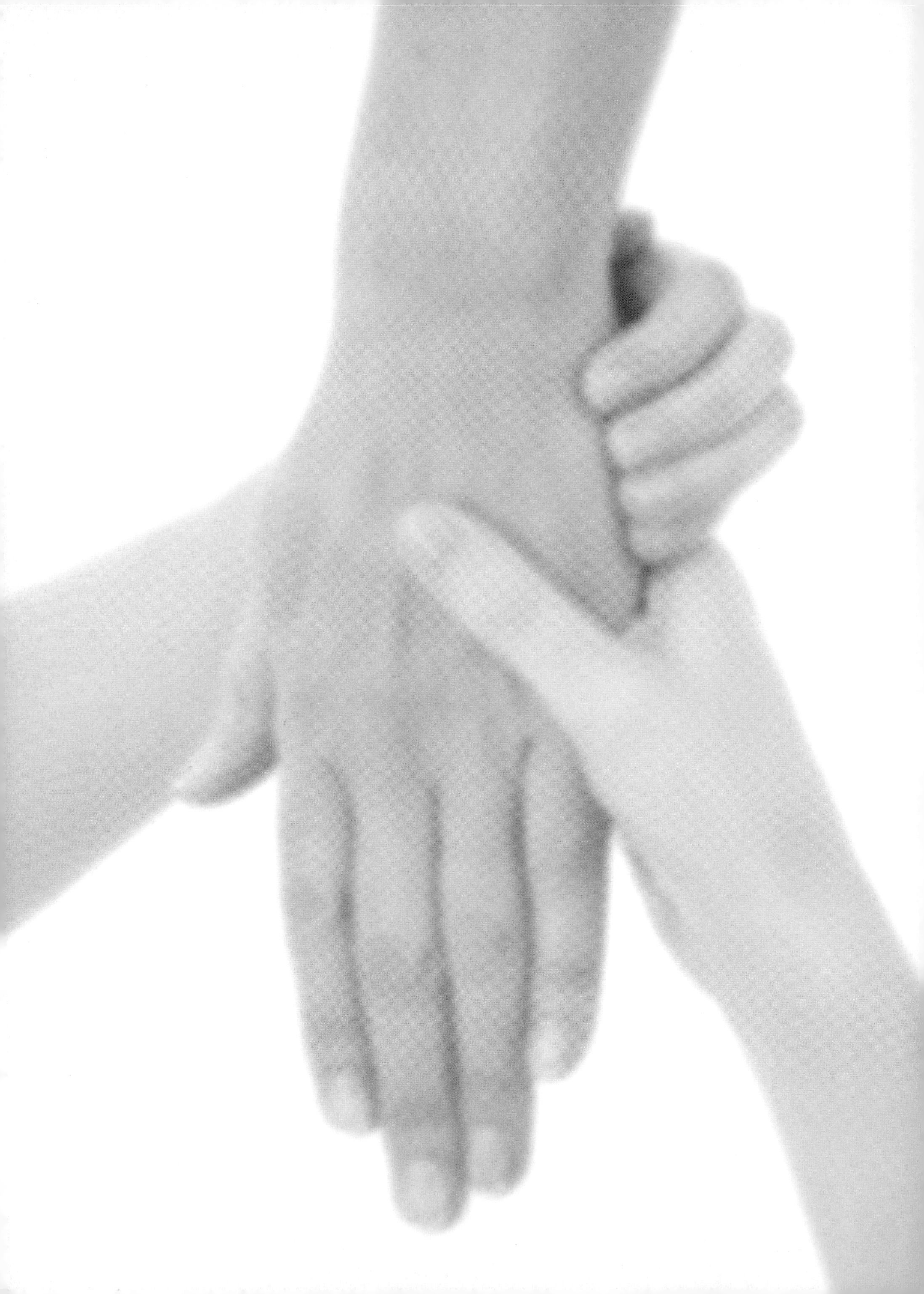

Hand reflexology

The feet and hands are the most usual and the most effective parts of the body for a reflexologist to treat. The hands are a particularly useful area to learn to work for two main reasons: they are a valid alternative if a foot cannot be treated for any reason (such as a broken bone), and they are an easier area to treat on yourself or for patients to work on themselves. The principles involved are the same as for foot reflexology, although the points on the hands are sometimes less easy to find.

Using reflexology on the hands

An understanding of the principles of hand reflexology comes into its own when a patient arrives in your practice with a strained ankle or an ulcerated foot, which makes treating the feet impossible. In these circumstances you can treat the hands instead.

The hands are far less sensitive than the feet. Try putting your feet into a very hot bath of water, then place your hands into the same bath. You will be able to sustain far more heat to your hands than you ever can to your feet. Your feet are such sensitive parts of your body that if you stub your toe the pain can be enough to make you feel quite sick.

It is easy to work on your own hands, and you can also show patients how they can work daily on theirs. This can bring relief from many conditions and helps patients to learn to take responsibility for their own health problems, which is an essential part of continued good health. I always show my patients the spinal area in the hand, which is quite easy to work on, as this in turn will stimulate the nerve connections to all parts of the body, as explained in 'The nervous system' (see page 112).

Looking at the charts on pages 166–167, you will see that it is quite straightforward to learn the locations of the hand reflex points once you have mastered those for the feet. They follow the same logical pattern as the feet: the reflex points for the upper body are found in the upper section of the hands (in the fingers); those for the mid body are in the middle part of the hand; and the intestinal, pelvic and urinary system points are in the lower areas and wrist.

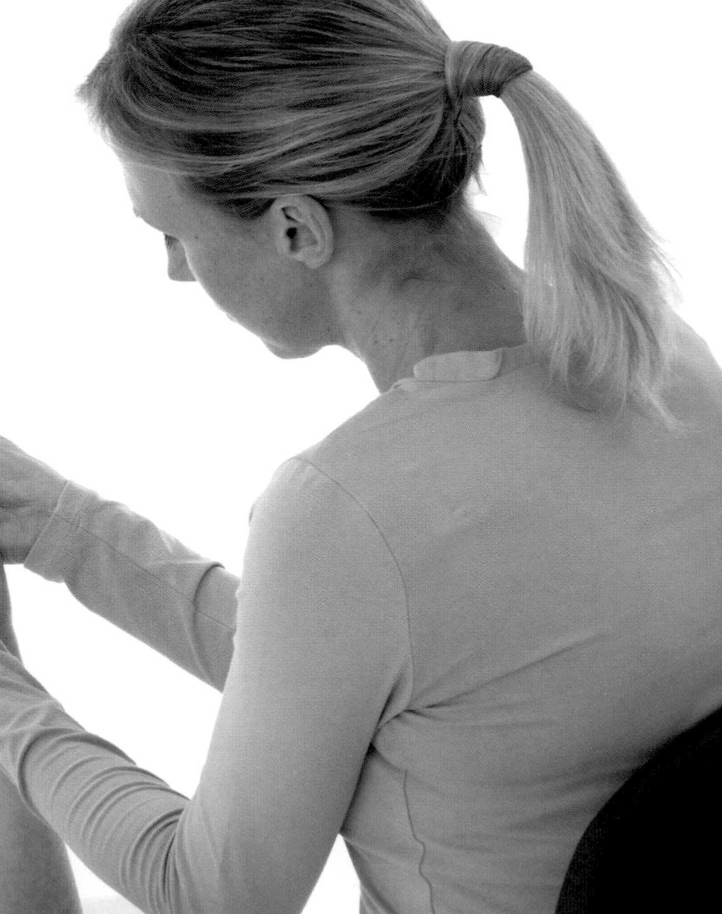

Hand reflexology Used by the practitioner when it is not possible for any reason to treat the patient's feet, hand reflexology techniques can also be adapted for self-treatment.

Anatomy of a hand

The human hand's ability to perform all manner of intricate and fine movements is quite remarkable. The articulation of the hand is more complex than that of the hands or paws belonging to any other animal, enabling humans to use a wide variety of tools and implements.

The human hand consists of 27 bones:

- 8 bones of the carpus or wrist, arranged in two rows of four
- 5 bones of the metacarpus or palm, one to each digit
- 14 digital bones or phalanges: 2 in the thumb and 3 in each finger.

The carpal bones fit into a shallow socket formed by the bones of the forearm.

Muscles and joints

The movements of the hand are achieved by two sets of muscles and tendons: the flexors for bending the fingers and thumbs and the extensors for straightening them out. The flexor muscles are located on the underside of the forearm and are attached by tendons to the phalanges of the fingers. The extensor muscles are on the back of the forearm and are similarly connected. The thumb has two separate flexor muscles that move the thumb in opposition to the other digits. This is what makes grasping possible.

Ligaments are fibrous tissues that help bind together the joints, and the sheaths are tubular structures that surround part of the fingers.

The surfaces of the joints of the hand, fingers and thumb are covered by cartilage. This shiny white material, which has a rubbery consistency, acts as a shock absorber and provides an extremely smooth surface so that all hand articulations are accomplished smoothly and easily.

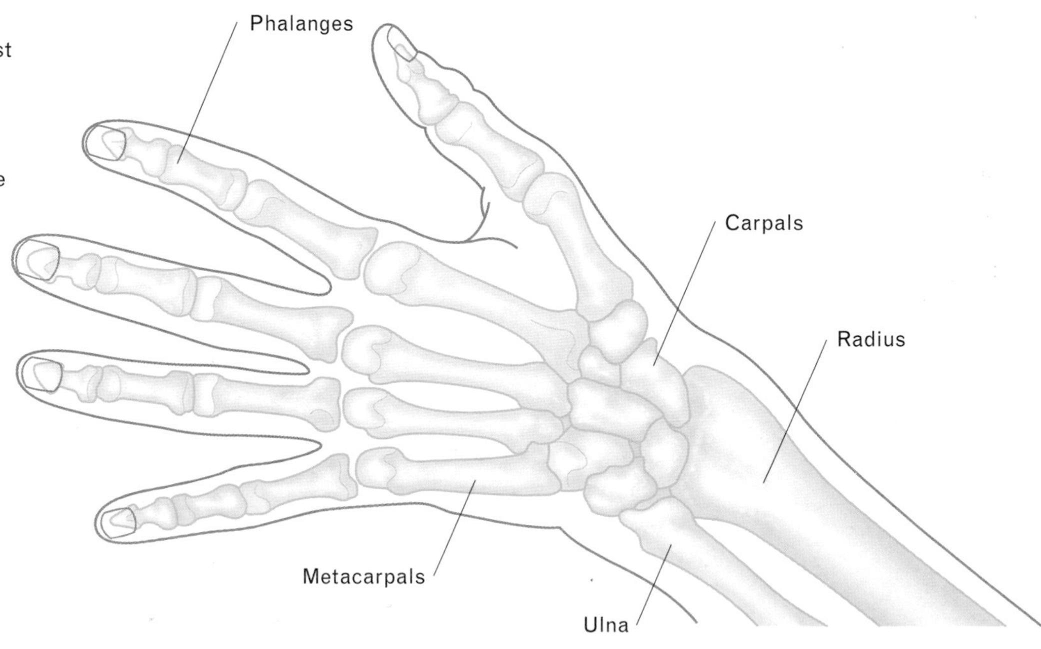

Bones of the hand The wrist and hand have a similar structure to the ankle and foot, with the metacarpals connecting the carpals to the phalanges. There are three phalanges on each finger, except for the thumb, which has only two.

Hand maps

All the reflex points relating to parts of the body are found on the hands and wrists as well as the feet. Because of the smaller size of the hand and the separation between fingers and thumb, the layout is more compressed and less obvious than on the feet.

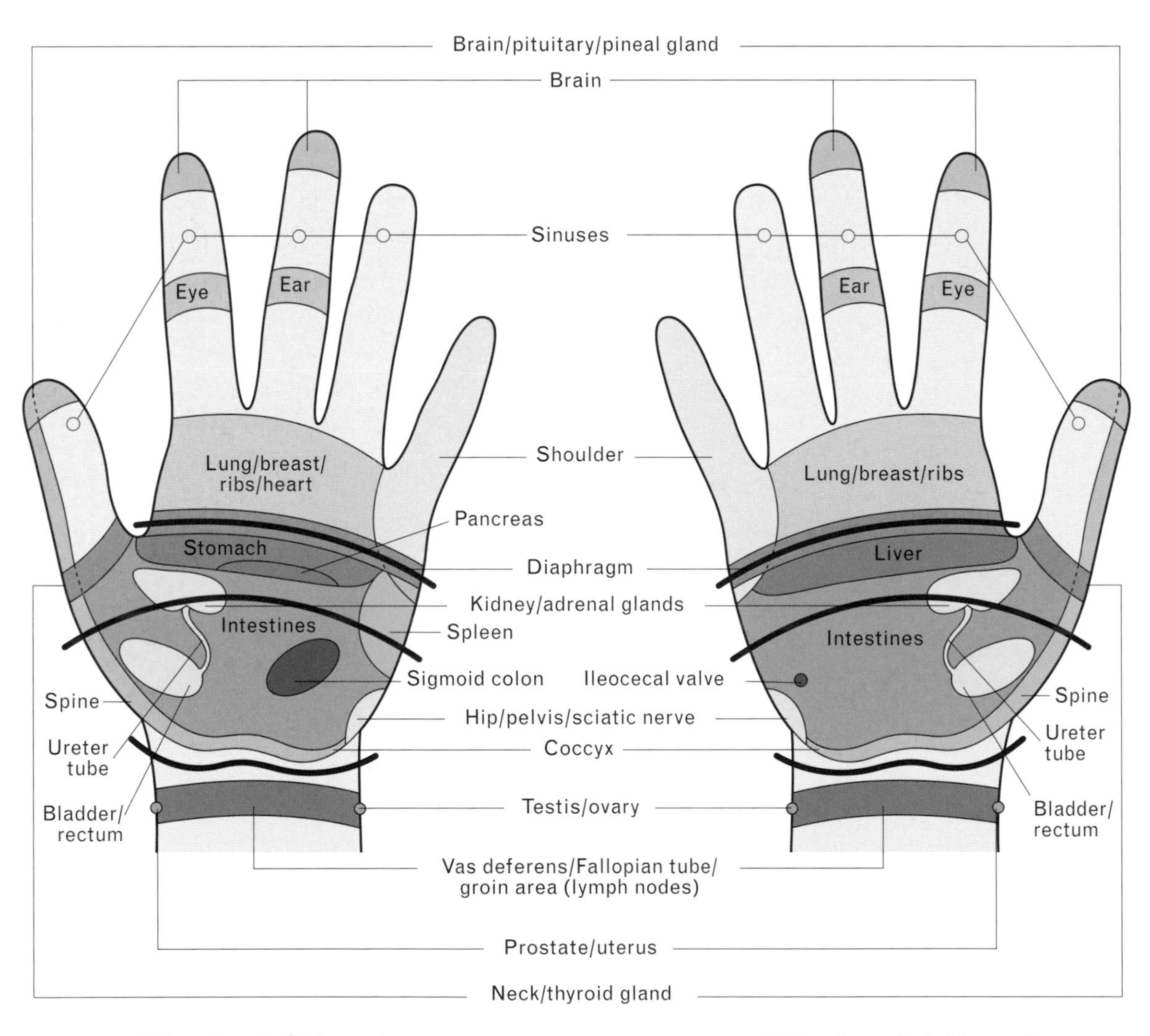

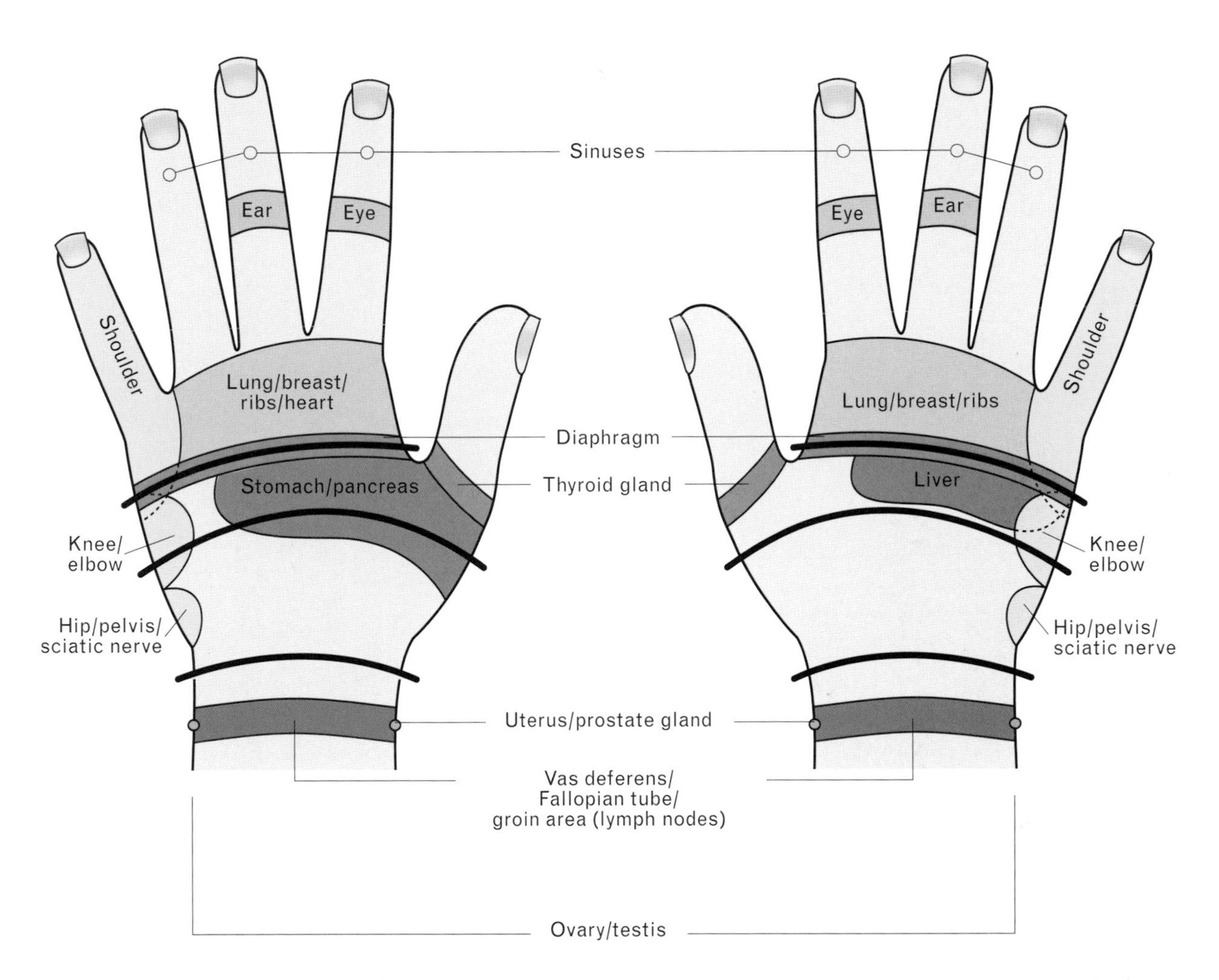

Dorsal left hand

Dorsal right hand

Hand relaxation exercises

Hand relaxation exercises are special techniques that are used at the beginning of a treatment session, during a treatment and at the end of the session. As in a foot reflexology treatment, the exercises are important because they relax the hand and create a contact between the patient and the practitioner.

The best position for you to start your treatment is sitting facing your patient with the patient's arm and hand resting on a table between you. Place the arm on a large pillow so that it has good but soft support.

Side-to-side relaxation

Right hand

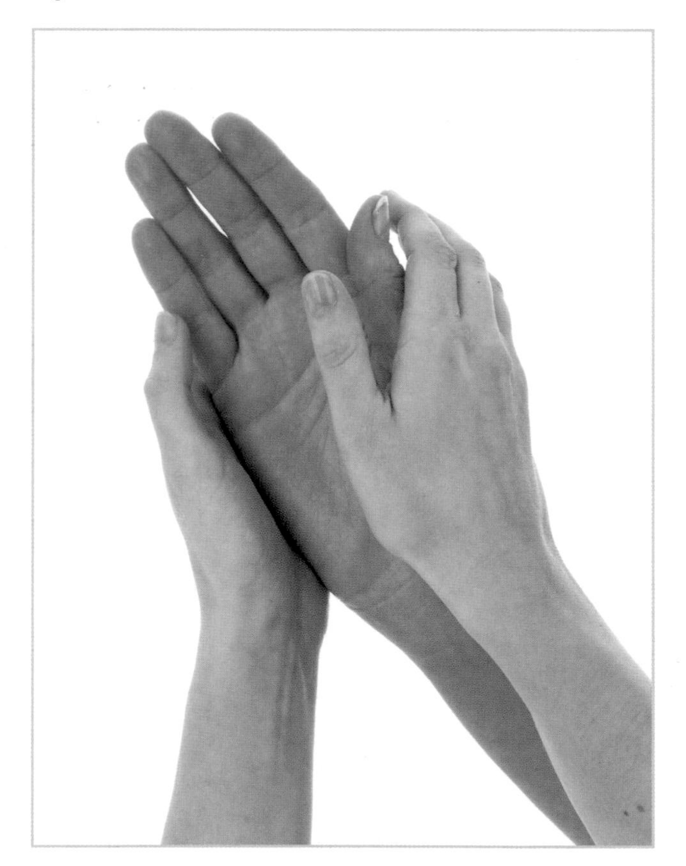

1 Supporting the right hand with both of your hands, move the hand gently from side to side.

Left hand

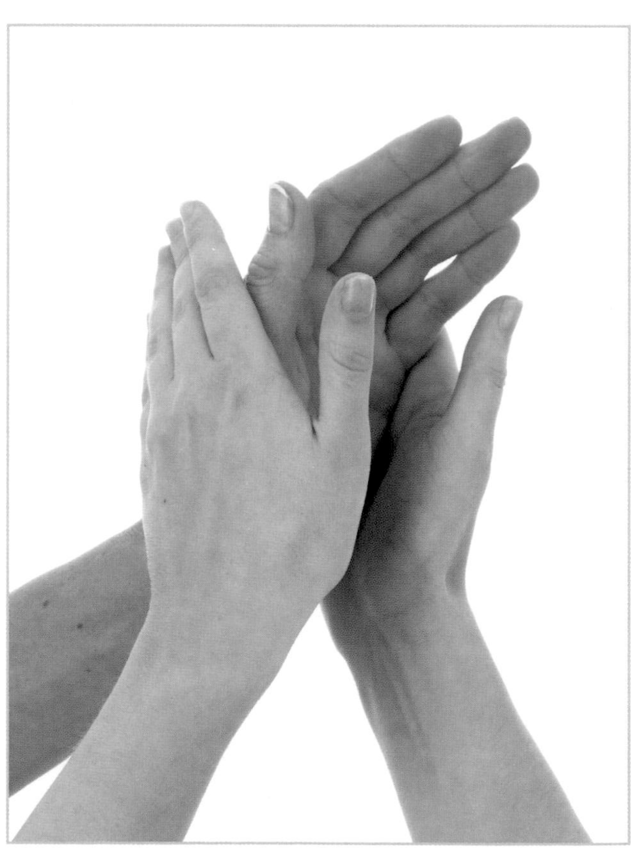

2 Supporting the left hand with both of your hands, move the hand gently from side to side.

Diaphragm relaxation

This exercise helps to relax the large diaphragm muscle, which is found at the base of the lung.

Right hand
Medial to lateral

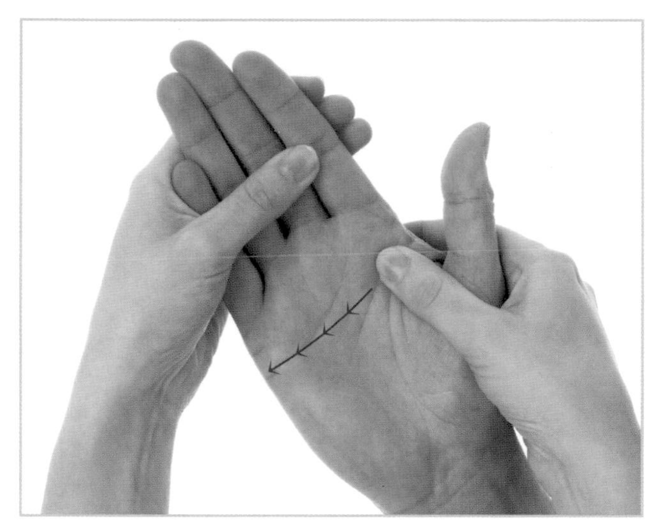

1 Place your right thumb on the diaphragm line and move it to the lateral edge, gently bending the fingers towards your thumb.

Right hand
Lateral to medial

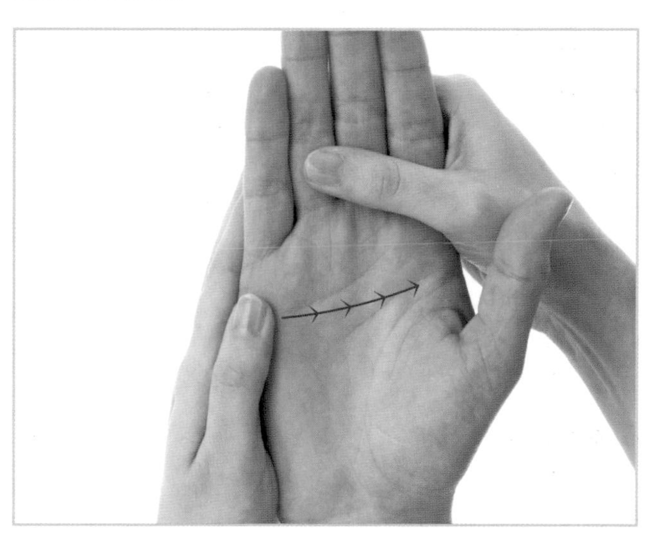

2 Place your left thumb on the diaphragm line and move it to the medial edge, gently bending the fingers towards your thumb.

Diaphragm relaxation

Left hand
Medial to lateral

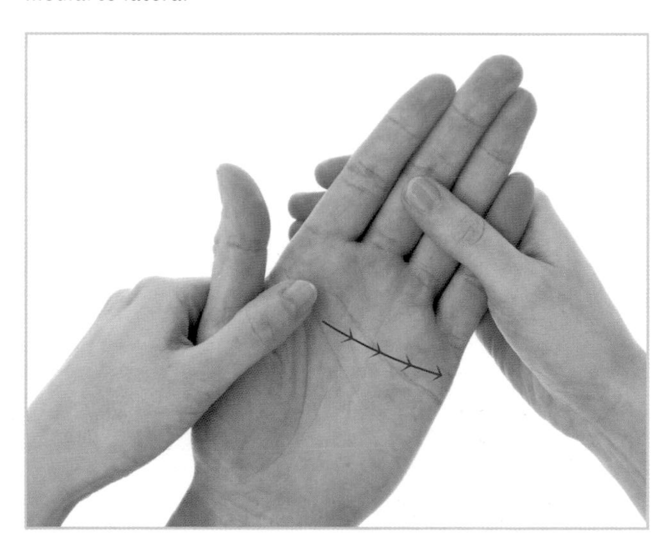

1 Place your left thumb on the diaphragm line and move it to the lateral edge, gently bending the fingers towards your thumb.

Left hand
Lateral to medial

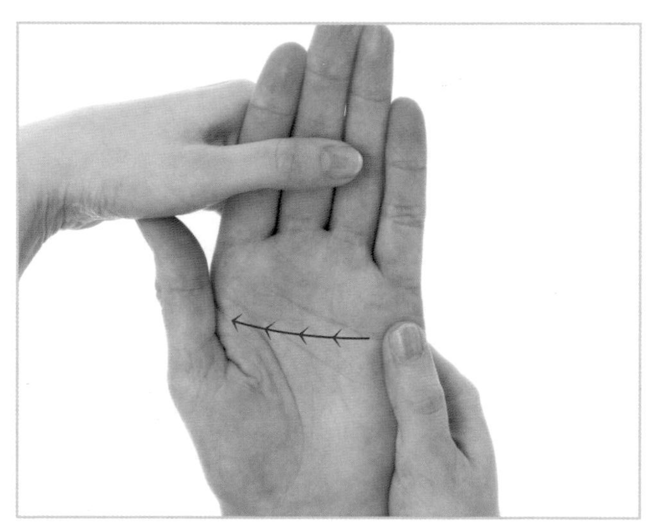

2 Place your right thumb on the diaphragm line and move it to the medial edge, gently bending the fingers towards your thumb.

Metacarpal kneading

Right hand

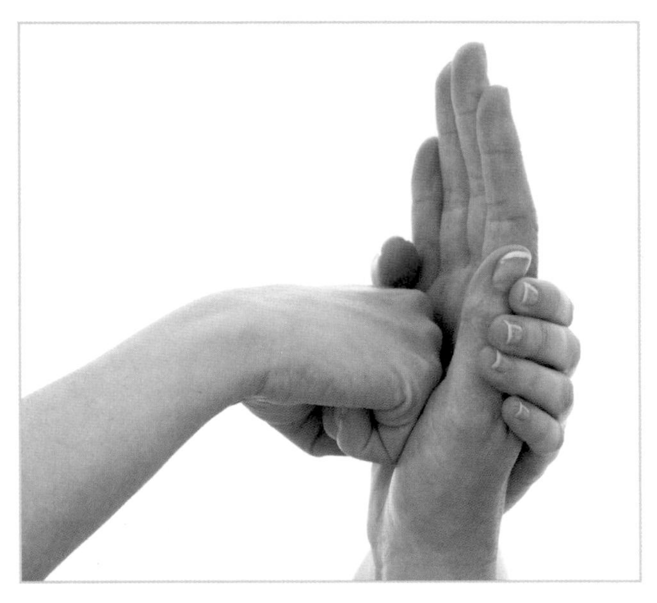

1 Supporting the right hand with your left hand, make a fist with your right hand and use it to knead the palm.

Left hand

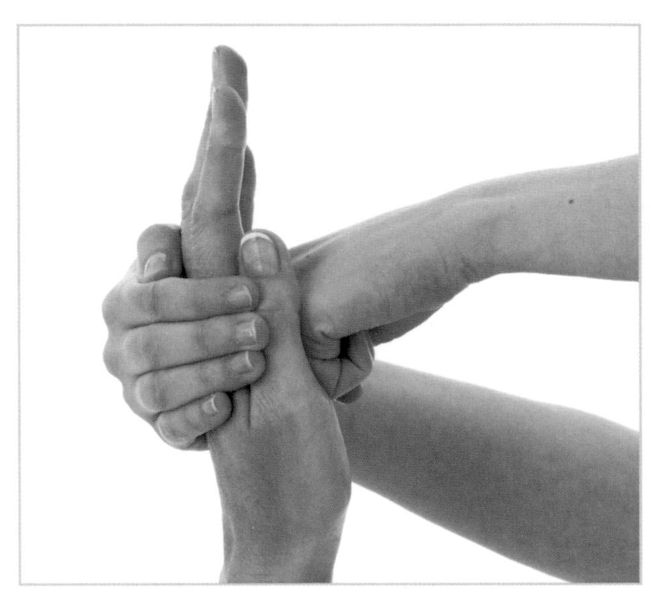

2 Repeat this exercise for the left hand, using your right hand as a support and making a fist with your left hand.

Wrist freeing

Right hand

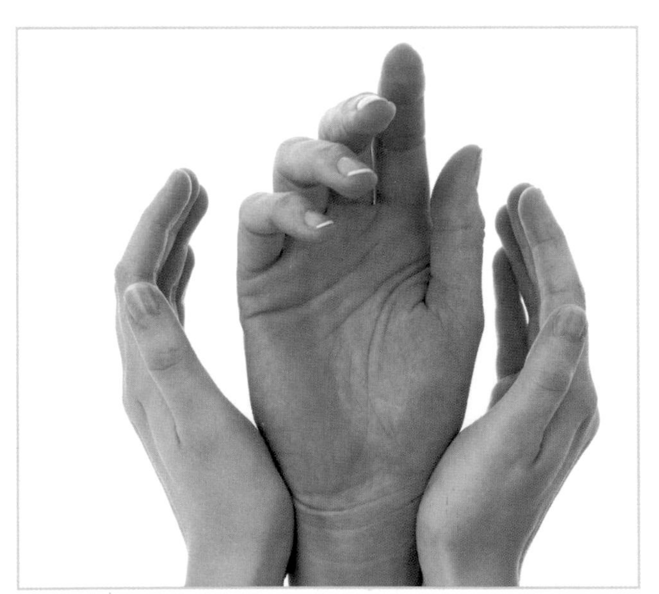

1 Support the right hand in front of the wrist and, with the heels of both your hands, rock the hand from side to side.

Left hand

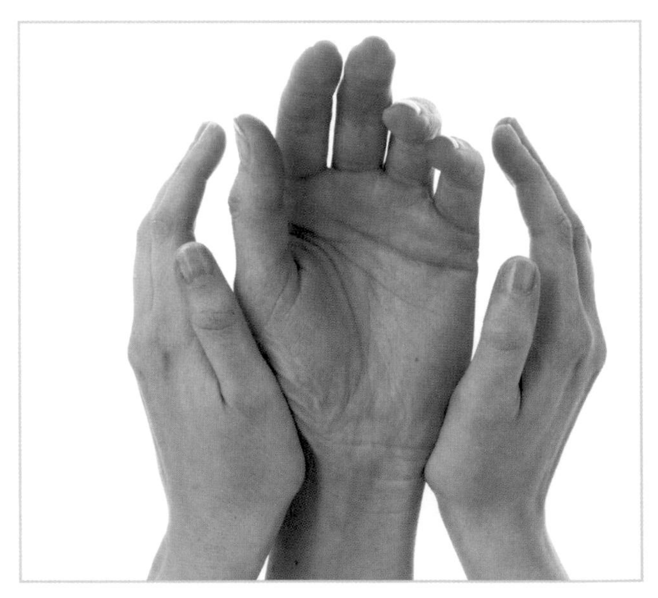

2 Repeat this exercise for the left hand, supporting it in front of the wrist and rocking it with the heels of both hands.

Undergrip

Right hand

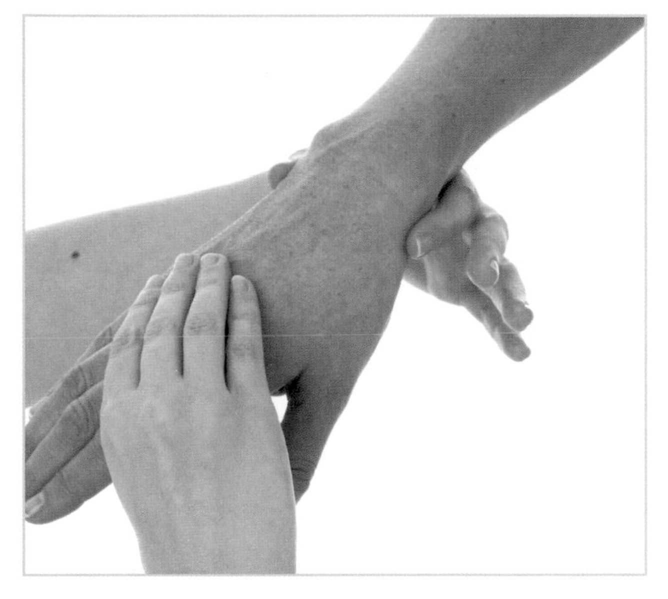

1 Supporting the hand with your left hand, use your right hand to turn it inwards in a rotating direction.

Left hand

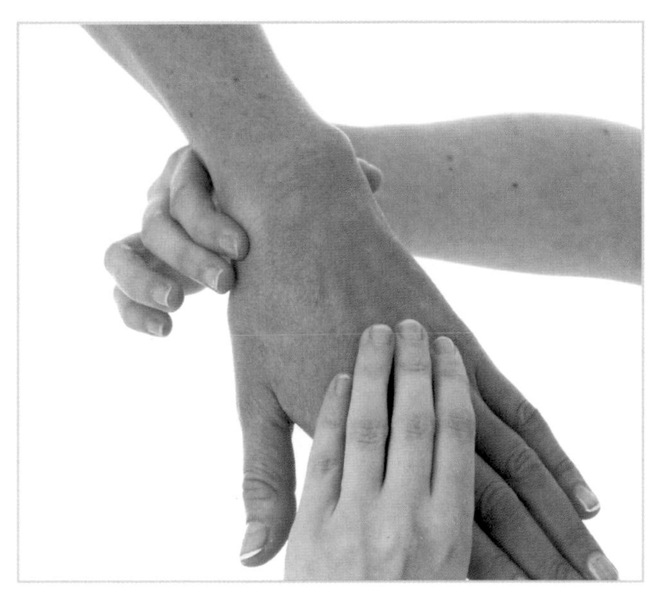

2 Supporting the hand with your right hand, use your left hand to turn it inwards in a rotating direction.

Overgrip

Right hand

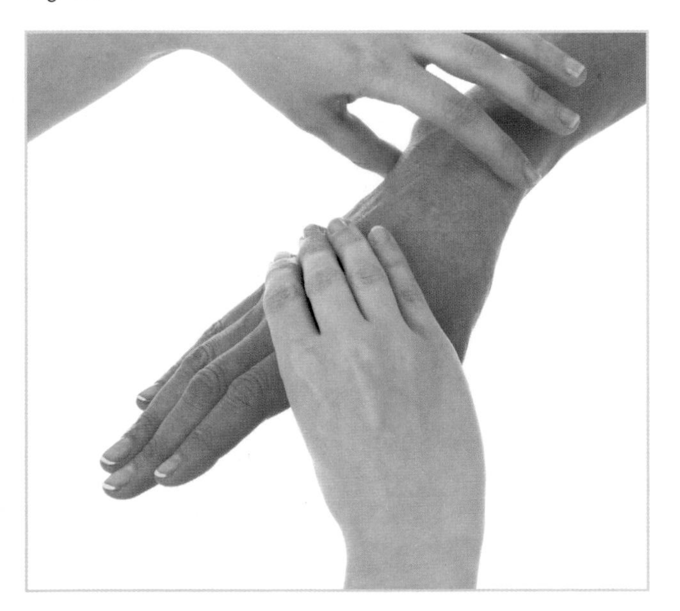

1 Support the hand by placing your left hand over the top of the wrist. Then use your right hand to turn the hand inward.

Left hand

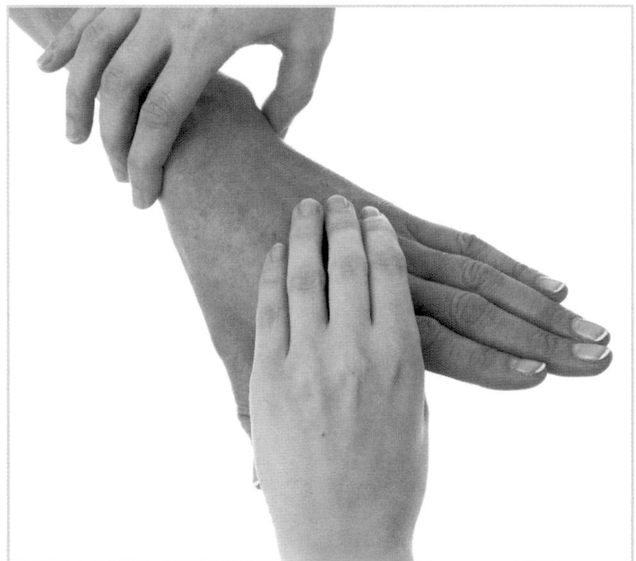

2 Repeat this exercise for the left hand, placing your right hand over the top of the wrist and using the left hand to turn the hand inward.

Hand moulding

Right hand

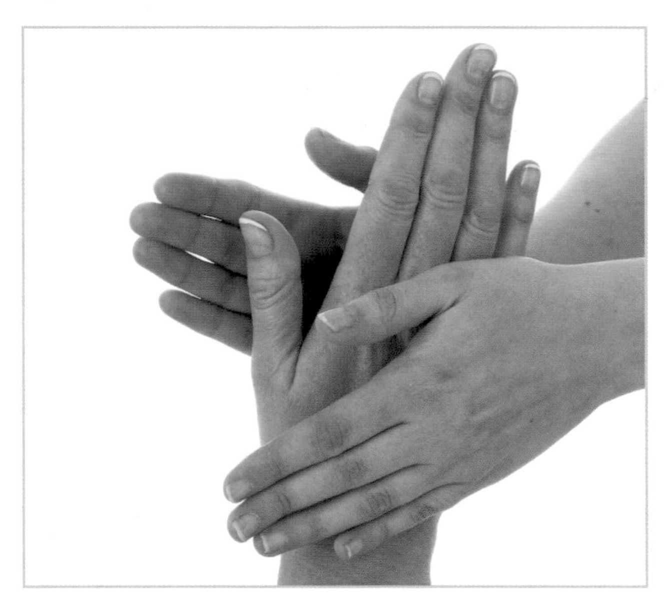

1 Cradle the right hand in the palms of your hands and rotate from the lateral side of the hand.

Left hand

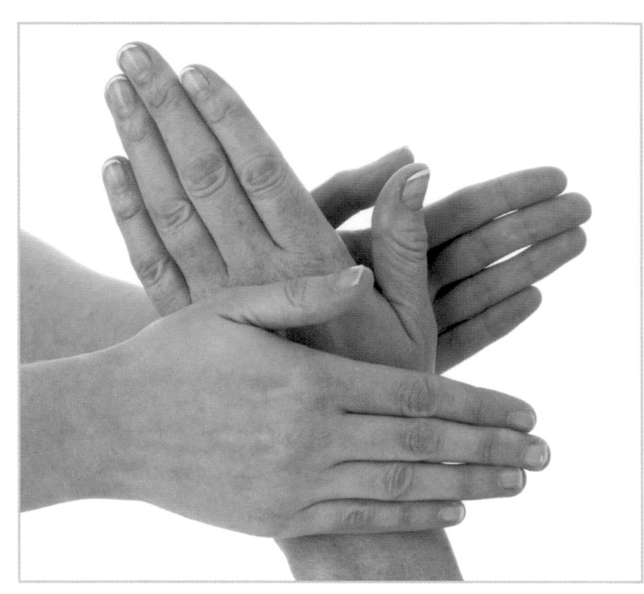

2 Cradle the left hand in the palms of your hands and rotate from the lateral side of the hand.

Ribcage relaxation

Right hand

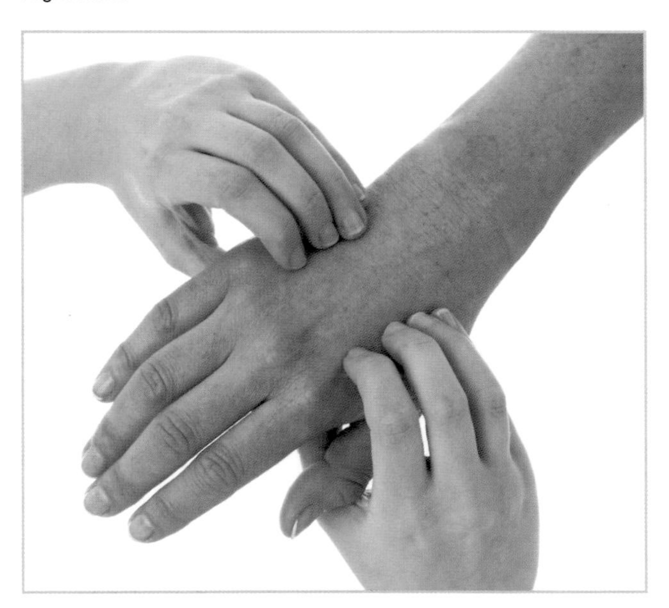

1 Working on the right hand, press in with the thumbs of both of your hands and creep around the dorsal side of the hand with the four free fingers of each hand.

Left hand

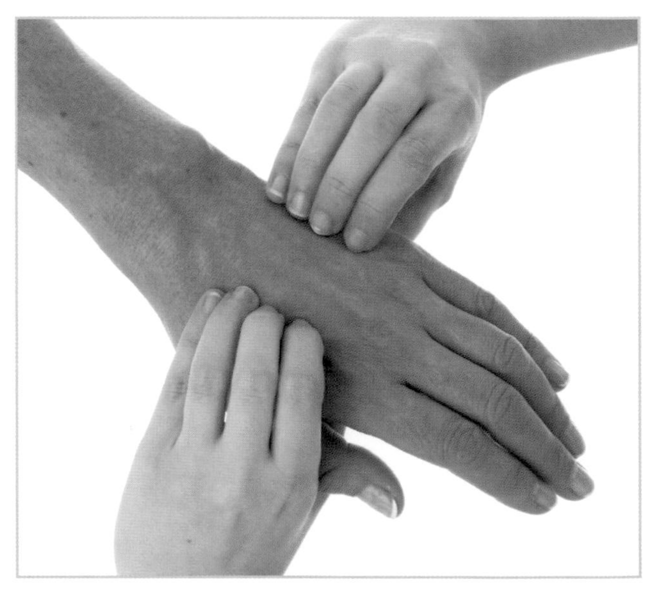

2 Repeat this exercise on the left hand, pressing in with the thumbs of both your hands and creeping around the dorsal side of the hand with the four free fingers of each hand.

Hand reflexology routine

This is the basic routine to adopt when giving a hand reflexology session or when working on your own hands. You will not, of course, be able to use the two-handed relaxation techniques described on pages 168–172 when treating yourself.

Lung area

Right hand – plantar
Medial to lateral

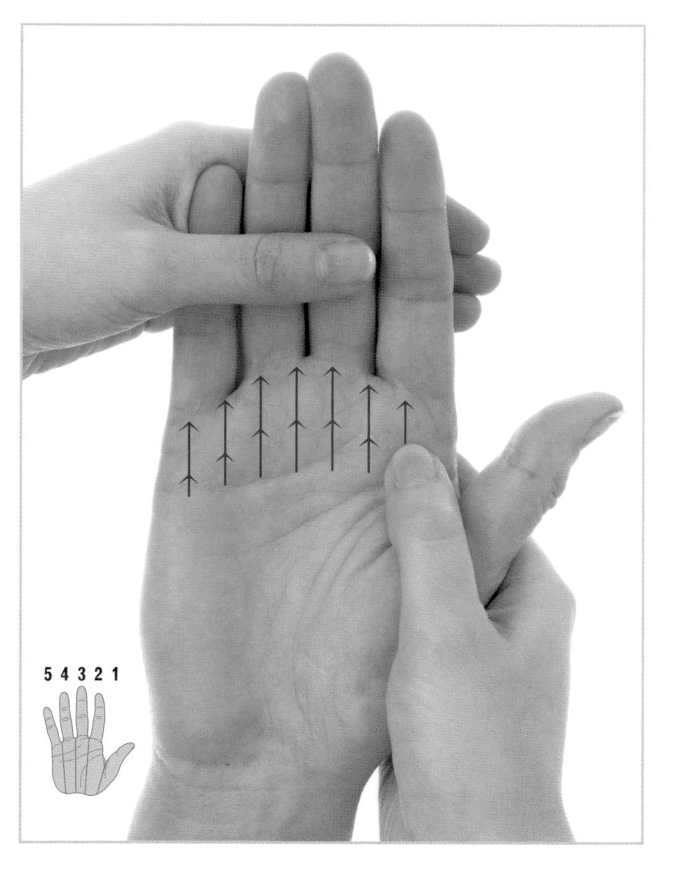

1 Place your right thumb on the diaphragm line of the right hand. Keep your thumb working up in straight lines to the base of the fingers from the medial to the lateral side of the hand.

Right hand – plantar
Lateral to medial

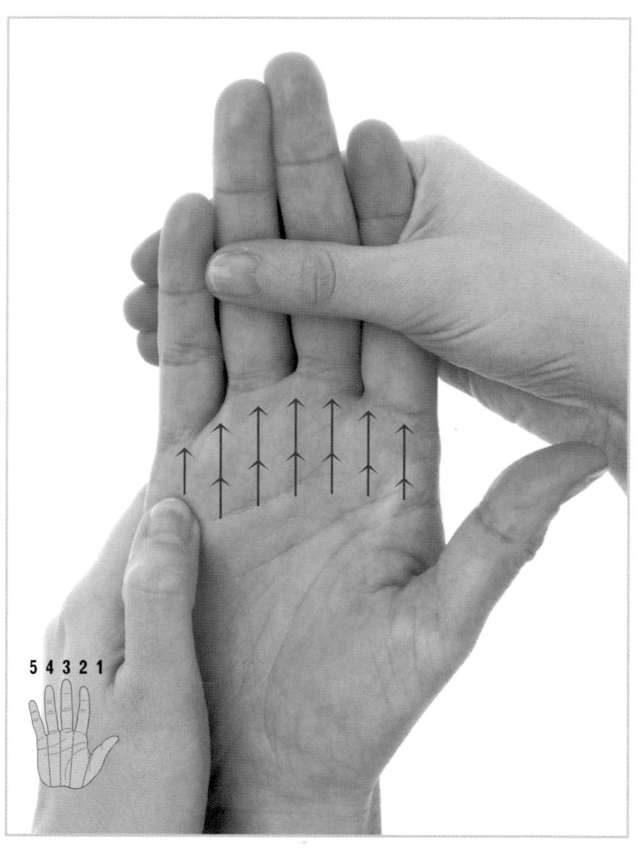

2 Using your left thumb, work up in straight lines from the lateral to the medial side of the hand.

Lung area

Right hand – dorsal
Medial to lateral

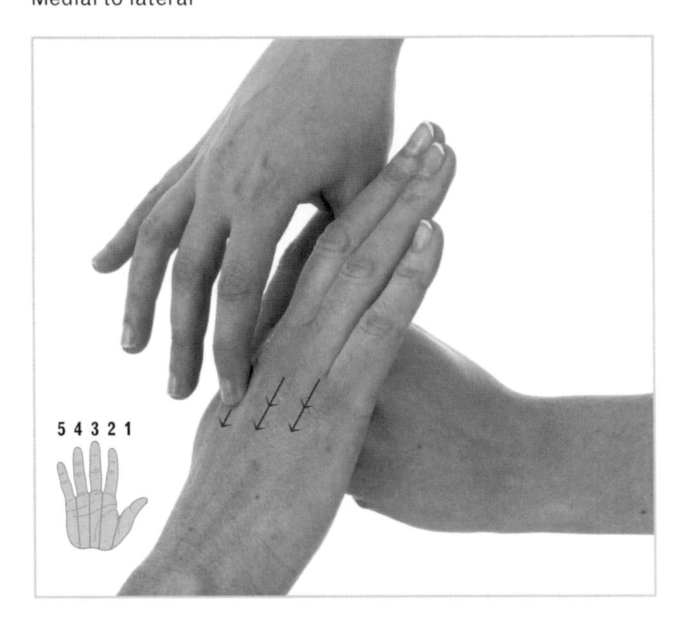

1 On the dorsal side of the right hand, place your right index finger where the fingers join the hand and work down the lines as indicated.

Right hand – dorsal
Lateral to medial

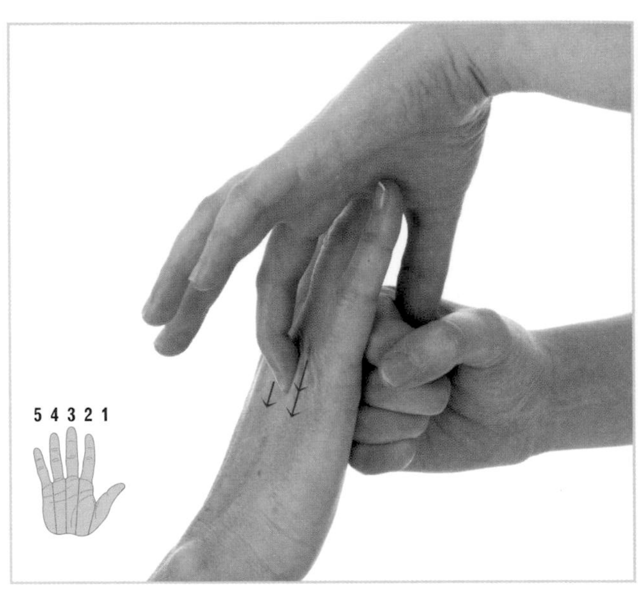

2 Work down the lines as indicated from the lateral to the medial side of the hand, using your left index finger.

Lung area

Left hand – plantar
Medial to lateral

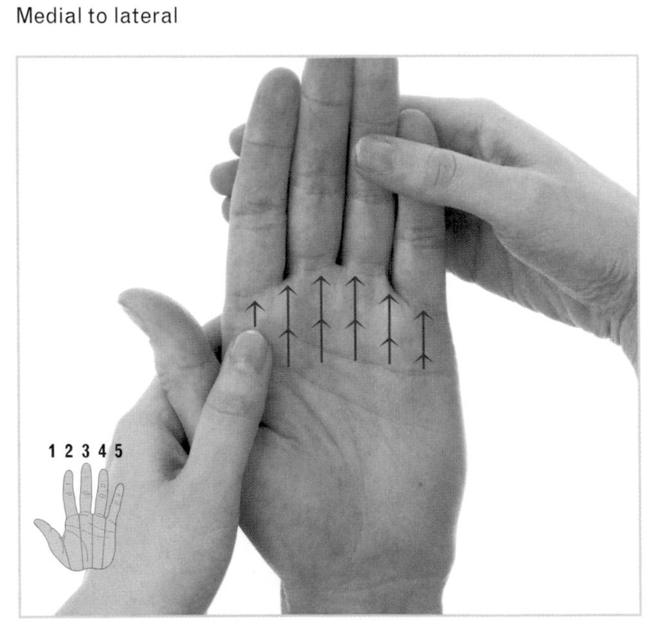

1 Place your left thumb on the diaphragm line of the left hand. Keep your thumb working up in straight lines to the base of the fingers.

Left hand – plantar
Lateral to medial

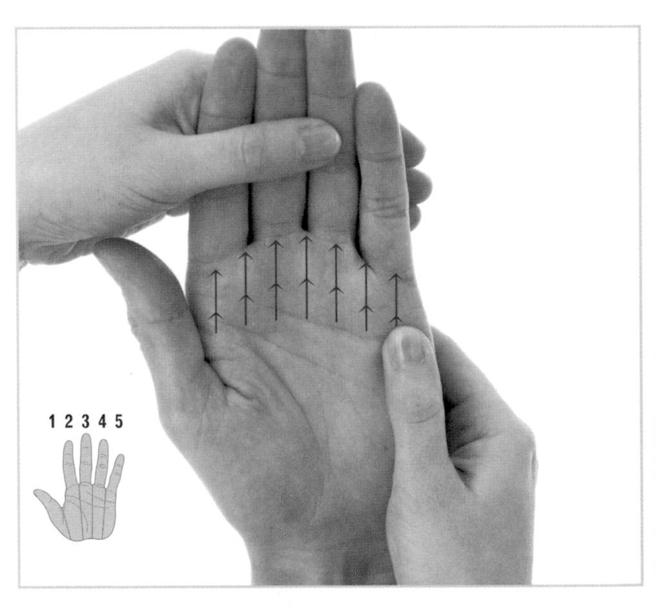

2 Work up in straight lines from the lateral to the medial side of the hand, using your right thumb.

Lung area

Left hand – dorsal
Medial to lateral

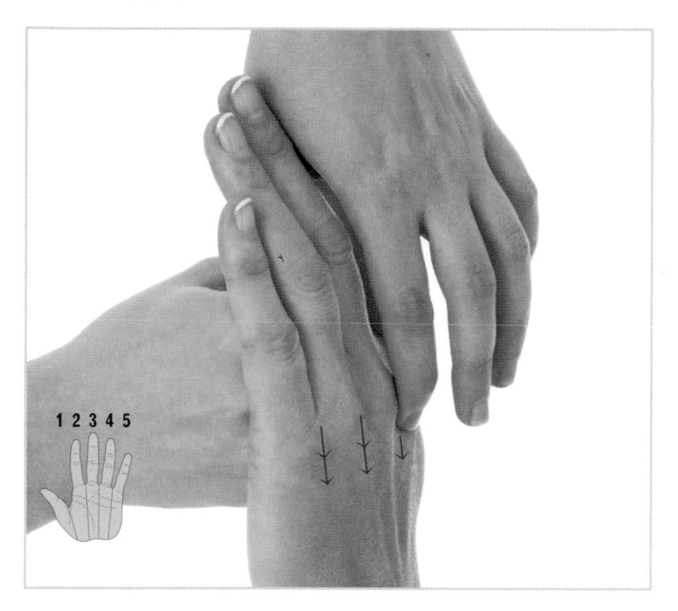

1 On the dorsal side, place your left index finger where the fingers join the hand and work down the lines as indicated.

Left hand – dorsal
Lateral to medial

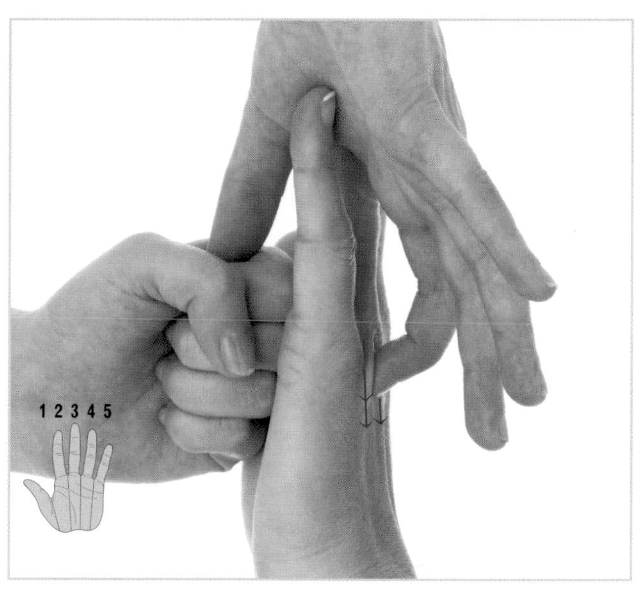

2 Work down the lines as indicated from the lateral to the medial side of the hand, using your right index finger.

The sinuses

Right hand – plantar
Medial to lateral

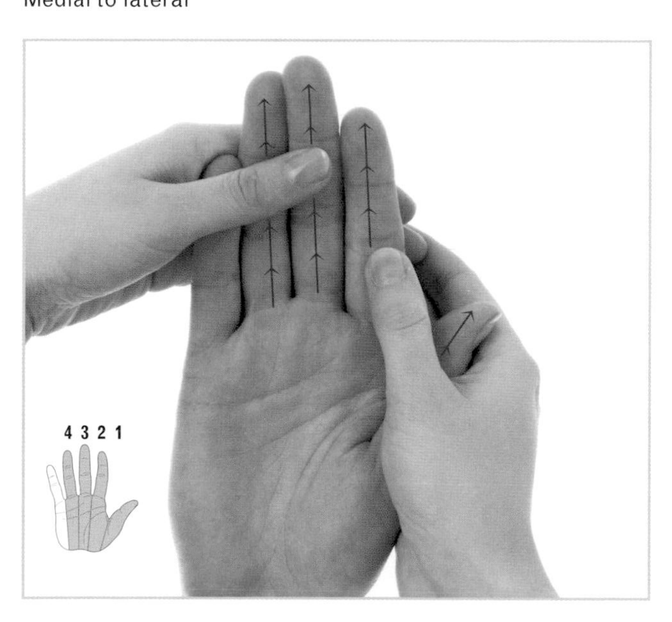

1 Use your right thumb to work out the reflex points as indicated, working in the direction of the arrows from the medial to the lateral side of the hand.

Right hand – plantar
Lateral to medial

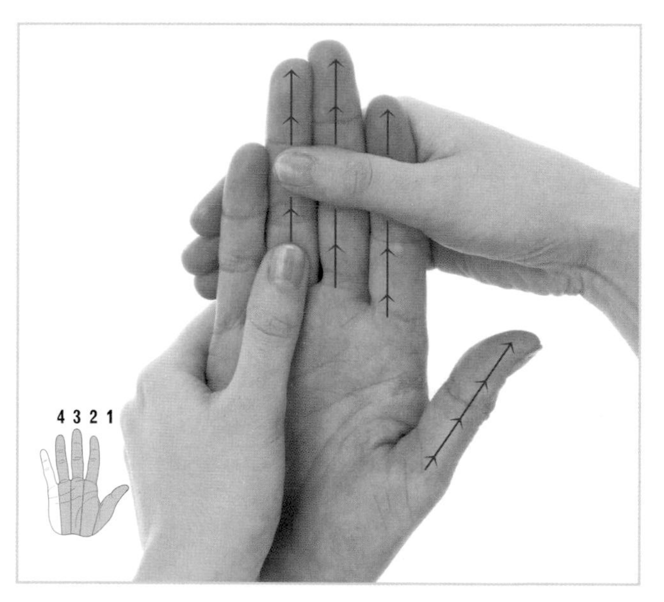

2 Use your left thumb to work out the reflex points as indicated, working from the lateral to the medial side of the hand.

The sinuses

Left hand – plantar
Medial to lateral

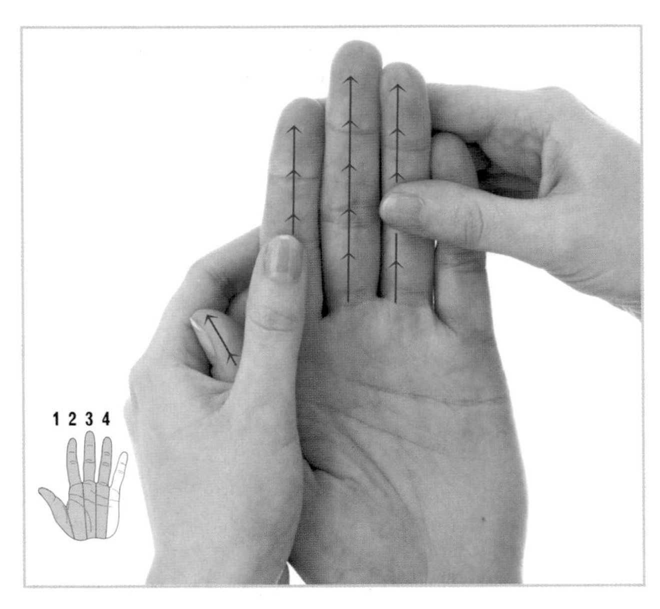

1 Use your left thumb to work out the reflex points as indicated, working in the direction of the arrows from the medial to the lateral side of the hand.

Left hand – plantar
Lateral to medial

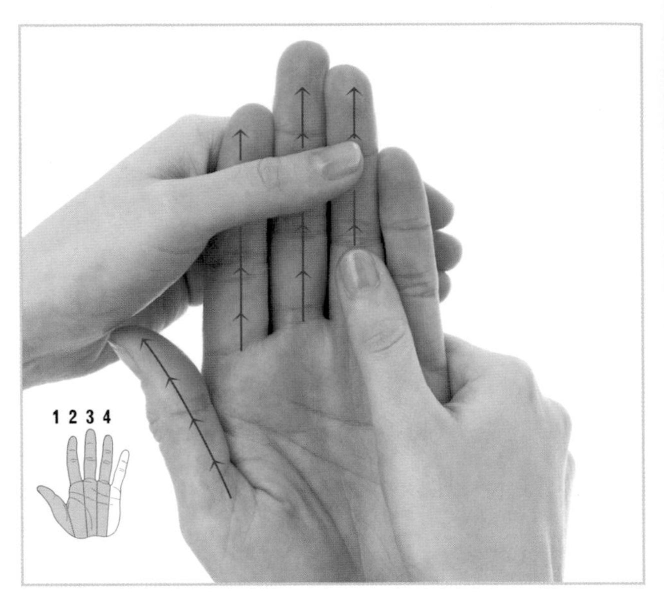

2 Use your right thumb to work out the reflex points as indicated, working from the lateral to the medial side of the hand.

The eye and ear

Right hand – plantar

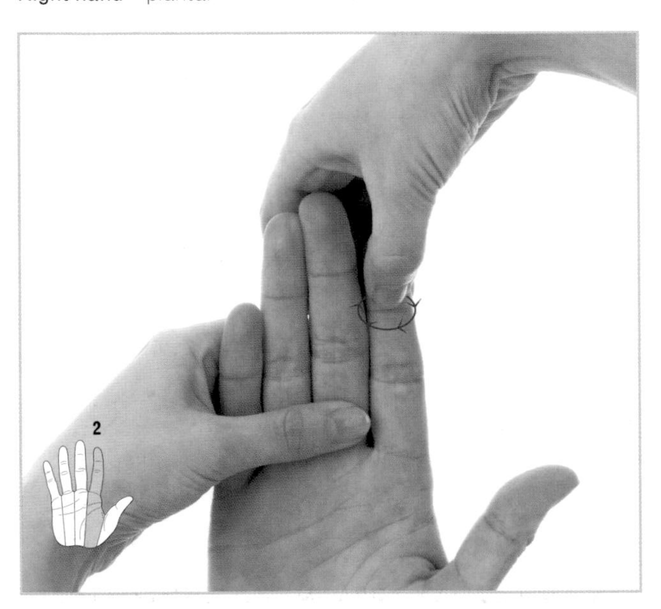

1 Using your right thumb, apply pressure to eye area at the top joint of the index finger; use a rotating movement.

Right hand – plantar

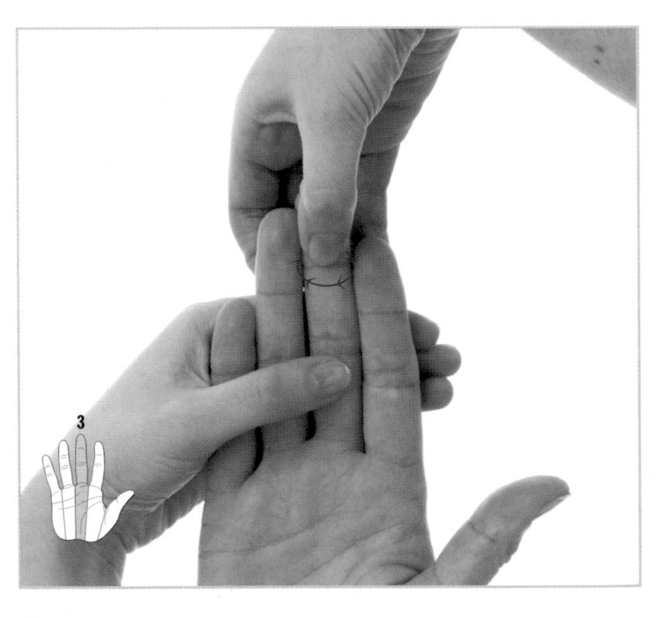

2 Using your right thumb, apply pressure to the ear area at the top joint of the third finger; use a rotating movement.

The eye and ear

Left hand – plantar

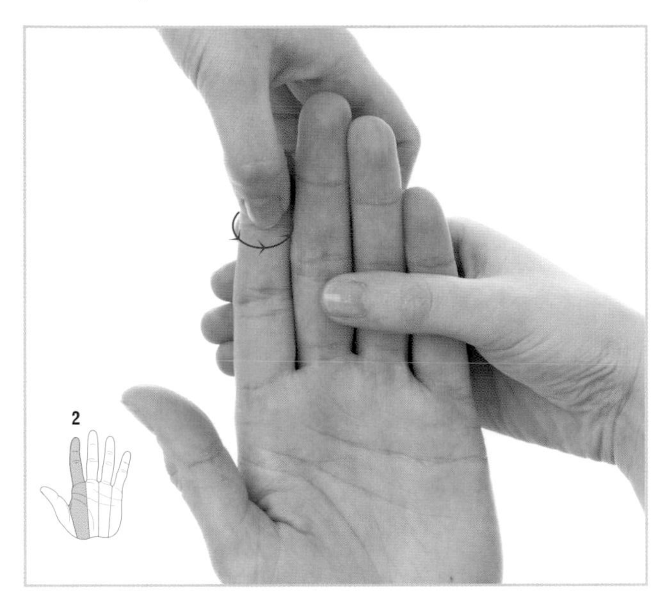

1 Using your left thumb, apply pressure to the eye area at the top joint of the index finger; use a rotating movement.

Left hand – plantar

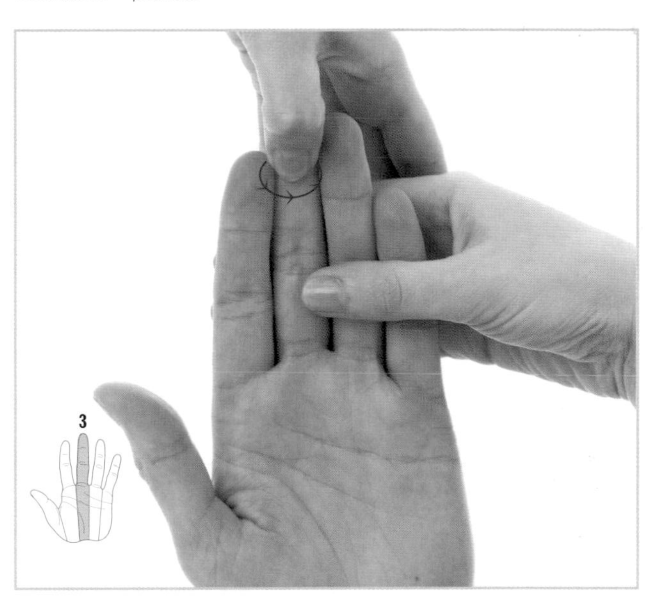

2 Using your left thumb, apply pressure to the ear area at the top joint of the third finger; use a rotating movement.

The neck and thyroid gland

Right hand – plantar

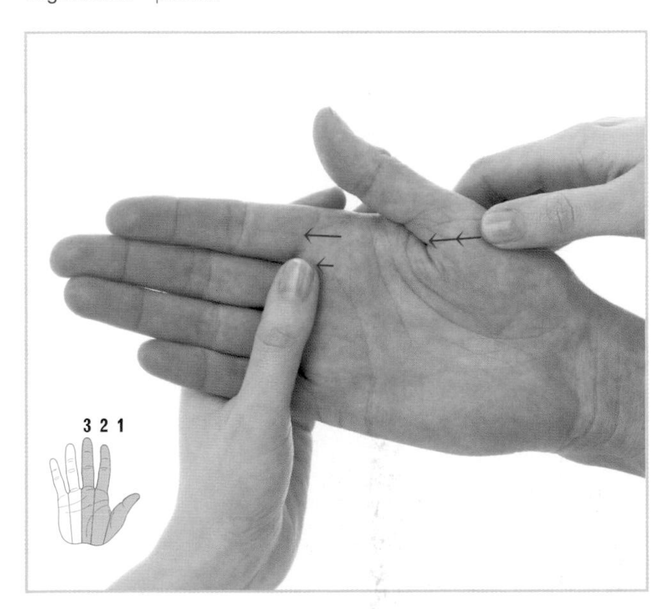

1 Using your right thumb, work the thyroid reflex at the base of the thumb on the right hand. You should also work the bases of the first two fingers, to help nerve and blood supply to the neck and relieve neck tension.

Right hand – dorsal

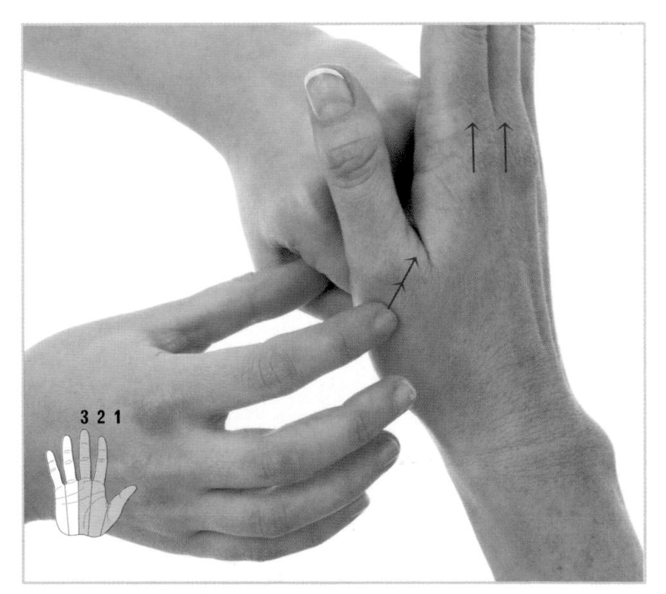

2 As you work the thyroid reflex on the dorsal side, support the hand with your left fist.

The neck and thyroid gland

Left hand – plantar

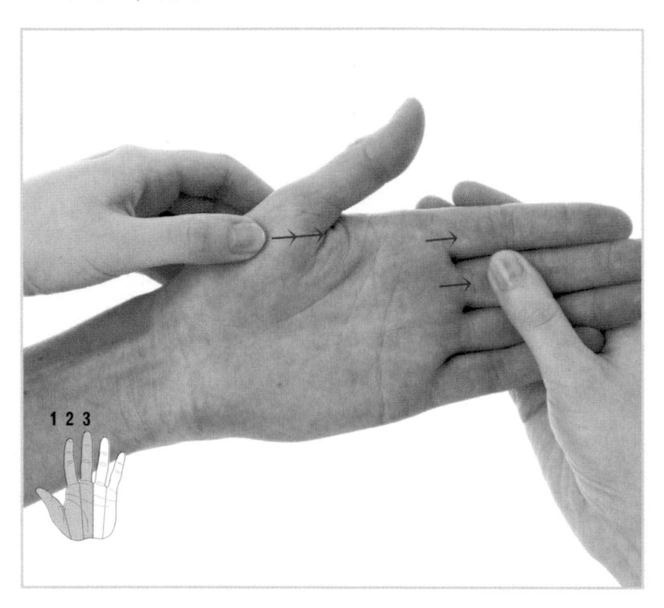

1 Using your left thumb, work the thyroid reflex at the base of the thumb on the left hand. You should also work the bases of the first two fingers, to help nerve and blood supply to the neck and relieve neck tension.

Left hand – dorsal

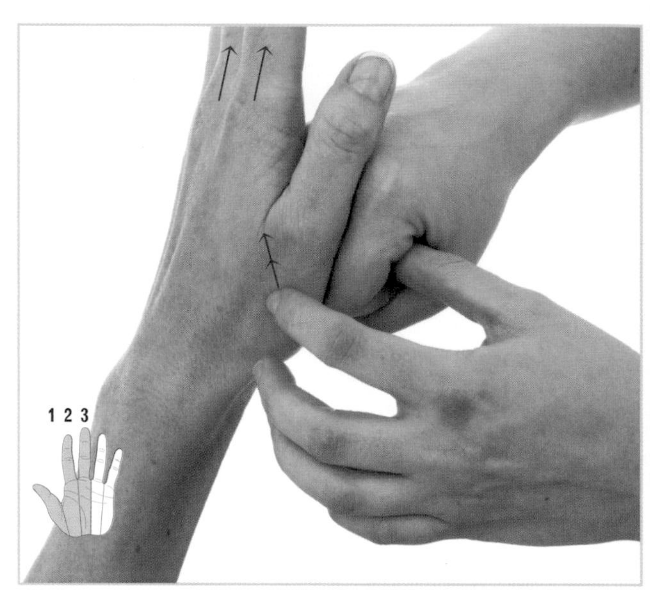

2 As you work the thyroid reflex on the dorsal side, support the hand with your right fist.

The coccyx

Right hand – plantar

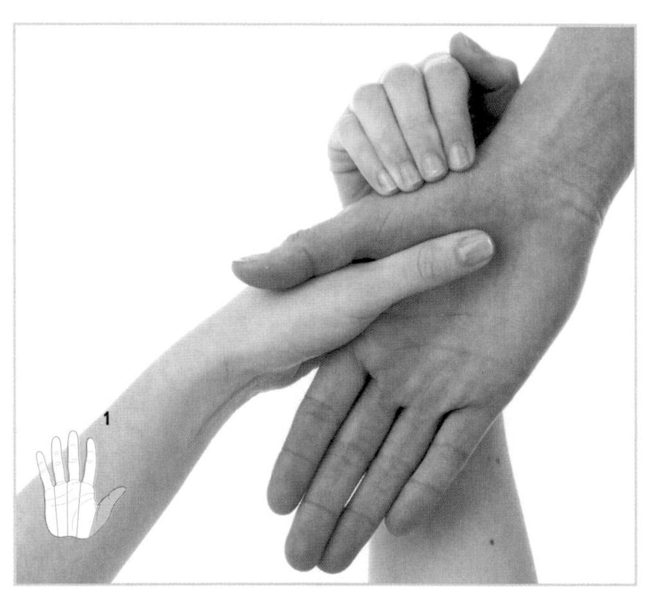

1 Apply pressure from the four fingers of your right hand to the area just in front of the thumb on the medial side of the right hand.

Left hand – plantar

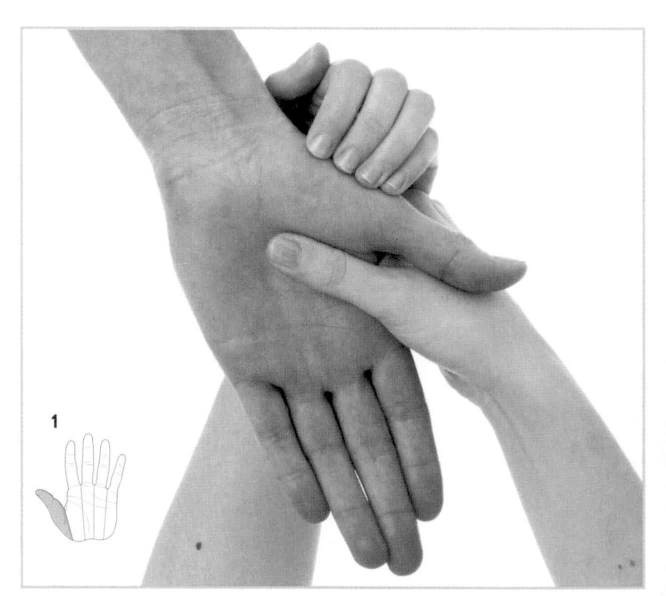

2 Apply pressure from the four fingers of your left hand to the area just in front of the thumb on the medial side of the left hand.

The hip and pelvis

Right hand – dorsal

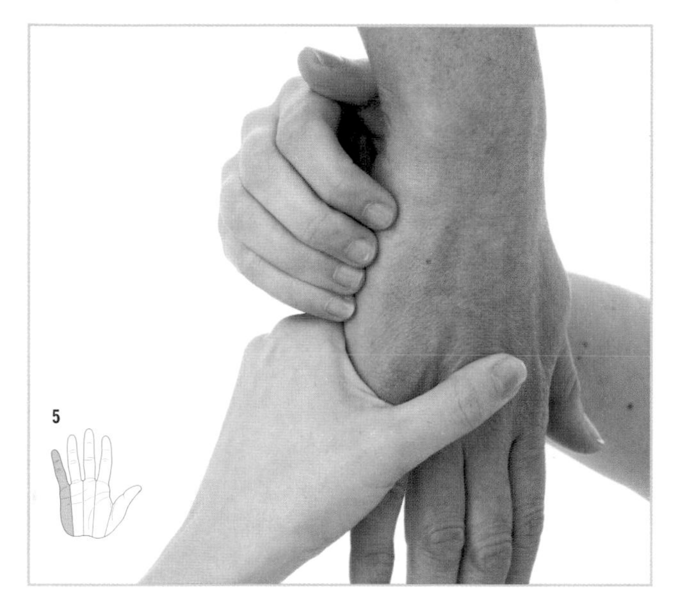

1 Apply pressure from the four fingers of your right hand around the hip and pelvis area on the lateral side of the right hand.

Left hand – dorsal

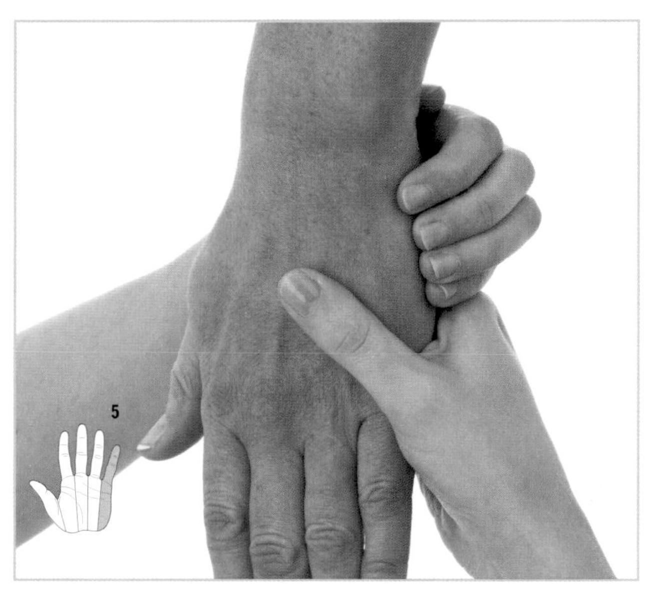

2 Apply pressure from the four fingers of your left hand around the lateral side of the left hand.

The spine

Right hand – plantar

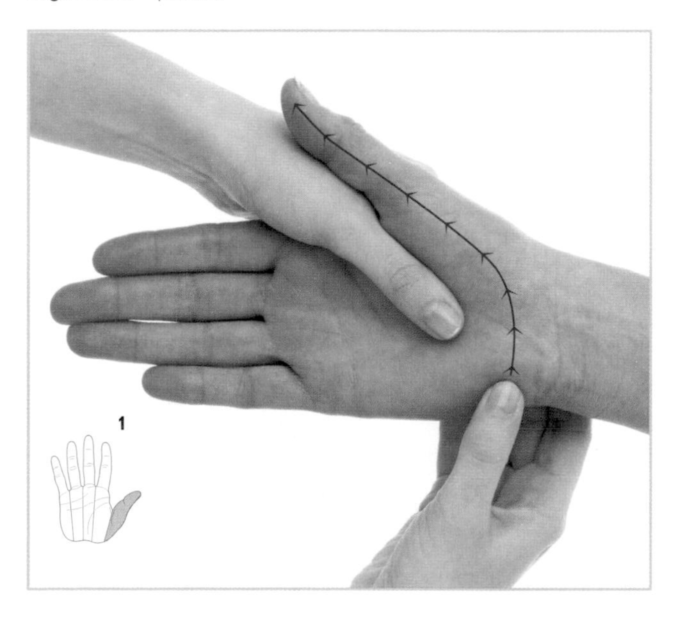

1 To contact the reflex points for the spine on the right hand, work up the line indicated with your right thumb.

Right hand – plantar

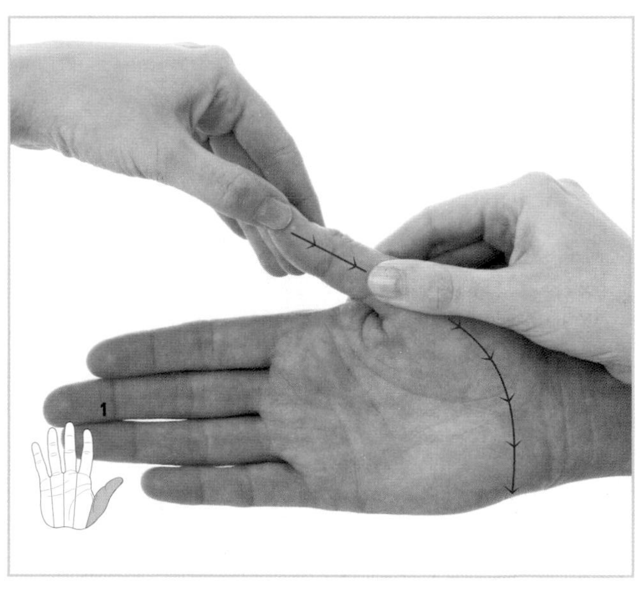

2 Use your left thumb to work back down the line of the spine as indicated.

The spine

Left hand – plantar

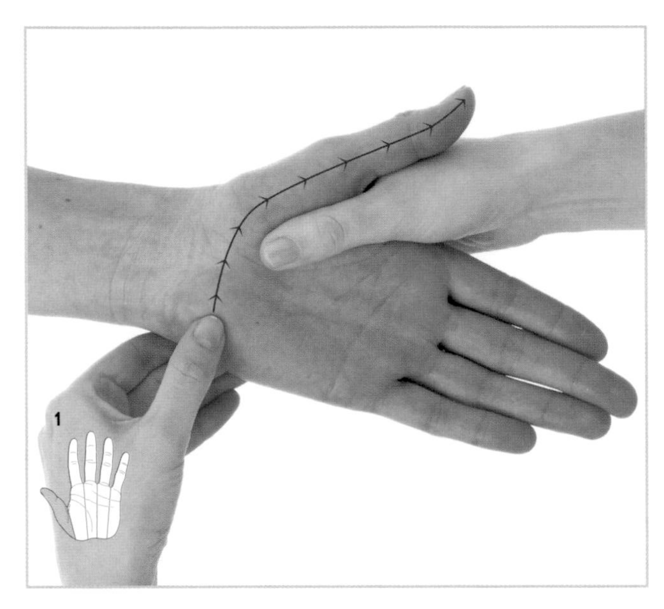

1 To contact the reflex points for the spine on the left hand, work up the line indicated with your left thumb.

Left hand – plantar

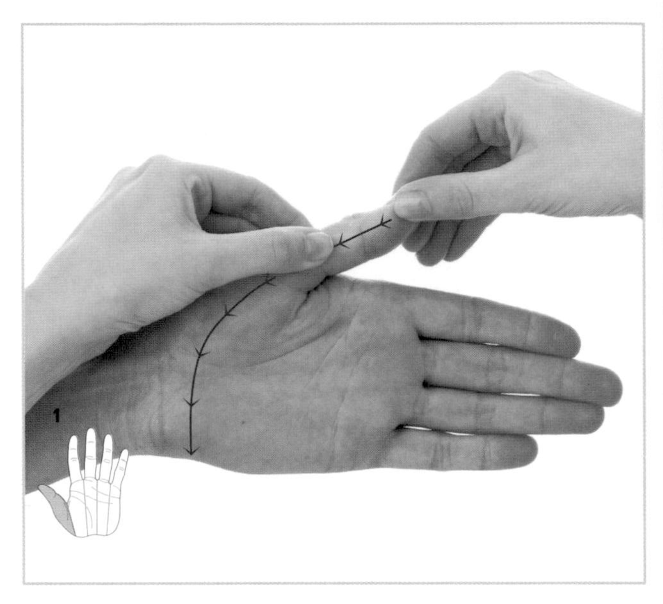

2 Use your right thumb to work back down the line of the spine as indicated.

The brain

Right hand

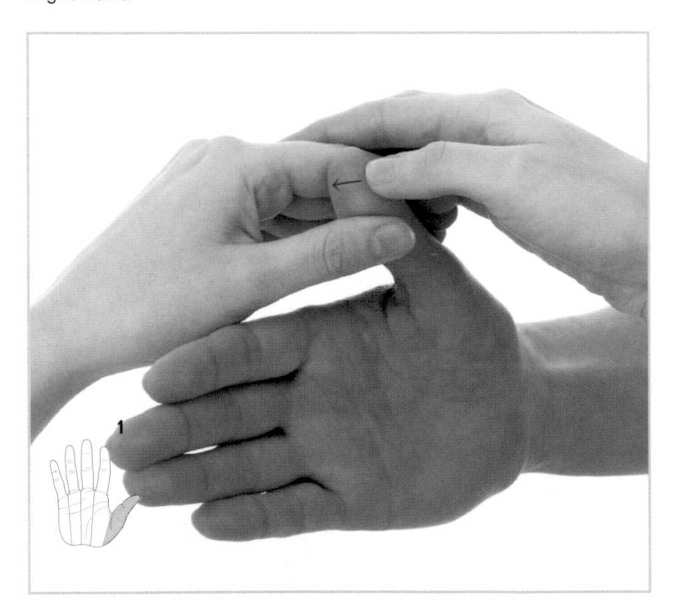

1 To work the right side of the brain, apply pressure with your right thumb directly to the top of the thumb.

Left hand

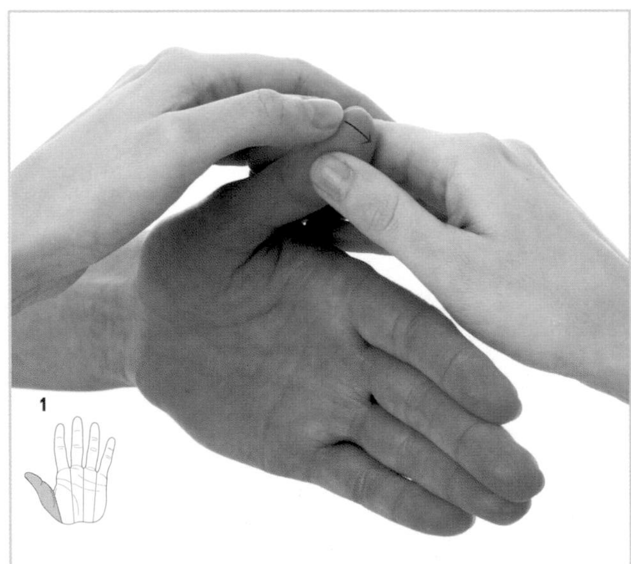

2 To work the left side of the brain, apply pressure with your left thumb directly to the top of the thumb.

The shoulder

Right hand – plantar
Medial to lateral

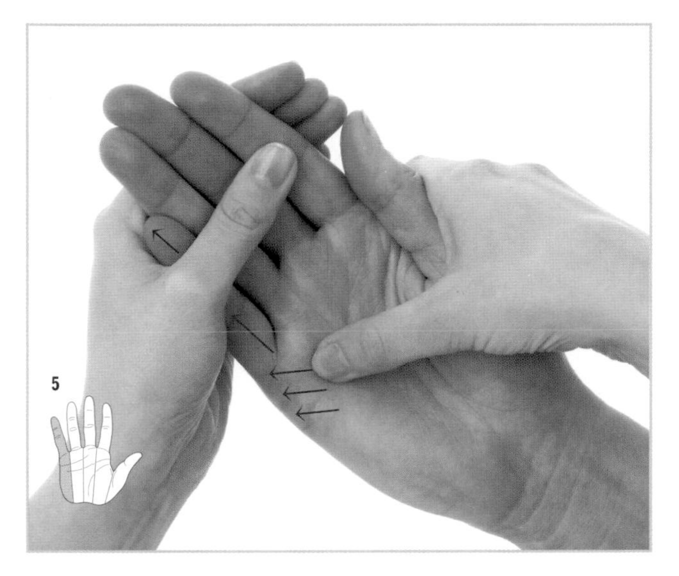

1 To work the right shoulder, use your right thumb to apply pressure to the area indicated, working from the medial to the lateral side and then continuing up the little finger.

Right hand – plantar
Lateral to medial

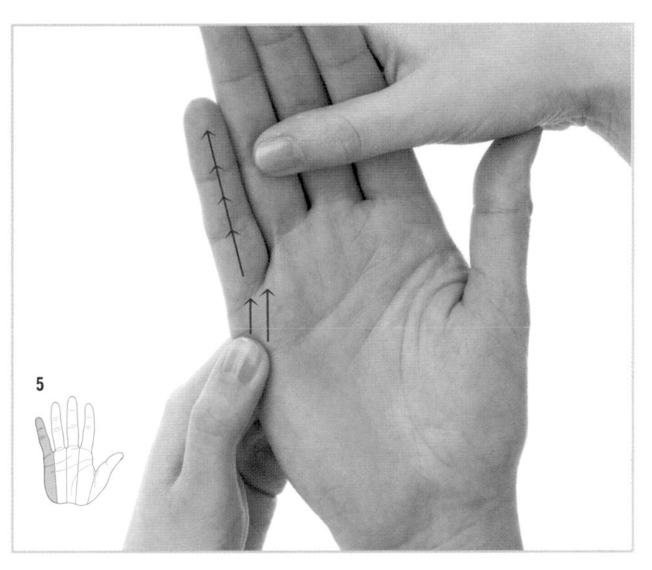

2 Use your left thumb to apply pressure to the area indicated, working from the lateral to the medial side of the hand and continuing up the little finger.

The shoulder

Left hand – plantar
Medial to lateral

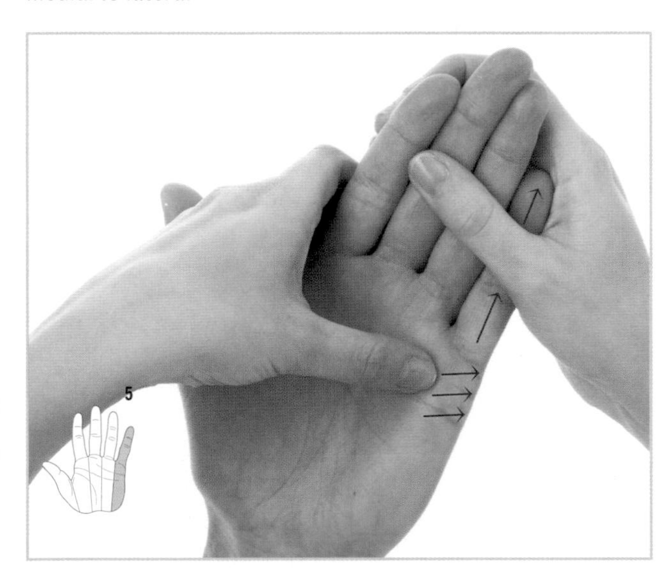

1 To work the left shoulder, use your left thumb to apply pressure to the area indicated, working from the medial to the lateral side and then continuing up the little finger.

Left hand – plantar
Lateral to medial

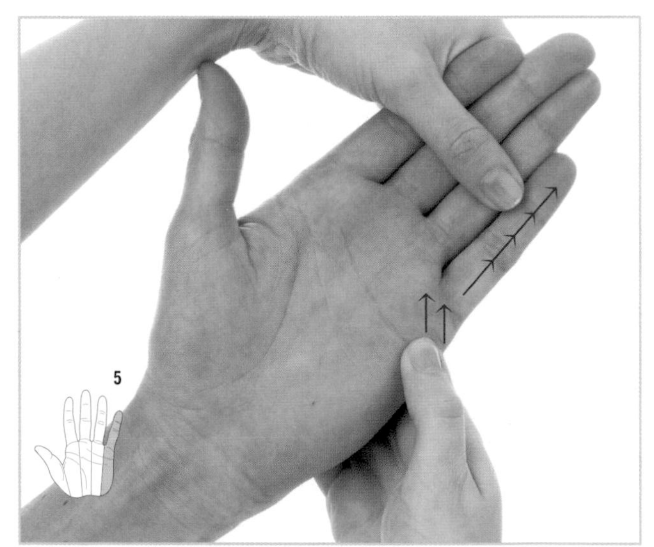

2 Use your right thumb to apply pressure to the area indicated, working from the lateral to the medial side of the hand and continuing up the little finger.

The knee and elbow

Right hand – dorsal

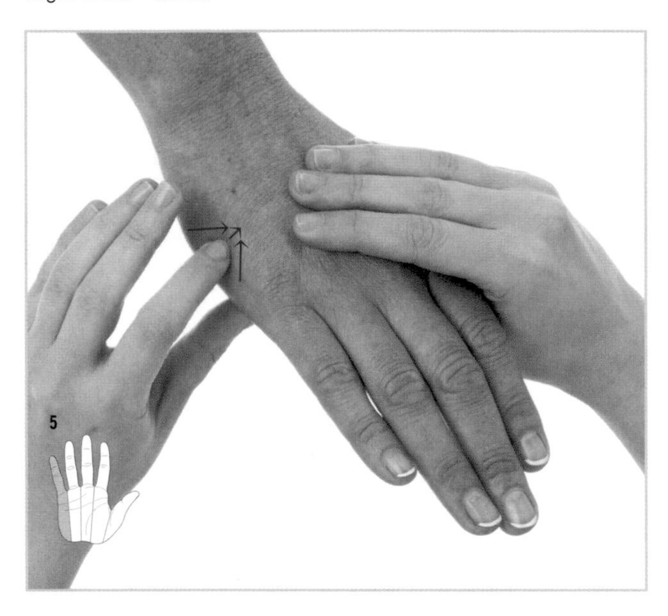

1 Work out the small triangular area indicated, using the index finger of your left hand.

Left hand – dorsal

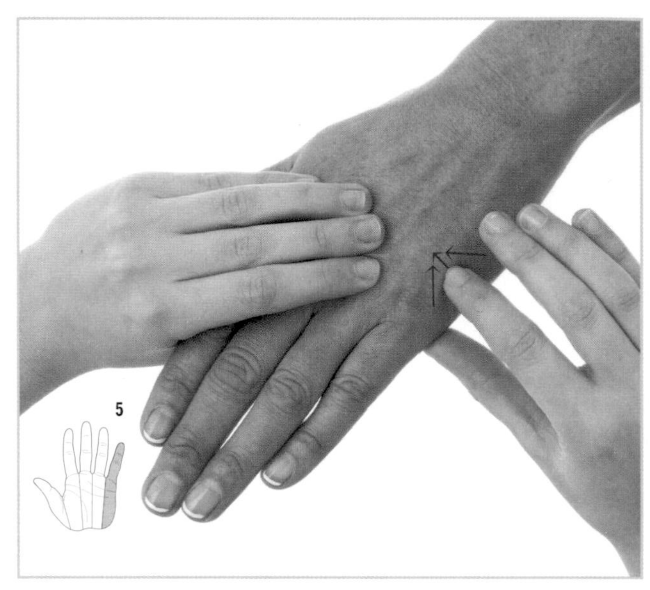

2 Work out the small triangular area indicated, using the index finger of your right hand.

The liver and gall bladder

Right hand – plantar
Medial to lateral

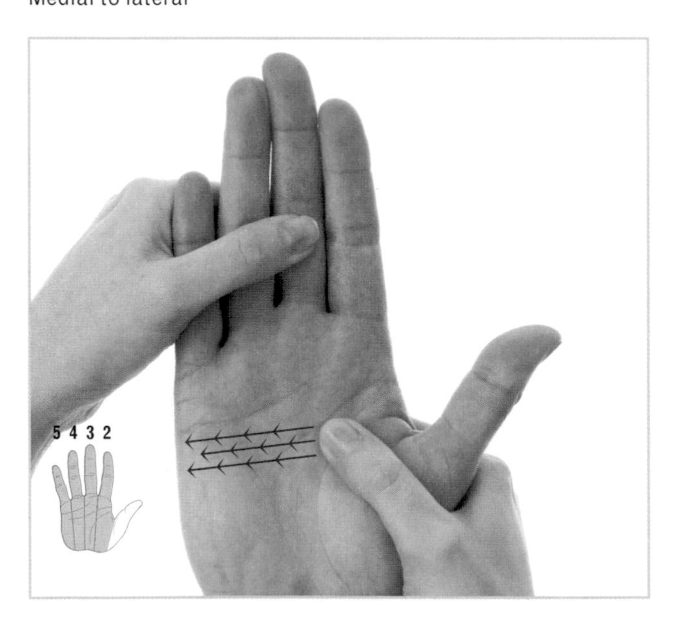

1 The reflex point for the liver and gall bladder are found on the right hand only. Use your right thumb to work over the area shown on the right palm in the direction indicated.

Right hand – plantar
Lateral to medial

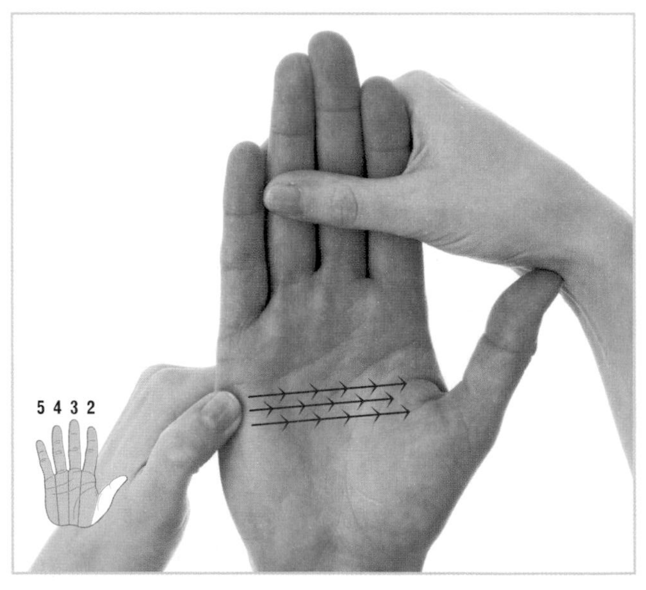

2 Use your left thumb to work over the area shown on the right palm in the direction indicated.

The stomach, pancreas and spleen

Left hand – plantar
Medial to lateral

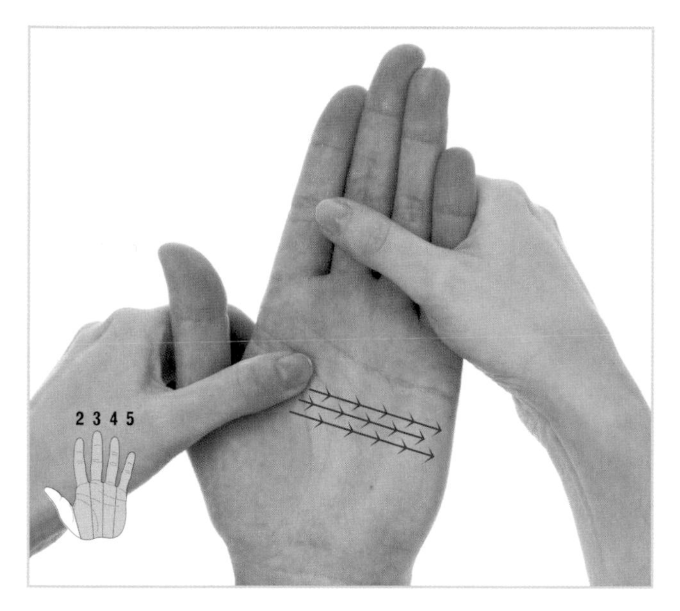

1 The reflex points for these parts of the body are found only on the left hand. Use your left thumb to work over the area shown from the medial to the lateral side of the left palm.

Left hand – plantar
Lateral to medial

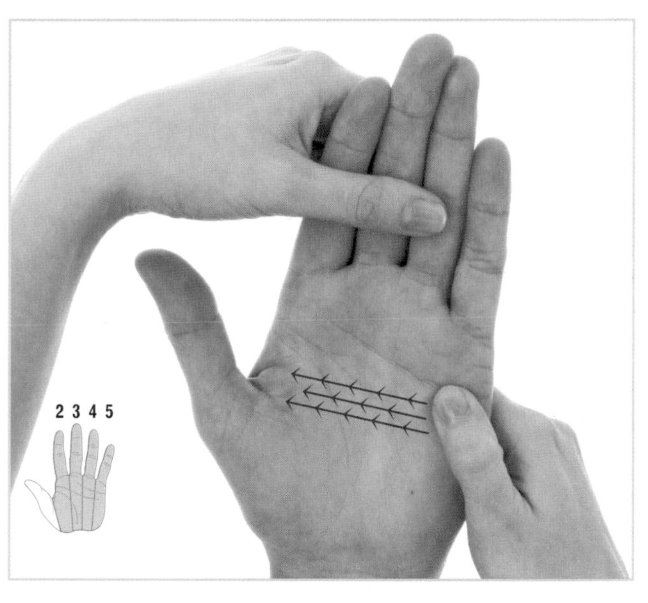

2 Use your right thumb to work over the area shown from the lateral to the medial side of the left palm.

The ascending, transverse and descending colon

Right hand – plantar
Medial to lateral

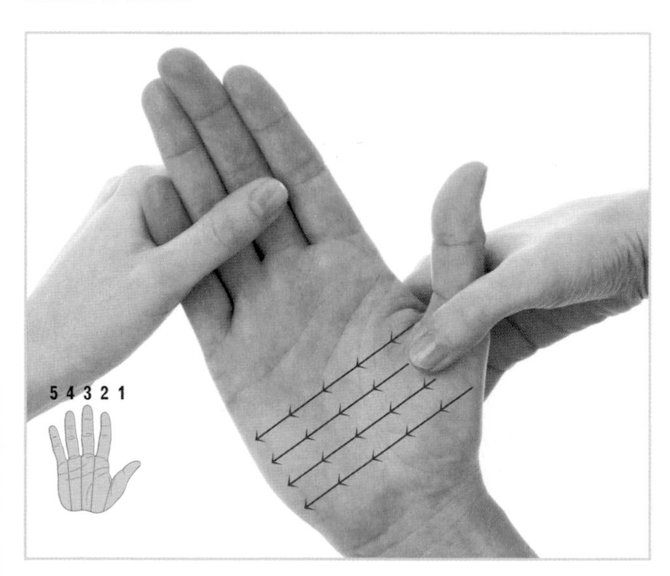

1 Using your right thumb, work across the area indicated on the right palm, working from the medial to the lateral side of the hand.

Right hand – plantar
Lateral to medial

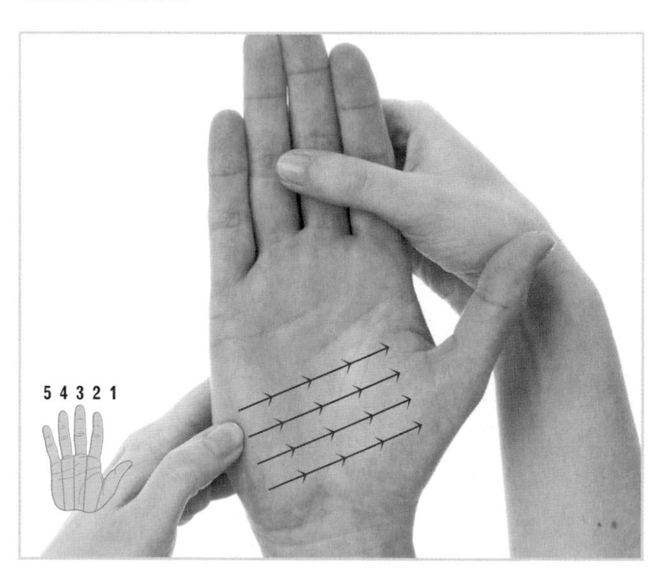

2 Using your left thumb, work across the area indicated on the right palm, working from the lateral to the medial side of the hand.

The ascending, transverse and descending colon

Left hand – plantar
Medial to lateral

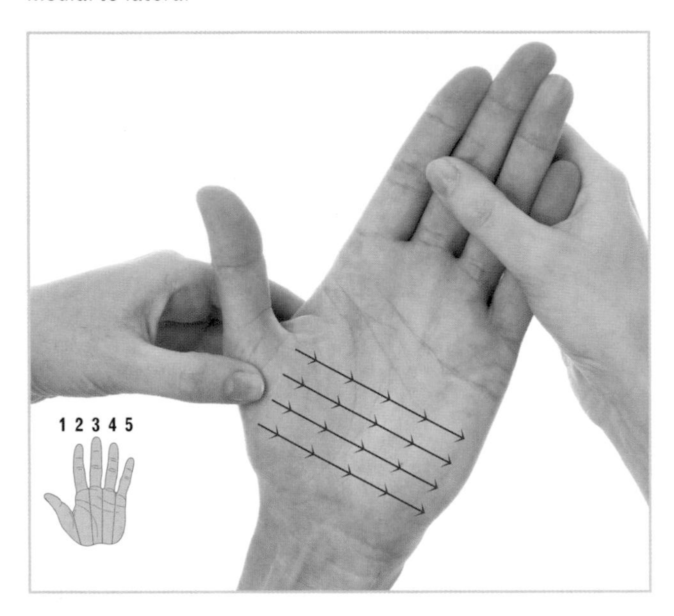

1 Using your left thumb, work across the area indicated on the left palm, working from the medial to the lateral side of the hand.

Left hand – plantar
Lateral to medial

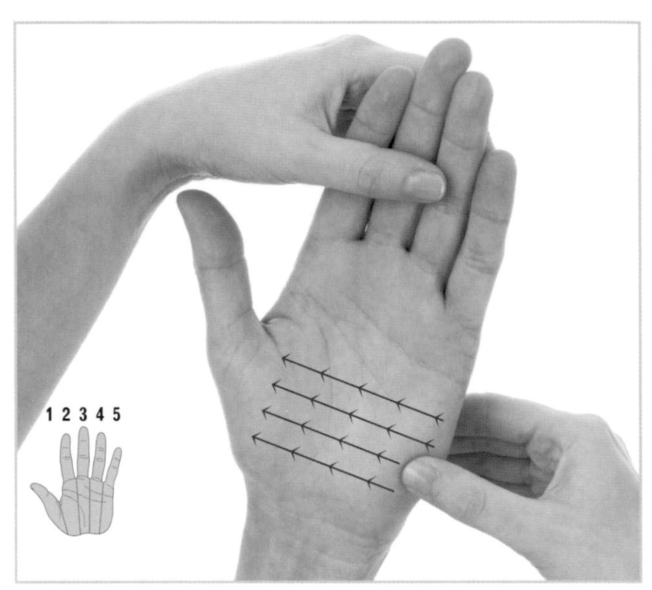

2 Using your right thumb, work across the area indicated on the left palm, working from the lateral to the medial side of the hand.

The bladder

Right hand – plantar

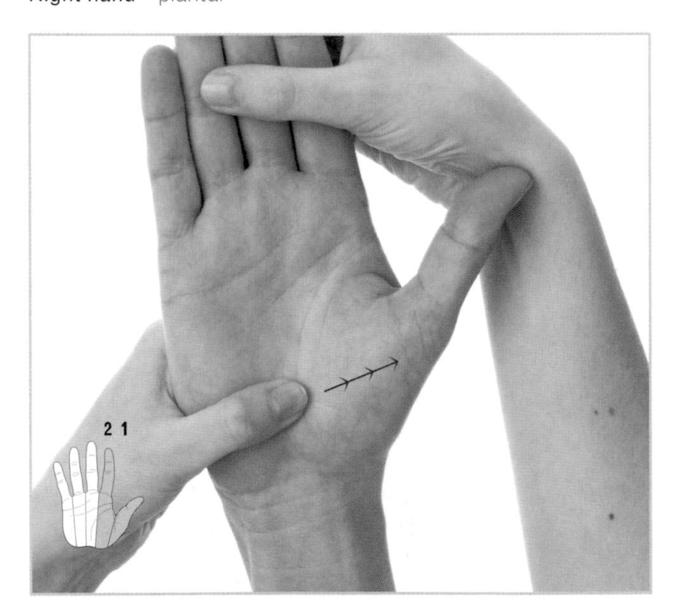

1 Supporting the hand with your right hand and using your left thumb, apply pressure to the fleshy pad just below the thumb.

Left hand – plantar

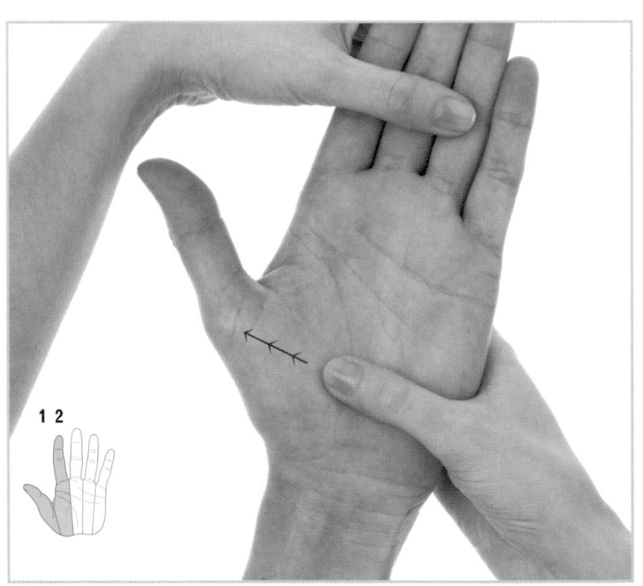

2 Supporting the hand with your left hand and using your right thumb, apply pressure to the fleshy pad just below the thumb.

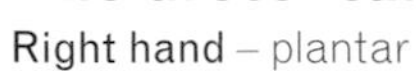

The ureter tube

Right hand – plantar

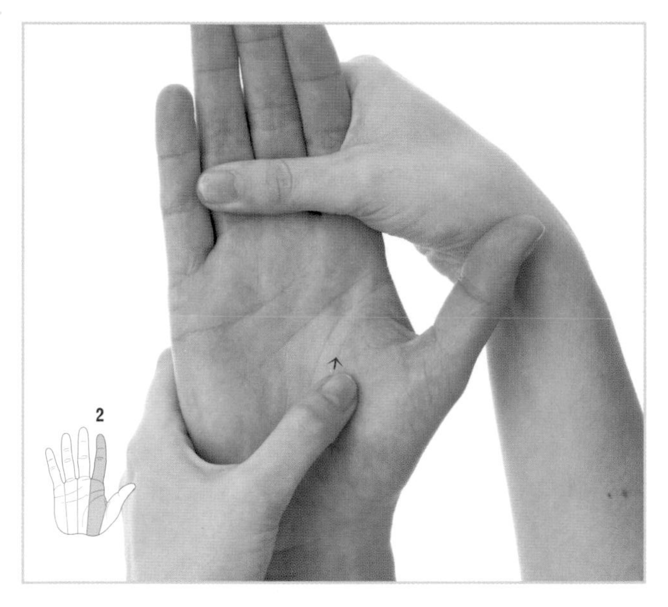

1 Working with your left thumb, continue from the bladder area (see above) towards the base of the index finger.

Left hand – plantar

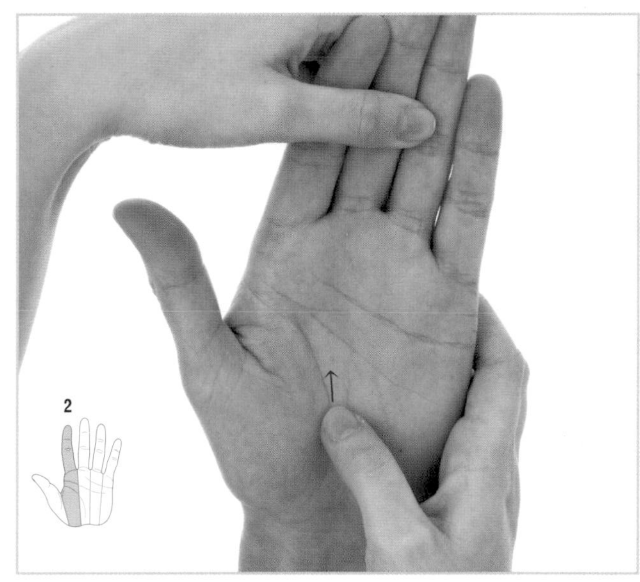

2 Working with your right thumb, continue from the bladder area (see above) towards the base of the index finger.

The kidneys

Right hand – plantar

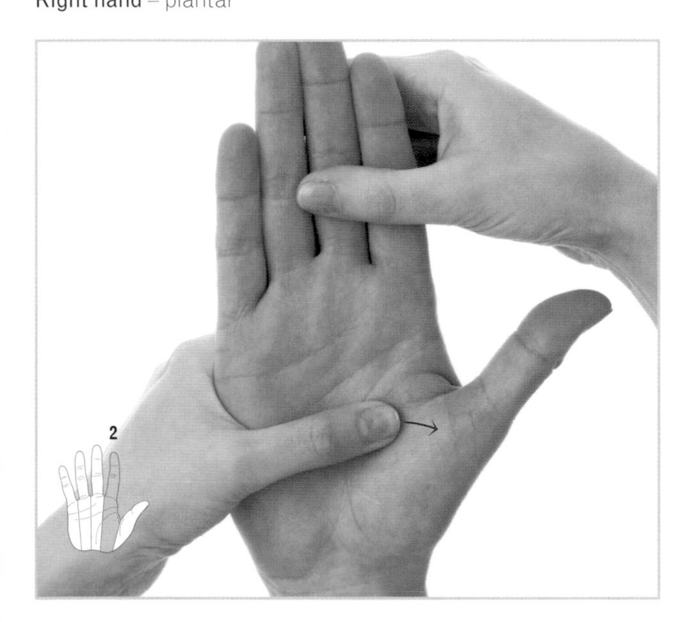

1 You will find the reflex point to the kidney just above the area to the ureter tube (see above). Work over this point with your left thumb.

Left hand – plantar

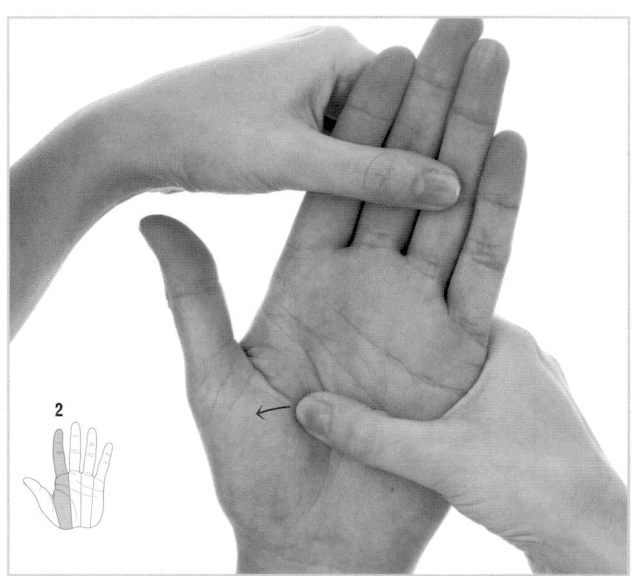

2 You will find the reflex point to the kidney just above the area to the ureter tube (see above). Work over this point with your right thumb.

The uterus/prostate

Right hand – dorsal

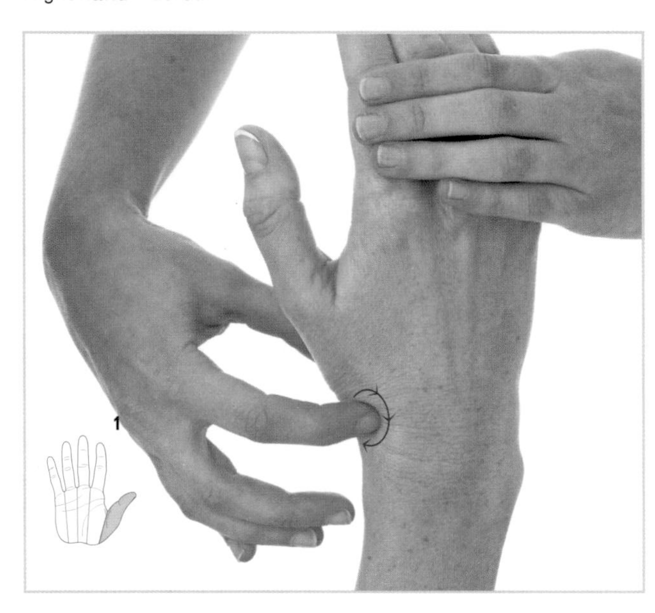

1 Using the index finger of your right hand, make contact with and work out the reflex points on the area of your wrist below the thumb.

Left hand – dorsal

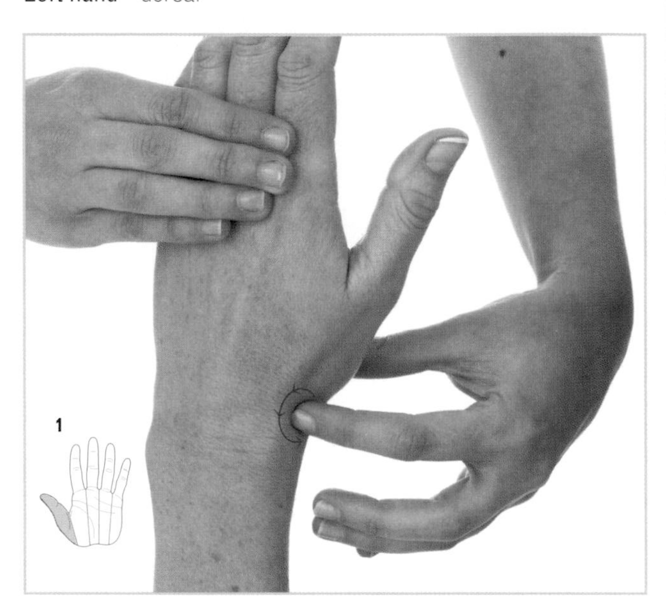

2 Using the index finger of your left hand make contact with and work out the reflex points on the area of your wrist below the thumb.

The ovaries/testes

Right hand – dorsal

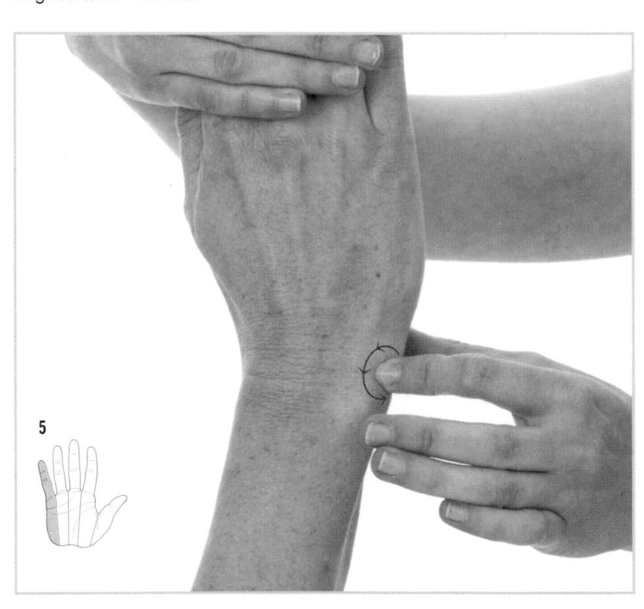

1 Use the index finger of your left hand to contact and work the reflex point just in front of the right wrist bone.

Left hand – dorsal

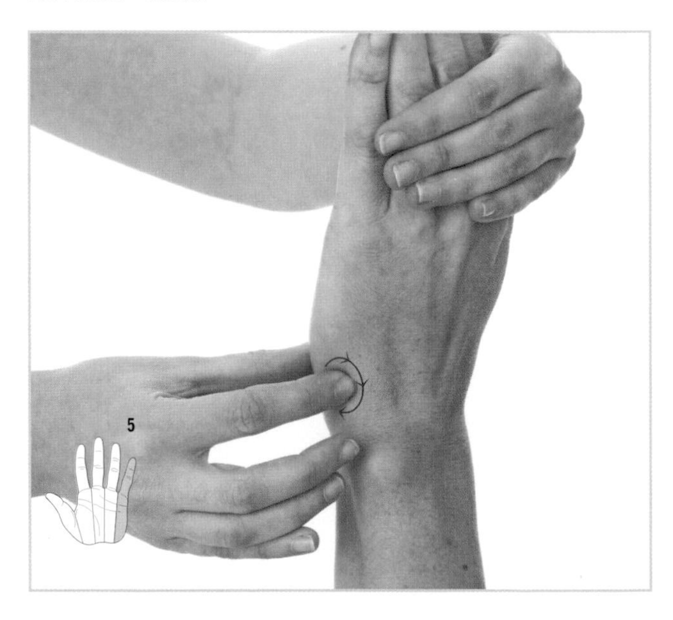

2 Use the index finger of your right hand to contact and work the reflex point just in front of the left wrist bone.

Fallopian tubes/vas deferens

Right hand – dorsal

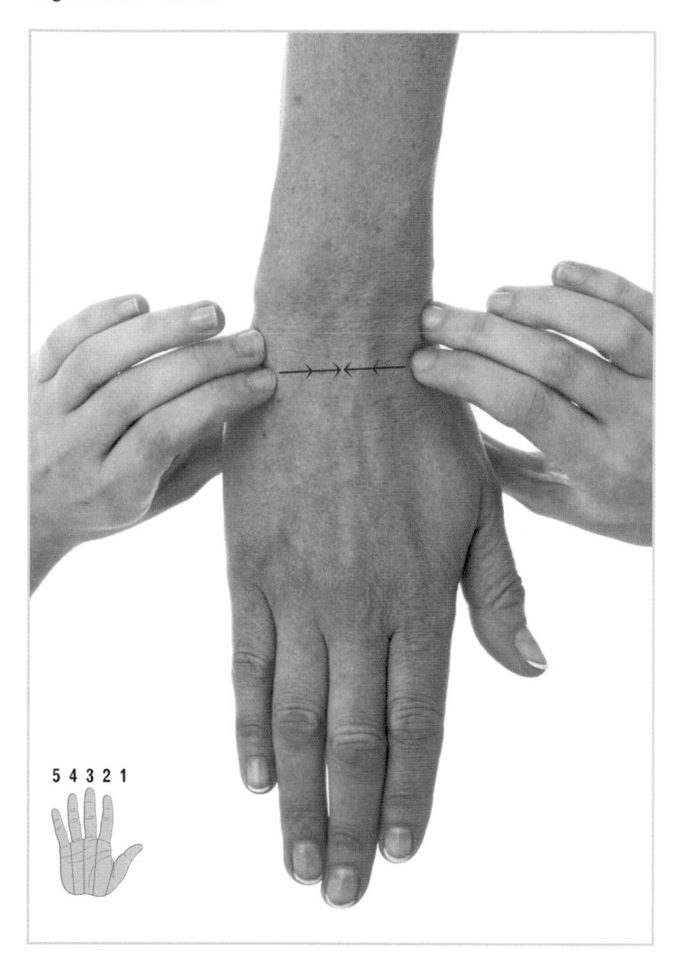

1 Applying pressure from the index and middle fingers of both hands, work out the area across the top of the wrist, as shown.

Left hand – dorsal

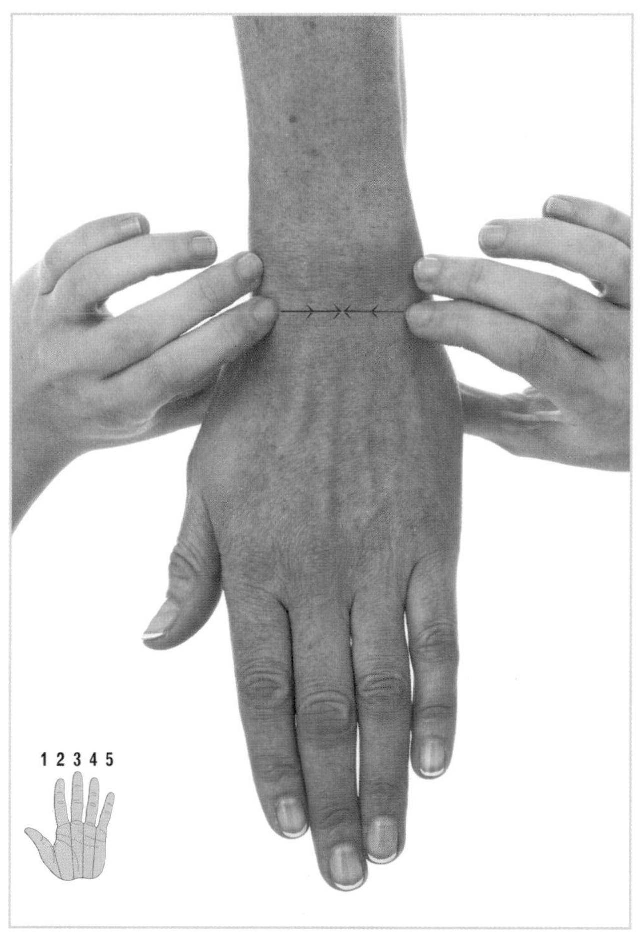

2 Applying pressure from the index and middle fingers of both hands, work out the area across the top of the wrist, as shown.

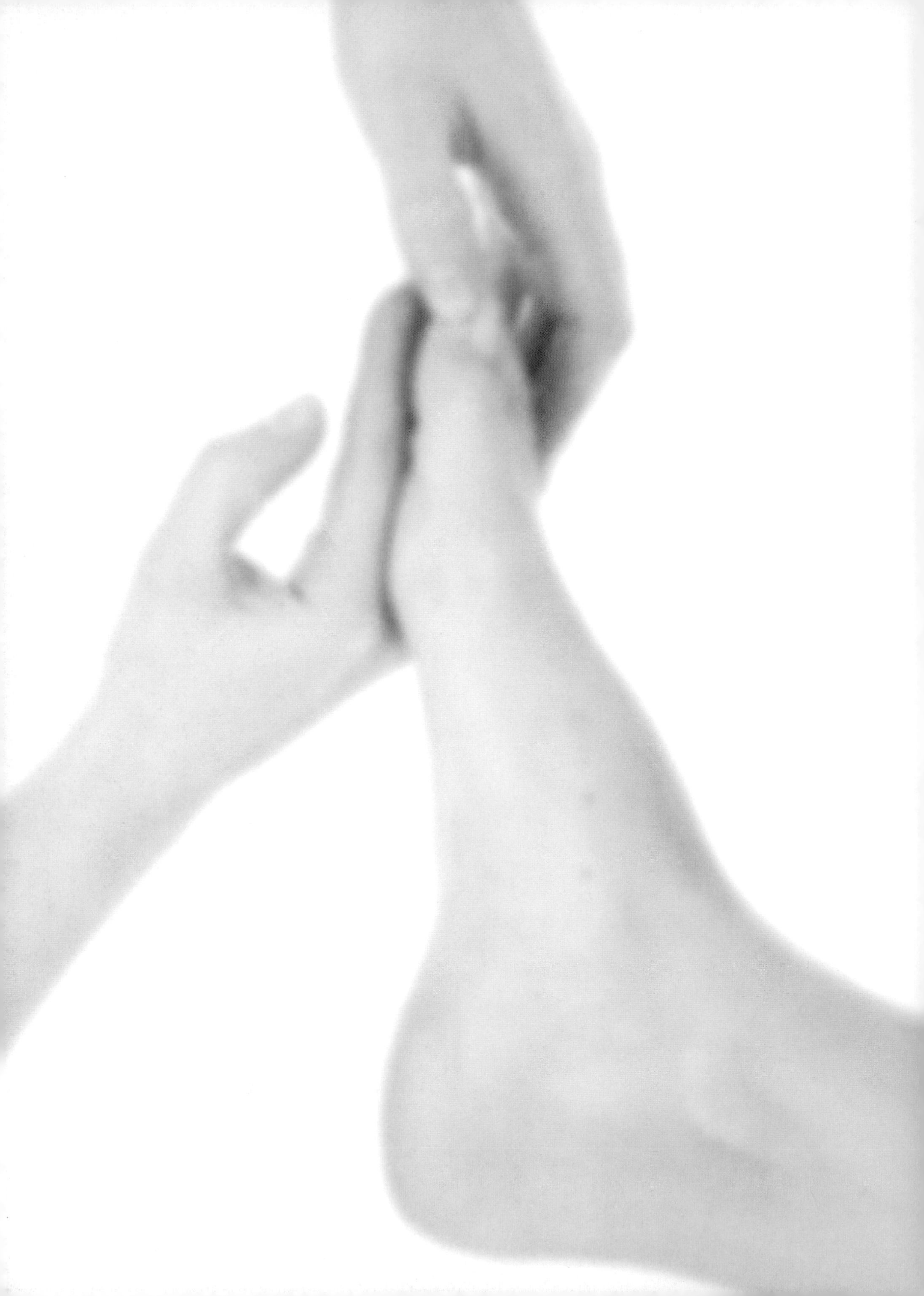

Reflexology for better health

Ailments and illnesses are often the result of a surprisingly complex combination of factors, but underlying most is a weakness in the immune system. If the body's immune system always functioned at its absolute optimum we would seldom be prey to illness, but lifestyle and stress reduce its effectiveness. As well as exploring how we can boost our immune system and reduce unwanted stresses on body and mind, this chapter includes useful checklists on which reflex areas it is especially effective to treat in different cases.

The immune system

Our resistance to illness, and how quickly and effectively we combat it, is controlled by our immune system. This complex system involves many different parts of the body and is strengthened and weakened by how we treat it from birth. Reflexology can boost the immune system, helping us get well and stay well.

A complex network, including the thymus gland, spleen, bone marrow, adenoids, tonsils and the lymphatic system, works to create the delicate system of checks and balances that is the immune system.

The body's warriors

As discussed in 'The lymphatic system', the thymus gland and bone marrow produce lymphocytes (see page 96), the specialized white blood cells that search for and destroy undesirable invaders such as bacteria, viruses and fungal parasitic infections. Under the influence of the nervous system, immune cells also carry receptors for brain hormones and transmitters, triggering the body's defensive responses whenever there is a need.

The immune system mounts an individualized response to each microorganism as it turns up. An acquired immunity to, for example, the measles virus will not help fight chickenpox: the immune system must make a specific response to deal with each specific invader.

NATURAL AND ACQUIRED IMMUNITY

We are born with an innate immunity, called natural, passive or first-line immunity. This is partly physical (beginning with the skin) and partly inherited. Early immunity can be boosted if a baby is breastfed, since this allows antibodies to be passed to the baby through the mother's milk. The body's adaptive immune system is often referred to as acquired immunity, as it evolves in response to specific microbial invaders encountered over the years. Once immunity to a specific organism has developed it remains 'on file', so that if we should contact that organism again, the body will be able to switch on a vigorous response to deal with the invader.

Successive lines of defence

The body's very first barrier against infection is the skin. Although many of us are most concerned about the quality of our skin from a cosmetic point of view, we should never forget that it plays a pivotal role in maintaining our overall health. In conjunction with keeping our various body parts contained, the skin also plays a central role in keeping undesirable visitors out. A cut or abrasion breaks this vitally important seal and potentially allows invaders to get in and set up the process of infection.

Protecting our various orifices are other buffers: the hairs in our nose and mucous membranes of the nose, mouth, throat and vagina. Infective material that makes its way past these first-line defences encounters a second line of defence, which includes the tonsils, adenoids and lymph nodes. This means that comparatively little gets as far as the bloodstream.

Vaccine-induced immunity

Modern medicine has also provided another form of defence: vaccination. Conventional medicine regards the process of vaccination as providing us with an effective defence against infectious diseases. However, many alternative therapists have pointed out that protection through vaccination may be subtly different from the strengthening effects of naturally acquired immunity.

Vaccines involve comparatively large amounts of antigens injected directly into the bloodstream, effectively by-passing the body's first-line defences. As a result the immune system registers this as an invasion. Alternative therapists regard this overly taxing assault on the immune system as being partly responsible for the

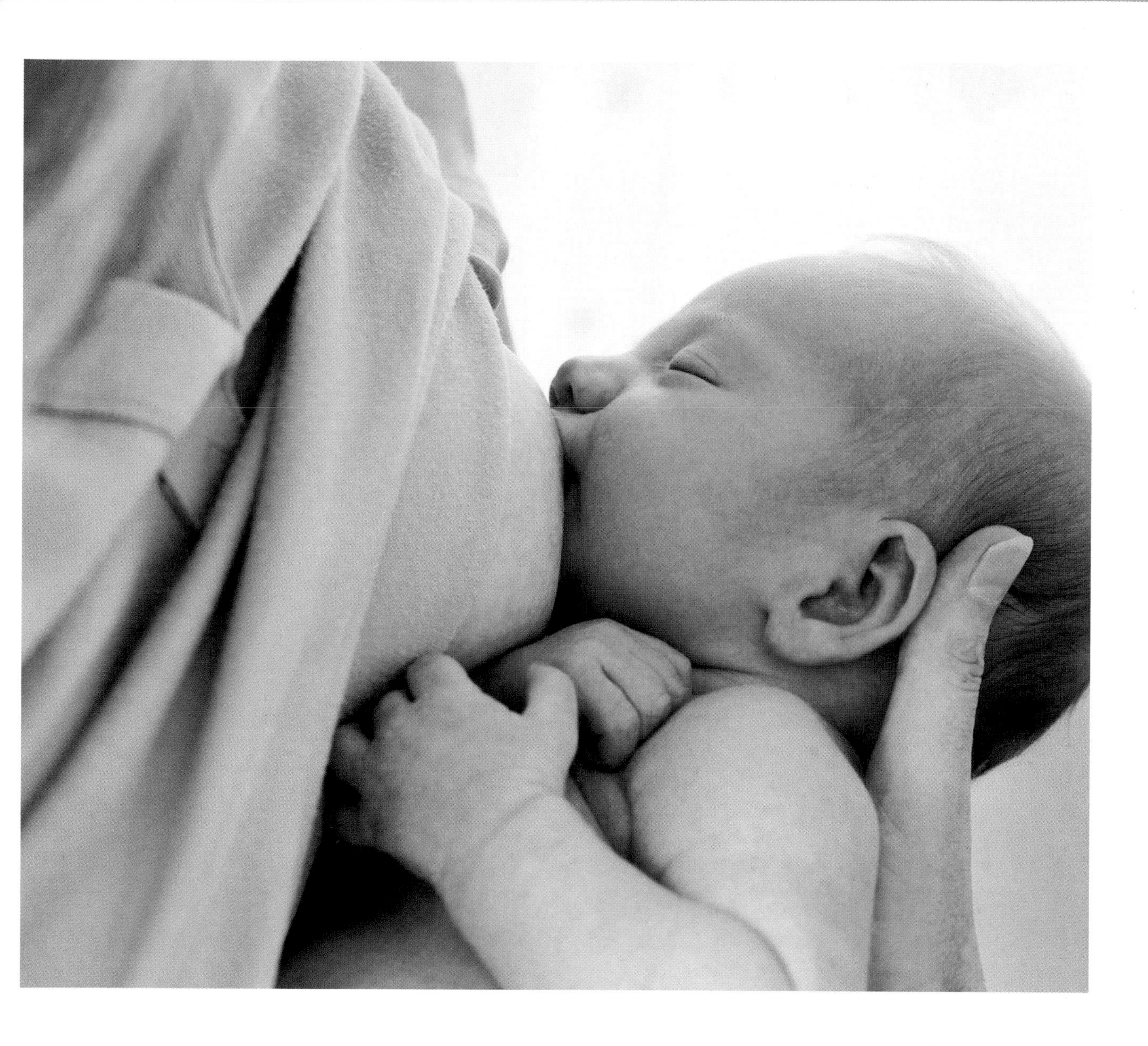

Boosting natural immunity A mother's antibodies are passed to the baby via her breast milk, strengthening the child's immune system.

symptoms some patients report. They will say that they have never felt fully well since a course of vaccination, and some will report additional problems after a severe reaction to vaccination, including allergies, persistent catarrhal problems, increased problems with asthma and recurrent chest or ear infections.

Antibiotics

Constant use of antibiotics reduces the effectiveness of the immune system and vaccinations have had a drastic effect on the ability to fight off childhood infections such as measles, mumps, chickenpox, rubella and whooping cough. These illnesses stimulate the immune system to cope with disease and encourage the spleen to work efficiently in producing antibodies that give natural immunity. Vaccination does not give this same natural protection and reduces natural immunity in the population at large.

We will never be without diseases; they are an integral part of life, but we can do much to help ourselves, if we make the effort to be responsible for what we do to our own bodies. I believe that prevention is a far better way than looking for ever more treatments to relieve disease.

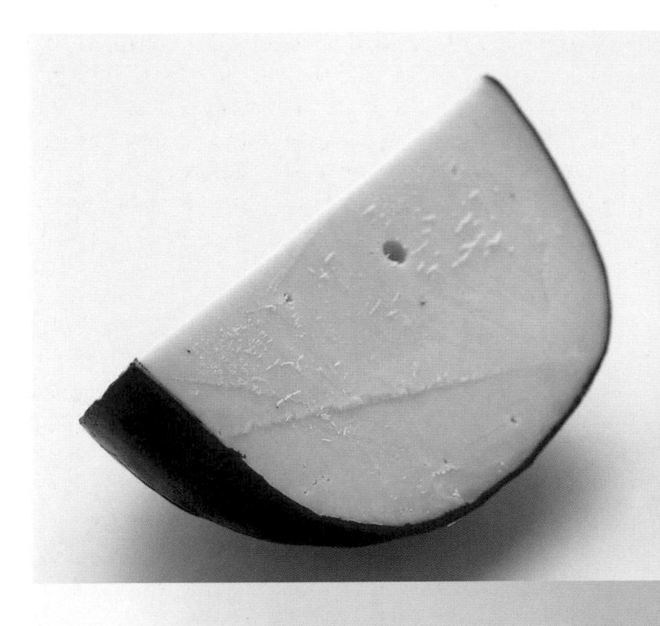

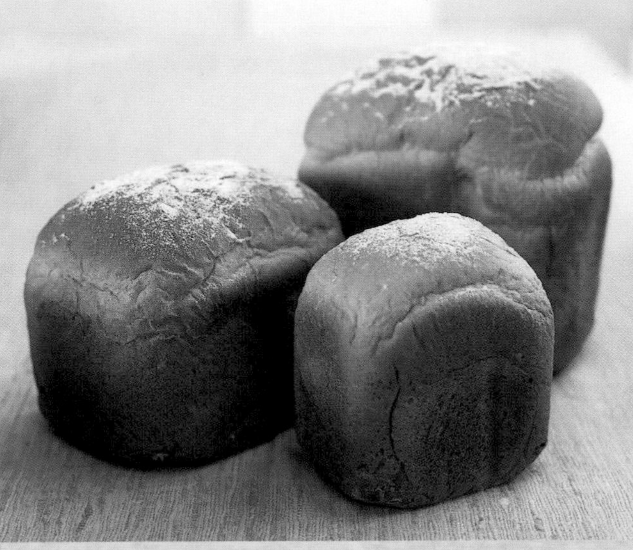

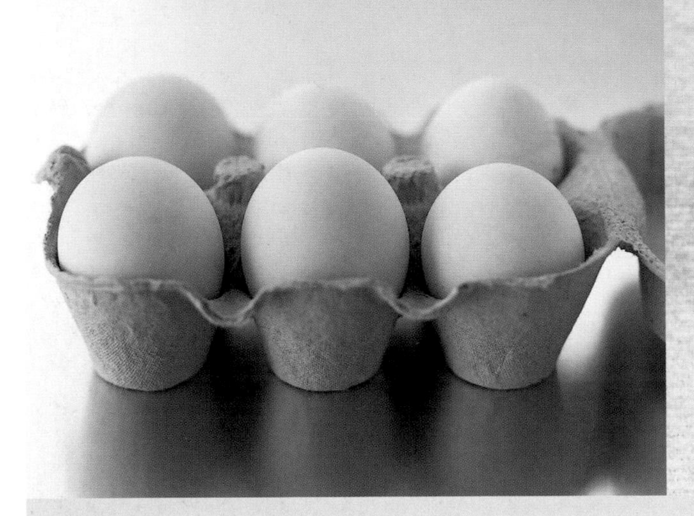

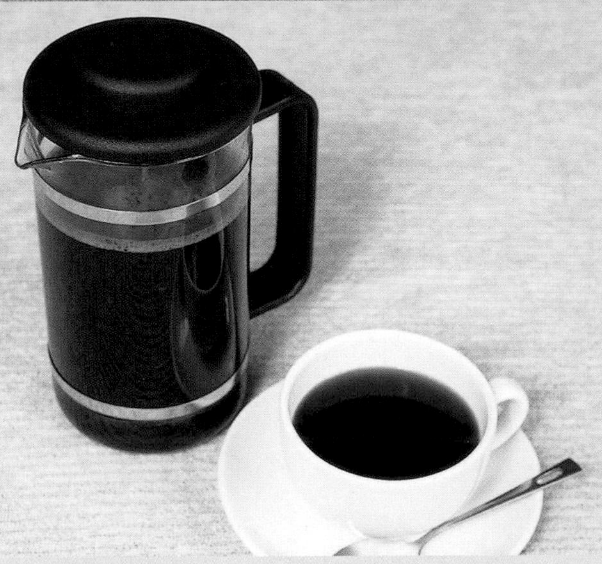

ALLERGIC RESPONSES

If the body's immune system becomes hypersensitive it can go into overdrive due to agents that are harmless under normal conditions. Such innocuous substances as pollen, dust, animal fur and certain foods can all cause such over-reaction in the body, resulting in asthma, hay fever, eczema, sickness or other allergic responses.

A classic allergic response is characterized by a rise in substances known as IgE antibodies. When an IgE antibody comes across an invader, it triggers a release of chemicals, including histamine. That is why a common conventional medical solution to allergic symptoms involves prescribing antihistamines.

An IgE reaction is swift in nature and easily defined, but a cell-mediated response may result in more subtle symptoms. These may not show straight away and can include anything from digestive disorders, such as irritable bowel syndrome, to hyperactivity and poor concentration in children. Symptoms may be triggered by exposure to a range of everyday foods, including sugar, tea, coffee, dairy products such as cheese, wheat, corn and eggs.

A robust immune system

An immune system that is functioning well will mount a rapid attack against any organism it recognizes from past experience. The response may be so efficient that we may not even realize we have been 'invaded' (indeed, we all have cancer cells circulating in our bodies, but fortunately in most cases the immune cells recognize and deal with them). However, if the organism is a new visitor to our body, full response may take a few days. During this interval we may notice that our glands are painful, inflamed and swollen and that our temperature rises. These are signs that the white blood cells are incubating a supply of antibodies in the lymph nodes and that our body is fighting an infection.

Most conventional drugs work by dampening down these signs. This brings short-term relief, but suppression means the infection is more likely to linger. The same is true of using medication designed to temporarily suppress a cough or dry up nasal mucus. The body has produced a cough or streaming nose to get as much toxic waste out as fast as possible, and interfering with the process is likely to mean that we are going to feel unwell for longer than we would if we supported the body's capacity for self-healing.

A weakened immune system

If an immune system is not in good shape we are likely to experience a variety of illnesses until our defence system is able to rebalance itself. If problems with the immune system continue in the long term, we run the risk of moving from minor health problems, such as allergies, recurrent infections or skin disorders, to more serious conditions, including various forms of cancer and auto-immune diseases such as rheumatoid arthritis.

Common problems that can arise as a result of a generally sluggish or poorly functioning immune system include recurrent colds, repeated bouts of urinary infections, poor resistance to any bug that happens to be around and a chronic weariness.

An immune system can be weakened not only by an onslaught of viruses, bacteria and toxins, but by lack of exposure to 'everyday' threats through which to build up a store of immune responses. In the Western world, most babies and children do not get the opportunity to build a strong immune system because they encounter so little in the way of bacteria and dirt. Today's immune systems are over-protected and often never learn to do their job.

Emotional troubles can also dangerously damage the immune system. An extreme example is that of a woman called Martina, who was born in Germany and had never had a day's illness in her life until, at the age of 35, she lost her only child, a much loved daughter aged just three years old, to leukaemia. Despite counselling and support from her husband and friends, Martina could not accept this loss and over the following year she too faded away and died of the same disease as her daughter. Her loss and grief had affected her immune system in such a way that it could no longer support her body's needs. This is a true example of how the power of the mind can affect the functions of the body.

HIV and AIDS

A healthy immune system depends on two types of T cells (helper and suppressor) working in harmony to protect the body. A serious problem can develop if the suppressor cells become dominant, making the immune system weak or deficient. This can occur as a result of a genetically inherited condition or when an opportunistic infection, such as the human immunodeficiency virus (HIV), moves in.

HIV attacks the helper T cells, destroying an essential link in the functioning of the immune system. The result is a cycle of infections, including chronically swollen glands, thrush, cold sores, genital herpes and extreme exhaustion. If untreated, most HIV-infected individuals go on to develop AIDS (acquired immune deficiency syndrome).

How reflexology can help

It takes a great deal of energy to fight off infection. We could do worse than learn from animals who, when they are sick, will stop eating (which avoids diverting energy to digesting food) and rest somewhere quiet and away from threat or stress. Resting induces a peaceful state of mind and is paramount in aiding the body's recovery.

Reflexology creates a great sense of relaxation for the body, mind and spirit, which supports an immune system fighting off disease. It helps to stimulate the elimination of toxic waste products from the liver, kidneys and bowel, improves nerve and blood supply and normalizes the body function.

The immune system has been shown to be profoundly influenced by severe emotional and physical shock, as well as by protracted stress. Our mental and emotional health can have a significant effect on the immune system; many people succumb to an illness after a period of extreme stress, the loss of a partner through bereavement or divorce, redundancy or worries about children. Reflexology's ability to induce relaxation and relieve tension is of immense value (see 'Stress', pages 194–196). We need reflexology on a regular basis, particularly when life is stressful and difficult, in order to assist the function of this vital system.

Stress

Stress is the most common cause of ill-health in modern society, probably underlying as many as 70 per cent of all visits to family doctors. It is vital to recognize when stress is affecting us adversely, and reflexology can be among the steps taken to counter its unhealthy effects.

Stress can be defined as any influence that interrupts or disturbs the functioning of the body: joints and muscles are put under stress when we run, for example, and exposure to the cold puts our whole body under physical stress. But whereas we will pay attention to a pulled muscle or frostbite, symptoms of mental or emotional stresses can all too often be overlooked or become accepted as a part of life, to the detriment of our physical and mental health.

Causes, effects and reactions

We can all reel off a number of well-known causes of emotional stress. These include bereavement, work problems, relationship difficulties, divorce, taking tests or examinations, moving house and financial worries, to name but a few.

A situation that makes one person emotionally or mentally stressed may have no effect at all on another, and everyone experiences stress a little differently. Some become angry or tearful or take it out on others. Others internalize it and develop eating disorders, start drinking too much or develop phobias. Someone who suffers from a chronic illness may find that the symptoms flare up under an overload of stress. People with underlying anxieties or insecurities may over-react, making even small difficulties seem like a crisis – the straw that breaks the camel's back.

Our early conditioning plays a part in this. A fearful mother who lacks self-confidence and sees doom and gloom in life situations will unwittingly teach her children to react in the same way. Friends, family background, teachers, education and religious beliefs all influence how we cope with what life throws at us. The threshold of a person's self-confidence often dictates how they react emotionally or mentally to an event and how many physical ill-effects they suffer as a result.

Chronic stress

The most insidious form of stress is that which, rather than being attributable to a particular dramatic event or pressure, takes the form of an ever-present underlying problem. This is exhausting, both mentally and physically, and can weaken the body's immune system, making you vulnerable to a variety of illnesses. Chronic stress can take the form of emotional worry, such as an unhappy relationship, but also external forces, such as pollution and noise.

Long-term or acute emotional and/or mental stress invariably takes its toll on the body with symptoms such as muscle stiffness, high blood pressure, excessive perspiration, headaches, poor immunity or a general lack of interest in life. These in turn affect other aspects of health: high blood pressure will lead to a susceptibility to coronary artery disease, strokes and heart attacks.

WHEN STRESS IS GOOD

Stress is not all bad, however. It is the body's way of rising to a challenge and preparing to meet a tough situation with focus, strength, stamina and a heightened state of alert (see page 102). Many human achievements would not have happened without the impetus of the 'adrenaline rush'. Few mountains would have been climbed, great athletic records set or discoveries made. Without 'good stresses' we would go through life like a limp lettuce leaf!

Stress By diminishing the efficiency of the immune system, the stress that many people encounter in their daily lives threatens the physical health of the body.

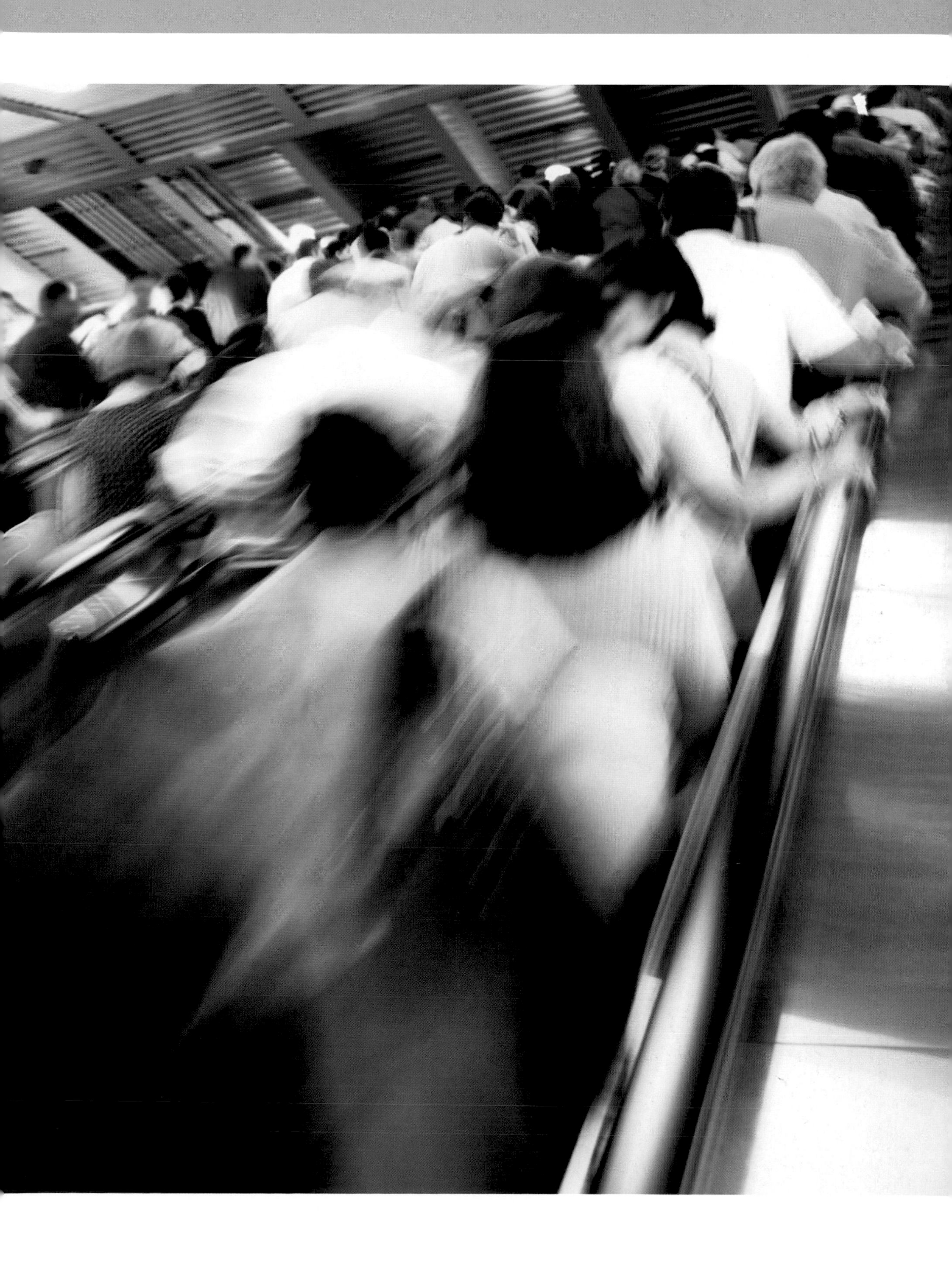

Hormones secreted by the adrenal glands reduce the activity of certain white blood cells that provide our bodies with resistance to infection and assist in other vital processes of the immune system.

In 'The endocrine system', the instinctive 'fight or flight' reactions set off by our adrenal glands was described (see pages 101–102) and some of the physical effects of inappropriate or chronic stress were listed. Stress can also bring on nervousness, irritability, anxiety, chronic fatigue or insomnia, and be at the root of other problems, such as:

- Allergies
- Eczema
- Loss of sex drive
- Cravings for sugar, caffeine, tobacco or alcohol
- Inability to concentrate
- General lack of interest in life
- Panic attacks
- Eating disorders
- Aggression.

Coping with stress

We need to build relaxation into our lives, whether that is through reflexology, meditation, breathing techniques, yoga, massage, tai chi, swimming or whatever form of relaxation takes your fancy. Just a walk in the country can be an excellent restorative.

Exercise in particular is highly recommended. When we are nervous we tend to pace around or strum our fingers: our body is trying to give us a message – it wants to move. Exercise has a stimulating effect on the body and burns up toxicity as well as increasing our oxygen supply. Nothing beats aerobic exercise for draining off stress energy and there are so many different types of suitable exercise to choose from, from running and cycling to dance classes and games such as badminton or football.

The body has a natural antidote to stress, called the 'relaxation response'. The chemical reactions it sets off create a sense of wellbeing and calm. You can help trigger the relaxation response just by learning simple breathing exercises and then using them when you are caught up in a stressful situation.

Try standing in front of an open window, taking a deep breath in through your nose (imagine your breath is reaching deep down into your lower abdominal area) and feeling your rib cage expanding. Hold your breath for a few seconds and then exhale as slowly as possible. Repeat this at least ten times. It is very difficult to feel stressed when you are breathing deeply.

Here are other good ways of counteracting the unhealthy effects of stress:

- Relaxation and meditation relieve stress by stilling the mind. This could be a recognized relaxation technique or something more personal that suits you: sitting quietly by a lake, watching logs burning in an open fire or gently stroking the family pet can generate a meditative state.
- Laughter is a real tonic, reduces stress and, it has been discovered, is a great stimulant to the immune system.
- Watch what you are thinking: a healthy dose of optimism can help you make the best of things.
- Burning the candle at both ends induces weariness and an inability to cope, so be sure to get sufficient sleep whenever possible. Sleep gives your body time to restore itself, and makes you better equipped to deal with negative stresses.
- Vitamin and mineral supplements can be helpful. Magnesium and calcium work in concert to maintain nerve function. Vitamin B6 can be helpful if there are symptoms of adrenal exhaustion, and zinc and vitamin C help to restore overworked adrenal glands.
- Cut back on, or cut out, caffeine, alcohol and sugar. These all stimulate the adrenals, and alcohol has a bad effect on the liver. Remember that the liver plays an important role in eliminating toxic substances from the body, including hormones released in large amounts during stress (see page 74).

How reflexology can help

Regular reflexology treatments are an excellent method of countering all forms of stress and aiding relaxation. It is not uncommon for patients to fall asleep during a treatment session and to report that they noticed a great improvement in their sleeping pattern afterwards. They can sleep longer and are no longer disturbed by anxiety dreams or frequent wakening because their mind is plagued by worry. During deep, restful sleep, the body is able to regenerate and restore the nervous system ready for the demands of the following day.

You will be able to feel if a patient is particularly stressed when you work on the solar plexus reflex (see page 109). Stimulation of the solar plexus area during a reflexology treatment will help the patient's ability to withstand the stresses and strains of modern-day life.

Fighting stress Relaxation through activities such as meditation is a gentle but effective way of releasing tension from the body.

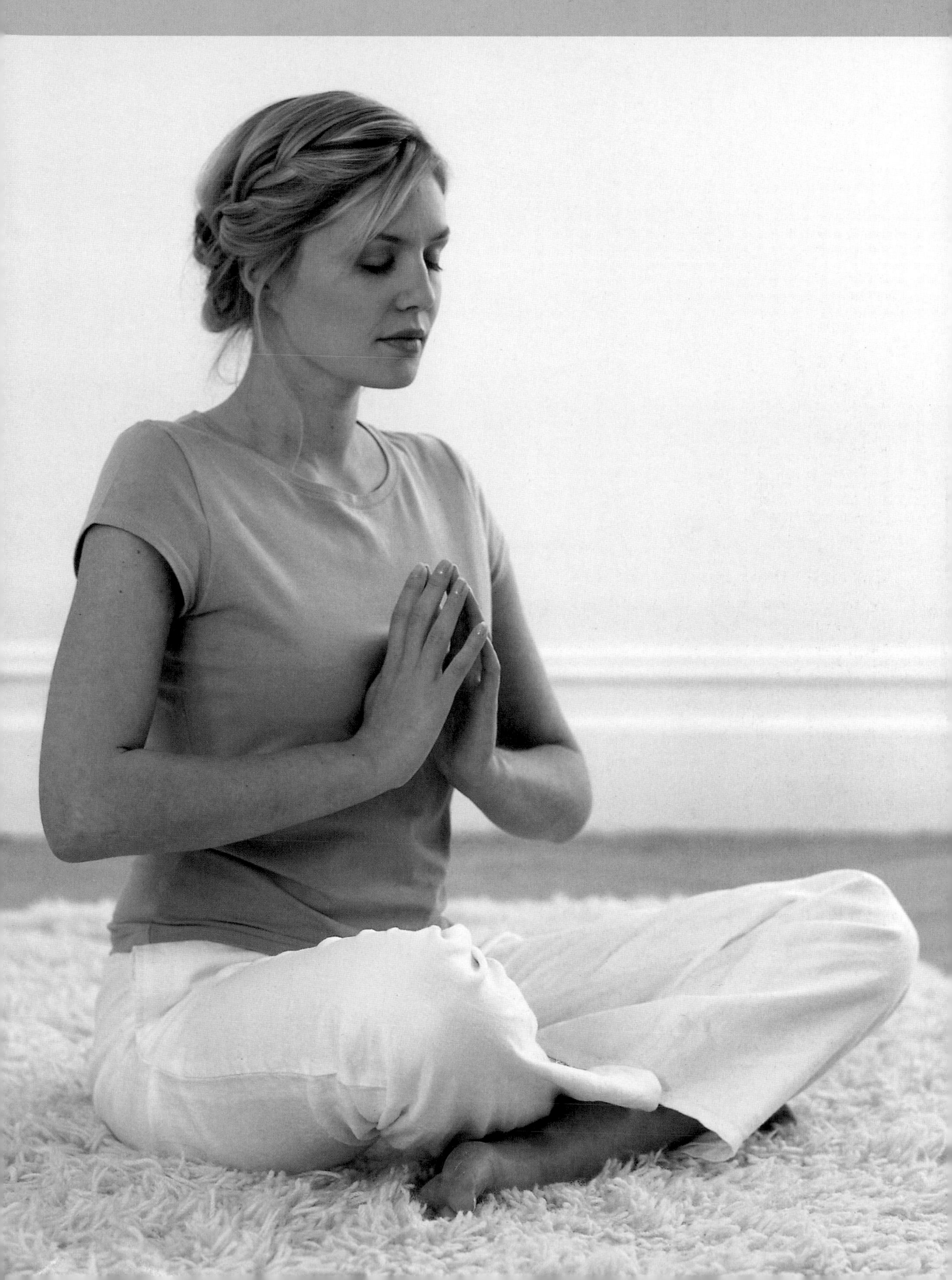

Areas of assistance

An area of assistance is an area or system of the body that is instrumental in helping to remedy dysfunctions in other parts, even though the area in question may seem to have no particular relationship to the illness. Frequently the assisted part is found to be in the same reflexology zone, details and examples of which are shown below.

Condition	Area of assistance	Why?
Shoulder conditions	Hip area.	Because they are in the same zone and treating this area of assistance balances the structure of the body.
Hip conditions	Shoulder.	As above
Asthma and all allergic and respiratory conditions, including eczema	Digestive system and adrenals.	Allergy usually starts in the digestive system in infancy. Also, the lung and digestive systems are in the same zones.
Knee conditions	Lumbar spine.	Most knee conditions other than specific troubles such as arthritis or knee injuries are caused by compression of the lumbar spinal nerves.
Eye and ear conditions	Kidney and cervical spine.	Because they are in the same zone. It is also accepted medically that the eyes are affected when there are dysfunctions in the kidney.
Infertility (if a hormonal imbalance)	Endocrine system.	Irregular cycles are often caused by hormonal imbalances.
Infertility (from organic causes)	Reproductive system.	Could have nothing to do with the hormonal system.
Pains in the calf	Lumbar spine and entire circulatory system.	Could be spinal compression in the lumbar area or a circulatory problem in the legs. This is a common symptom in diabetics and in those with arteriosclerosis when the heart can not pump blood efficiently to the extremities. This condition is commonly known as intermittent claudication.

Condition	Area of assistance	Why?
Weakness in the hands and tingling in the fingers	Cervical spine.	Compression in the neck causes these symptoms.
Underactive condition such underactive thyroid	Pituitary and adrenal glands.	To stimulate the body and encourage extra activity in the thyroid.
Any overactive condition	Solar plexus.	To bring about a calming and relaxed effect. Avoid the adrenal glands.
Vertigo (dizziness)	Cervical spine.	Improves nerve and blood supply to the head.
Lumps and cysts in the breast	Endocrine system.	These symptoms are frequently caused by an endocrine imbalance.
Palpitations (racing heart)	Stomach area.	Unless there is a known heart condition, these symptoms can be a result of indigestion causing the stomach to exert pressure on the heart.
Depression	Endocrine system.	Depression is often a hormonal imbalance.
Exhaustion	Thyroid and adrenal glands.	Helps stimulate the body.
Heart conditions	Liver and thoracic spine.	The liver has a responsibility in the circulatory system, controlling the clotting factor and cholesterol levels. Nerves in the thoracic spine help heart muscle function.
Constipation	Liver and lumbar spine.	Gall lubricates the bowel and the lumbar spinal nerves stimulate nerve function to the pelvic area.
Indigestion	Liver and thoracic spine.	Thoracic spinal nerves improve blood supply to the liver.
Migraine	Liver and cervical spine.	Helps detoxification and relaxes tension in the neck.
Fluid retention in the legs	All the main lymphatic areas plus the urinary system.	Helps balance the fluid levels and assists in elimination of excess fluid.
Varicose veins	Intestines and lumbar spine.	Any pressure in the intestinal area (such as constipation or prolapsed bowel) can cause varicose conditions of the legs. Working on the lumbar spine can improve nerve and blood supply to the pelvic areas.

Reference guide for treating specific conditions

Condition	Symptoms/description	Main areas to treat
Addison's disease	Adrenal insufficiency.	Whole of the endocrine system.
Alzheimer's disease	Degeneration of cerebral cortex. Loss of memory and paralysis.	Extensive work on whole of spine and brain, preferably daily.
Ankylosing spondylitis	Disease of joints, destruction of joint space, followed by sclerosis and calcification, resulting in rigidity of spinal column and thorax.	Spine, brain, shoulder, hip, knee, coccyx and pelvis. Adrenals to help break down inflammation.
Arteritis	Inflammation of arteries.	Heart/lung, thoracic spine, adrenals.
Asthma, *see* Bronchitis		
Bronchitis and asthma	Inflammation of bronchial tubes. Spasm of the bronchioles, resulting in difficulty in exhalation.	Heart/lung, adrenals, thoracic spine (to help nerve supply to thoracic area), digestive system (often, a weakness in the digestive system causes excessive mucus in the system.
Bursitis	Inflammation of bursa in a joint.	Work the relative joint, such as knee/elbow, plus lumbar spine in the case of knee; cervical spine for elbow. Helps the nerve supply to the affected part.
Cancer	Depends on the organ involved.	The whole of the body, especially the spleen to help the immune system.
Candida	A fungus causing thrush.	The whole of the intestinal and reproductive area.
Carpal tunnel syndrome	Numbness and tingling in the fingers and hands, the result of compression of the median nerve of the wrist.	Cervical spine and elbow area to aid nerve supply to the wrist.
Cataract	Opacity of lens of eye.	Eye, sinuses, cervical spine.

Condition	Symptoms/description	Main areas to treat
Cerebral haemorrhage (stroke)	Rupture of an artery of the brain due to either high blood pressure or disease of artery.	Entire spine, brain, respiratory, circulatory and kidney (to help renal blood supply and, ultimately, blood pressure).
Cerebral palsy (spasticity)	Condition in which the control of the motor system is affected due to a lesion resulting from a birth defect or deprivation of oxygen at birth.	Spine and brain. Work this area frequently during a treatment, six or seven times up and down each foot.
Cervical spondylosis	Degenerative changes in the intervertebral discs in the cervical spine.	Entire spine and chronic neck area.
Cholecystitis	Inflammation of the gall bladder.	Liver and gall bladder area.
Chronic fatigue syndrome, *see* ME		
Colic	Waves of abdominal pain fluctuating in severity.	Digestive system, solar plexus.
Colitis, diverticulitis and irritable bowel syndrome	Inflammation of the colon.	Entire digestive system and lumbar spine to help nerve and blood supply to the pelvic area.
Conjunctivitis (eye condition)	Inflammation of the conjunctiva.	Eye/cervical spine and all sinus areas.
Constipation	Difficulty in passing a motion.	Entire intestines and liver/gall bladder (bile helps lubrication of the bowel) and lumbar spinal nerves.
Crohn's disease	Chronic form of enteritis affecting terminal parts of the ileum.	Entire intestines and lumbar spine to help blood supply to pelvic area.
Cystitis	Inflammation of the urinary system, mainly affecting the bladder.	Urinary system. Coccyx, pelvis and lumbar spine.
Depression	A feeling of gloom.	Entire endocrine system to help balance hormonal output. Lots of work on relaxation techniques.
Diabetes	Caused by a deficiency of insulin production of the pancreas.	Digestive, endocrine, circulatory and respiratory systems and thoracic spine.
Down's syndrome	A chromosomal deficiency.	Cannot help condition but work respiratory system as this area is prone to illness.

Condition	Symptoms/description	Main areas to treat
Dysmenorrhoea	Painful or difficult menstruation.	Urinary and reproductive, coccyx/ pelvis and lumbar spine.
Ear infection	Infection and inflammation of the inner ear.	Digestive system (trying to eliminate excess mucus), sinus, ear and eye.
Eczema and all skin diseases	Inflammation of the skin.	Treat as for asthma: comes from the same source. Digestive system and adrenals.
Emphysema	Over-distension of the lungs by air. Alveoli of the lungs distended due to atrophy of the alveolar walls.	Treat as for asthma.
Endometriosis	Inflammation of the lining of the uterus (endometrium).	Reproductive and endocrine, as can be a hormone imbalance.
Epilepsy	Disorder of brain marked by the occurrence of convulsive fits.	Brain and spine.
Fever	Rise in normal body temperature.	Pituitary, hypothalamus, thyroid.
Fibroid	Tumour composed of mixed muscular and fibrous tissue in uterus.	Reproductive system.
Glandular fever	Fever with enlargement and tenderness of the lymphatic glands.	Lymphatic system.
Gout (excessive uric acid)	Inflamed red area; usually toes, elbow and knee.	Digestive system, liver and kidneys.
Haemorrhoids	Varicose veins in rectum.	Descending colon and rectum, pelvic and coccyx.
Hay fever	Allergic rhinitis.	Sinus, ear, eye, adrenal, digestive system.
Headache	Pain in head.	Entire spine, brain.
Hepatitis	Inflammation of liver causing nausea, upper abdominal discomfort, jaundice, itching of skin.	Liver, digestive system and adrenals.
Hiatus hernia	Acid reflux after eating; pain in stomach.	Digestive system, stomach, solar plexus.
HIV	Failure of the immune system.	Adrenals, spleen and respiratory system.

Condition	Symptoms/description	Main areas to treat
Hypertension	High blood pressure.	Circulatory, respiratory and kidney. Do not work on the adrenals when treating high blood pressure.
Hypotension	Low blood pressure.	As above, but work on adrenals to increase blood pressure levels.
Incontinence	Absence of voluntary control of the passing of urine or faeces.	Urinary/intestinal areas, lumbar spine, coccyx, pelvis.
Indigestion (dyspepsia)	Failure of the digestive processes.	Digestive and intestinal areas.
Infertility	Inability to conceive.	Entire endocrine and reproductive system.
Insomnia	Inability to sleep.	Spine, brain (pituitary), respiratory, circulatory and general treatment.
Iritis	Inflammation of the eye.	Eye, kidney, neck (urinary problems affect the eyes).
Lumbago	Painful condition of the lumbar muscles due to inflammation. May be caused by displaced invertebral disc.	Coccyx, pelvis, lumbar spine.
Mastitis	Inflammation of the breast.	Breast, shoulder, endocrine system.
Mastoiditis	Inflammation of the mastoid bone in the ear.	Head, neck, ear, cervical spine.
ME (myalgic encephalomyelitis) and chronic fatigue syndrome	Extreme, debilitating fatigue and poor immunity to infection.	Spleen and nervous system.
Ménière's disease	Attacks of vertigo, nausea, tinnitus and hearing loss.	Ear, head, sinuses, cervical spine and chronic neck.
Migraine	Paroxysmal attacks of headache, usually with nausea also preceded by disorders of vision	Head, cervical neck and cervical spine; liver (this is often digestive in origin and the liver is usually affected).
Multiple sclerosis	Degeneration of the myeline sheath in nerves.	Spine, brain.
Myocarditis	Inflammation of the myocardium.	Respiratory, circulatory and thoracic spine.
Nephritis	Inflammation of kidney.	Urinary system, lumbar spine.

Condition	Symptoms/description	Main areas to treat
Neuralgia	Pain in the nerves of face.	First three toes, eye, ear, facial area, sinuses, cervical spine.
Oedema	Abnormal amount of fluid in the tissues causing swelling, particularly in the ankles and legs.	Urinary and circulatory systems, lumbar spine, lymphatic area surrounding groin.
Orchitis	Inflammation of testicles.	Reproductive, coccyx, pelvis, lumbar spine.
Osteoarthritis	Disorder due to excessive wear and tear of joint surfaces, affecting mainly weight-bearing joints, hips, knees and spine.	Work out thoroughly prime joint or part of body affected, spine and urinary system, to encourage good elimination.
Ovarian cysts	Hormonal imbalance. Abdominal discomfort.	Reproductive, endocrine, spine.
Palpitations	Racing heart and anxiety.	Chest, heart, solar plexus.
Pancreatitis	Inflammation of pancreas.	Digestive system.
Parkinson's disease	Shaking of limbs, fixed, staring expression, poor coordination.	Central nervous system, spine and brain.
Phlebitis	Inflammation of the veins.	Circulatory, respiratory.
Pleurisy *See* Bronchitis and asthma		
PMT (pre-menstrual tension)	Mood swings, bloating, swollen hands, depression, food binges.	Endocrine, also reproductive systems.
Prostatis	Prostate inflammation.	Urinary and reproductive, also the lumbar spine.
Rheumatoid arthritis	Pain, stiffness, swelling in joints such as knee, foot, hand, elbow, shoulder.	Digestive, hip, pelvis, spine, elbow, shoulder, knee, thyroid/parathyroid.
Rhinitis or hay fever	Inflammation of nose.	Sinuses, nose/throat, adrenals to reduce inflammation, digestive system (this is often a food allergy).
Salpingitis	Inflammation of Fallopian tubes.	Entire reproductive and endocrine systems plus coccyx. Pelvic/hip.
Sciatica	Compression of the sciatic nerve causing pain.	Lumbar spine, coccyx, pelvic/hip, sciatic area.

Condition	Symptoms/description	Main areas to treat
Shingles	Inflammation of nerve endings in spine.	All spinal areas.
Sinusitis	Inflammation of facial sinuses.	Sinuses, eye and ear, cervical spine, facial area.
Spondylitis	Inflammation of a vertebra, occurring characteristically in young men. Origin unknown – see Ankylosing spondylitis	Entire skeletal system.
Tennis elbow	Inflammation of bursa of joint affecting the insertion of the extensor tendon of the forearm muscles.	Cervical spine, shoulder, elbow.
Thrombosis (clot in circulatory system)	Coagulation of blood in the vessels.	Respiratory and circulatory systems, thoracic spine.
Thyrotoxicosis (Hyperthyroidism)	Excess production of thyroxine.	Thyroid and all endocrine glands.
Tinnitus	Ringing in the ears.	Neck, ear, sinuses, cervical spine.
Tonsillitis	Inflammation of the tonsils.	Throat, sinuses, cervical spine, thymus gland in young children to help immunity.
Trigeminal neuralgia	Pains in the face of unknown cause.	Face, sinuses, eye/ear, neck.
Urticaria	An itchy rash caused by emotions or allergy.	See asthma and eczema.
Varicose veins	Caused by chronic constipation and pressure during pregnancy.	Intestinal area, lumbar spine.
Vertigo	Dizziness.	Ear, head, sinuses, cervical spine.

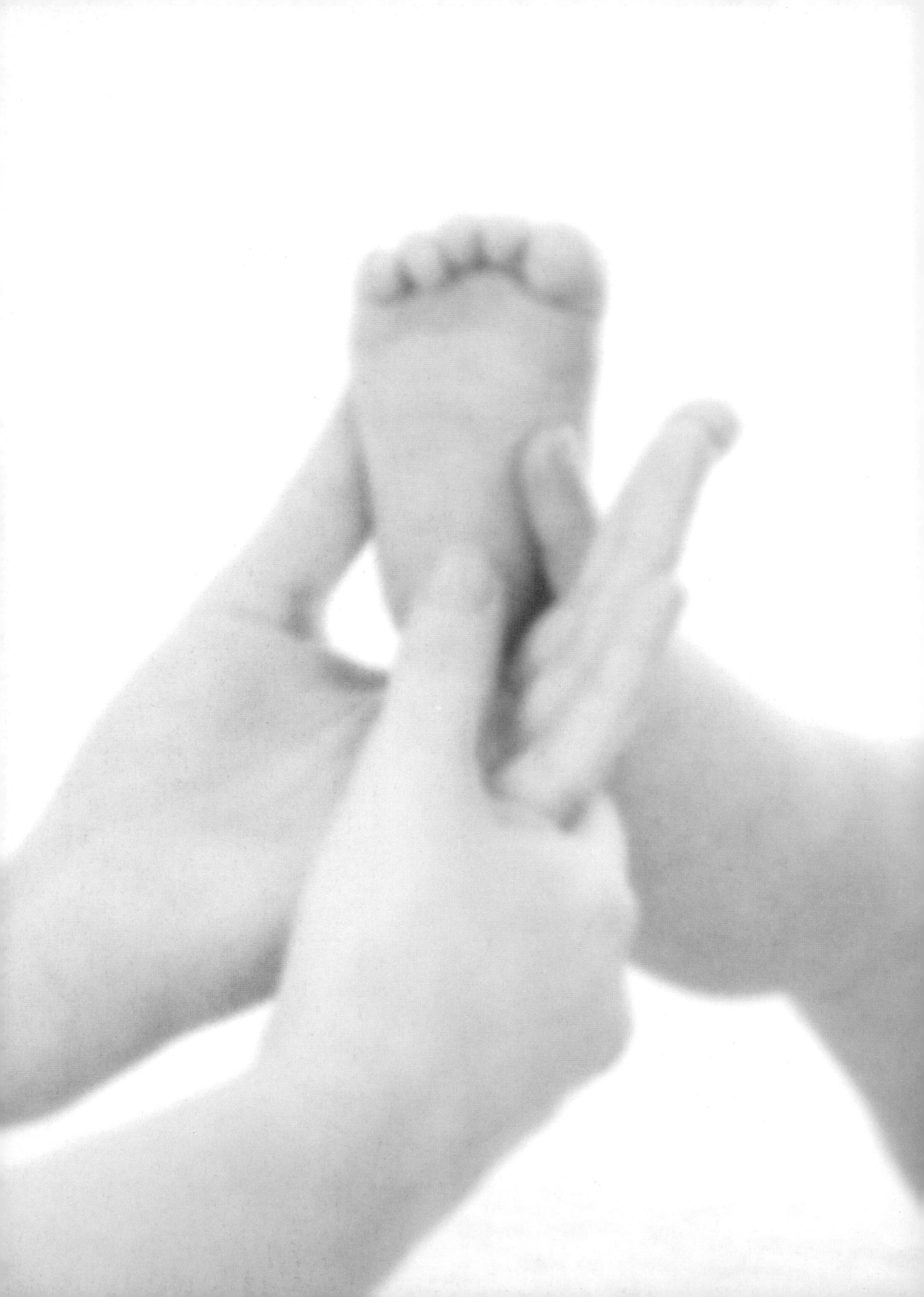

Specialized reflexology

Most patients you see will be seeking your help to alleviate one of the physical or psychological problems covered in the previous chapter, but reflexology can be valuable in other circumstances. It is enormously helpful to women during pregnancy and childbirth, as well as later in life to relieve menopausal symptoms. Its relaxing techniques are therapeutic for everyone, from babies to the terminally ill, and it also has its place in assisting sufferers of two of our biggest killers: heart disease and cancer.

Pregnancy

Pregnancy is a time of major physical and psychological adjustments. A woman's body not only undergoes hormonal and physiological changes as she nurtures her unborn child for 40 weeks, but also has to cope with the emotions associated with a major change in life.

IS IT SAFE?

Women often ask whether reflexology is a safe treatment during pregnancy. The answer is definitely yes: the sense of wellbeing it engenders and the alleviation it can bring can only be positive and there is no negative side. The only caution I would advise is in the first trimester for women with a history of miscarriage (see page 64).

Nine months may seem like a long time, but a pregnant woman's body changes very fast as the baby inside her grows, and her skeleton, muscles and hormones are making constant adjustments.

Many women experience back and leg pain for the first time when they are pregnant. Aches and pains at this time can be caused by the shifting balance of weight, and also by hormones that soften the ligaments of the body in preparation for childbirth. This can cause strain in the lower back. Another common problem is sciatica, brought on by extra weight at the front of the body putting pressure on the sciatic nerve. Sciatica that starts during pregnancy usually disappears once the baby has been born.

Reflexology can provide a very effective way of easing common problems associated with these changes, such as back pain, morning sickness and general discomfort.

Pregnancy is a time of emotional adjustment as well. The hormonal changes during pregnancy are enormous, and these often account for mood swings from feelings of depression and anxiety to elation. Worries are very usual: about being able to cope as a mother, about finding time for the rest of the family, about the birth itself (particularly for a first-time mother) and about whether the baby will be healthy. Happily, most women have a normal pregnancy and a healthy baby, but these very normal anxieties are emotionally tiring.

This is an emotionally taxing time for fathers-to-be as well, for many of the same reasons. Some may even develop symptoms associated with pregnancy, such as nausea resembling morning sickness and mood swings. Reflexology can help both expectant mothers and fathers with treatment that is both relaxing and restorative.

Reflexology during pregnancy Many babies become extremely active while their mothers are indulging in a reflexology treatment session.

Treating minor problems during pregnancy

Reflexology is an ideal non-invasive therapy for dealing with the minor ailments that many pregnant women experience. Treatment will help the mother-to-be and do no harm to the growing baby. It will also assist general relaxation during pregnancy, lifting mood and easing the anxieties that some mothers-to-be have about the prospect of labour and giving birth.

Morning sickness

Work the areas relating to the pituitary gland and the stomach.

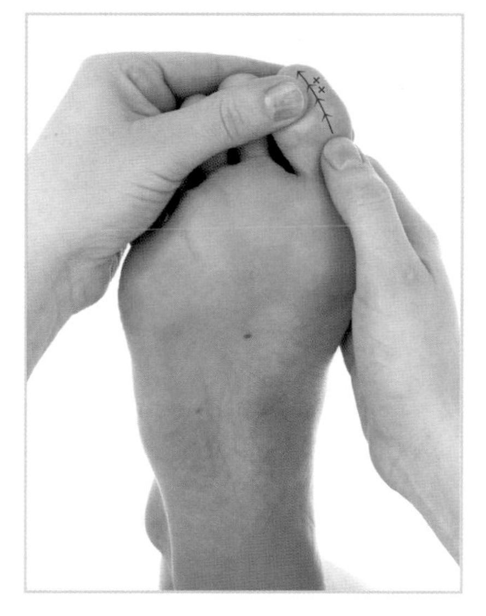

1 Use your right thumb to work the pituitary area of the right foot three times up the medial side of the big toe (see page 105).

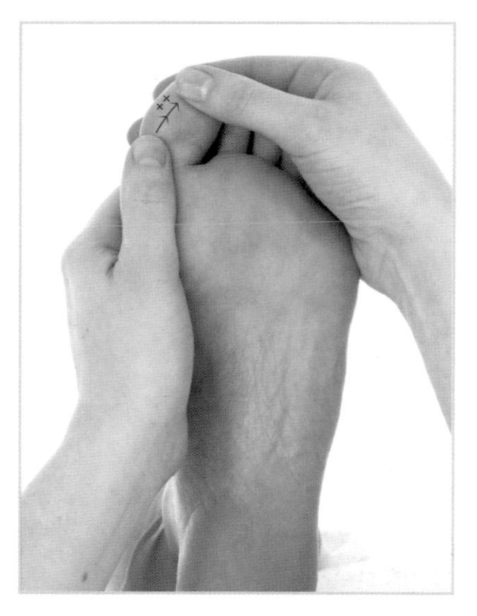

2 Use your left thumb to work the pituitary area of the left foot three times up the medial side of the big toe.

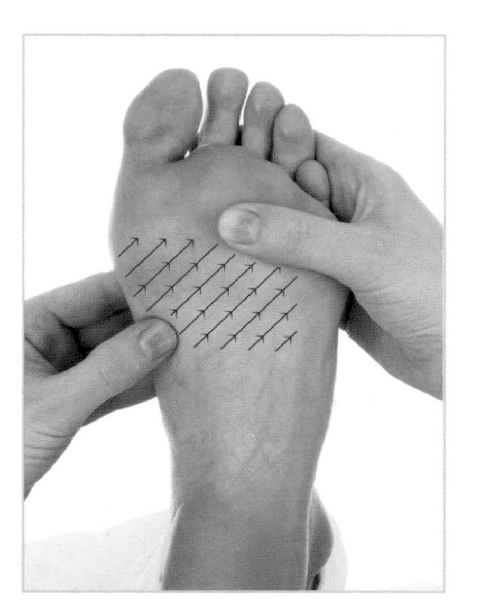

3 Use your left thumb to work the stomach area on the left foot in a criss-cross direction from medial to lateral (see page 79).

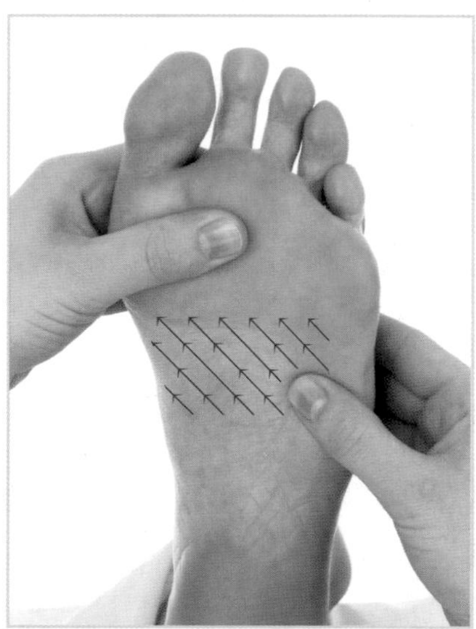

4 Use your right thumb to work the stomach area on the left foot from lateral to medial.

Constipation and haemorrhoids

Work the areas relating to the intestines, sigmoid colon and rectum.

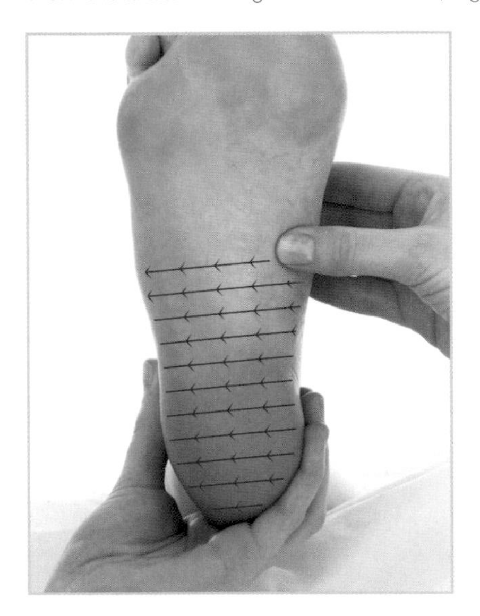

1 Use your right thumb to work the intestinal area of the right foot in straight lines across the foot from medial to lateral (see page 80).

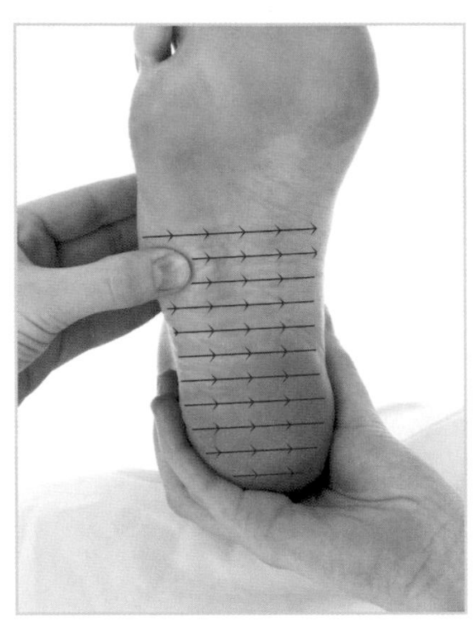

2 Use your left thumb to work the intestinal area of the right foot in straight lines from lateral to medial.

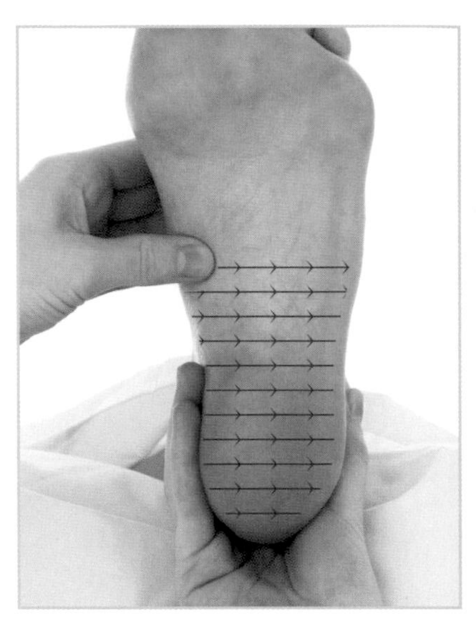

3 Use your left thumb to work the intestinal area of the left foot in straight lines across the foot from medial to lateral (see page 81).

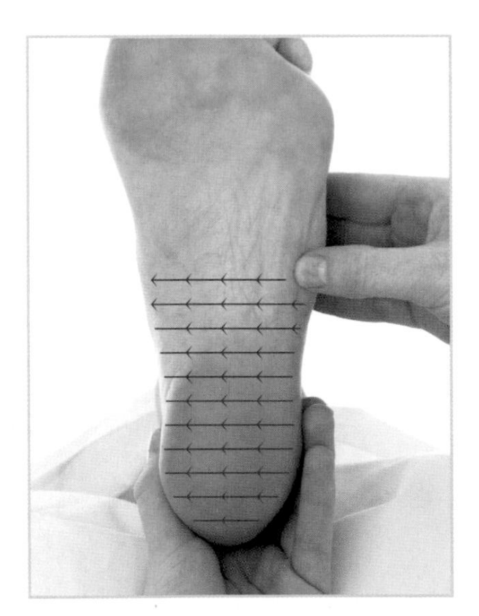

4 Use your right thumb to work the intestinal area of the left foot in straight lines from lateral to medial.

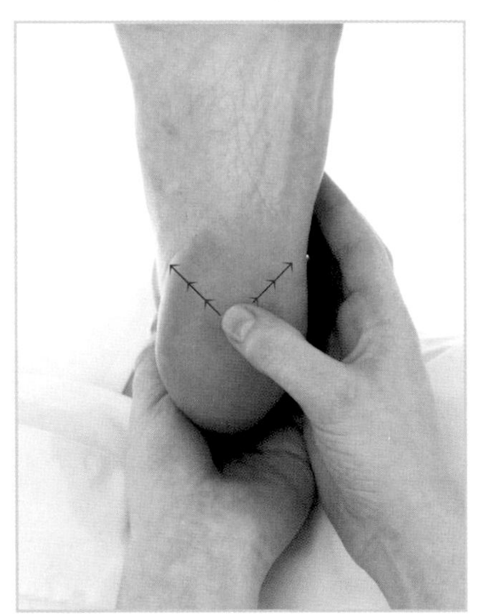

5 To work the sigmoid colon area of the left foot, place your right thumb on the mid point and work towards the medial edge and then the lateral edge (see page 81).

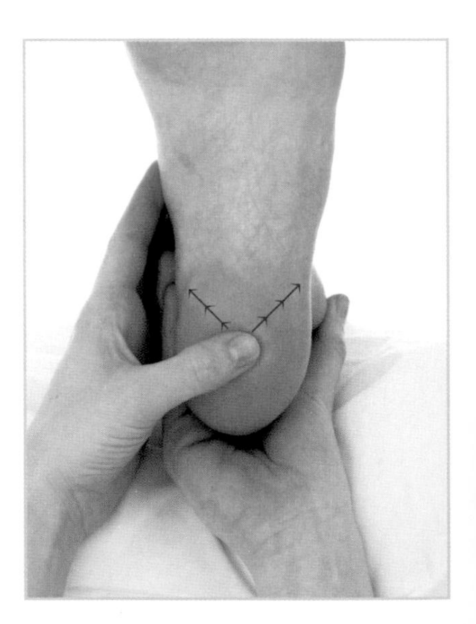

6 Then place your left thumb on the mid point of the right foot and work towards the lateral and then the medial edge as indicated.

Heartburn

Work the area relating to the stomach area and do a diaphragm relaxation.

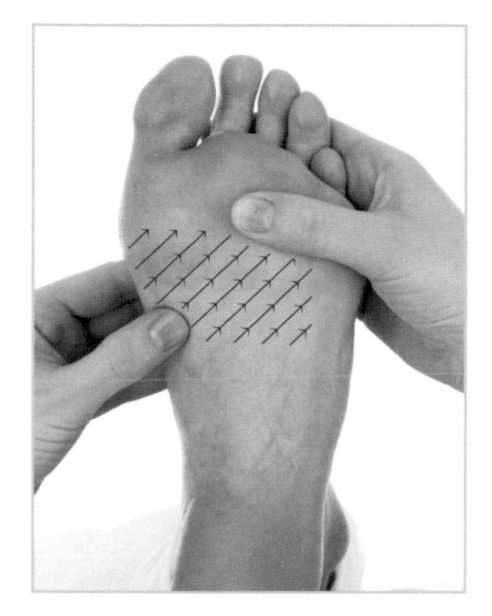

1 Use your left thumb to work the stomach area on the left foot in a criss-cross direction from medial to lateral (see page 79).

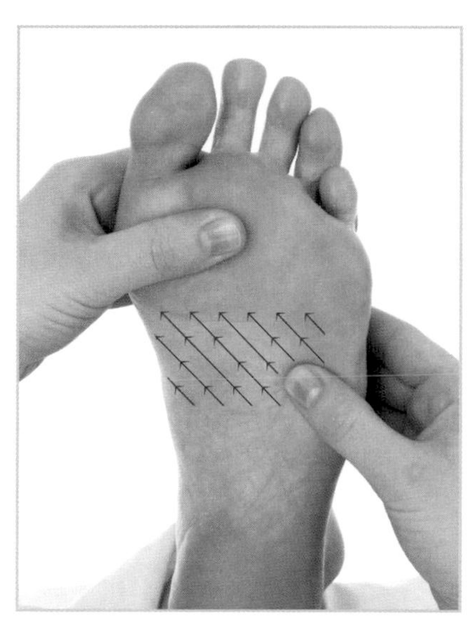

2 Use your right thumb to work the stomach area on the left foot from lateral to medial.

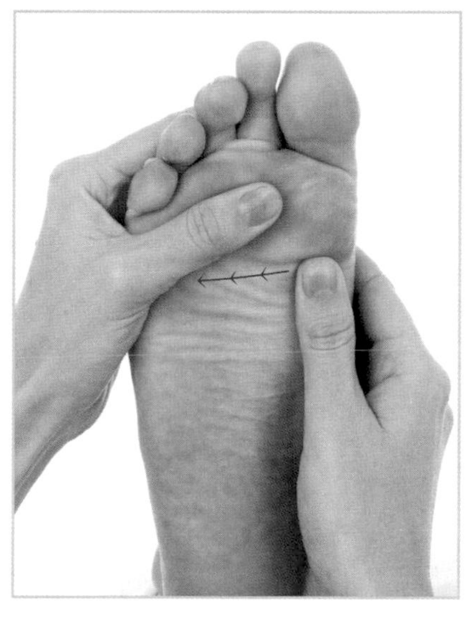

3 For a diaphragm relaxation exercise (see page 55), place your right thumb on the start of the diaphragm line on the right foot. As you move it to the lateral edge, bend the toes downwards towards your thumb.

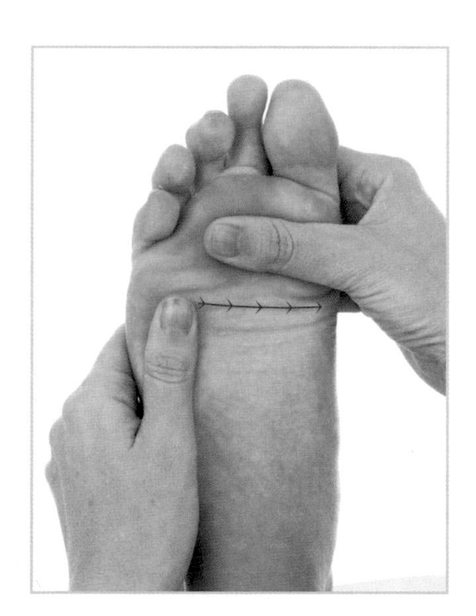

4 Place your left thumb on the diaphragm line. As you move it to the medial edge, bend the toes downwards towards your thumb.

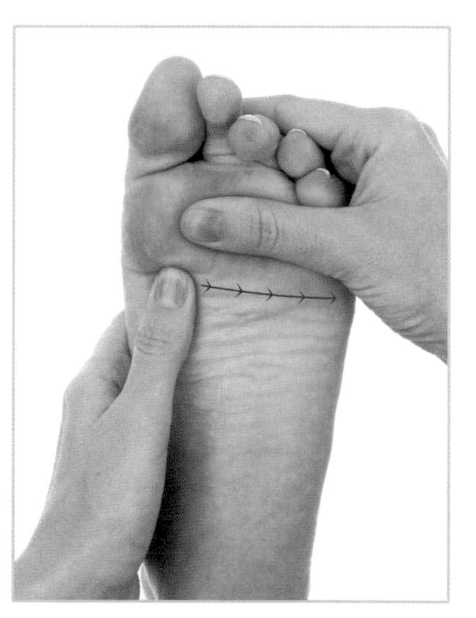

5 Place your left thumb on the start of the diaphragm line on the left foot. As you move it to the lateral edge, bend the toes downwards towards your thumb.

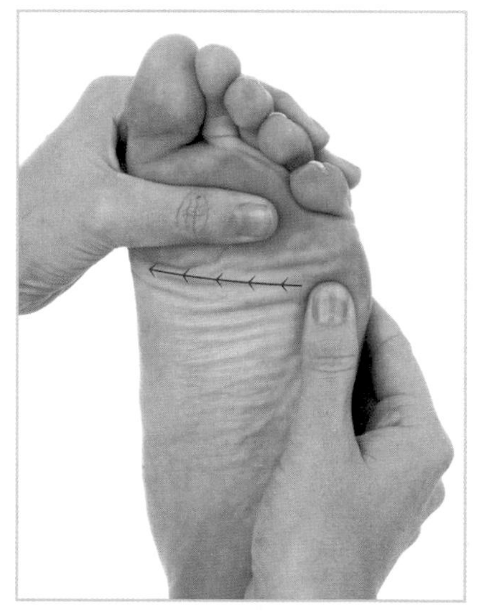

6 Place your right thumb on the diaphragm line. As you move it to the medial edge, bend the toes downwards towards your thumb. At no time during the diaphragm relaxation should your thumb leave the surface of the foot.

Leg and back pain

Work the coccyx, hip and pelvis, spine, cervical spine and side of neck areas.

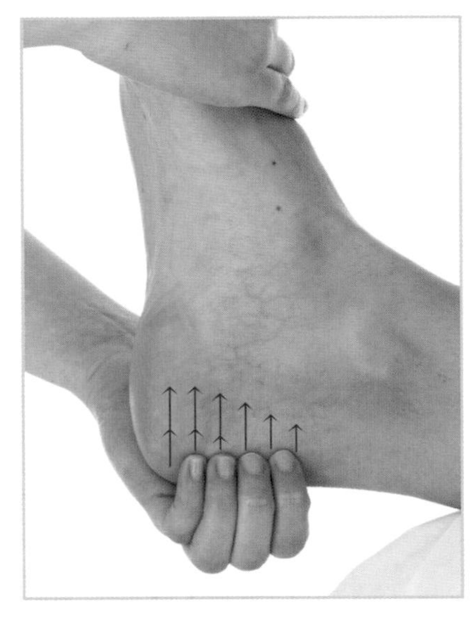

1 Use pressure from the four fingers of your left hand on the coccyx area of the right foot (see page 134). Repeat two or three times.

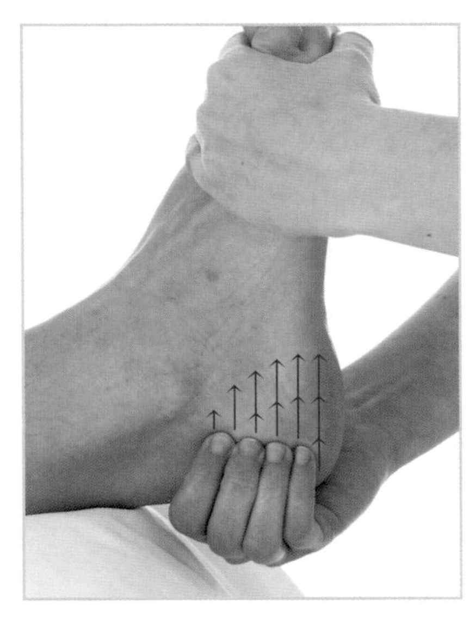

2 Use pressure from the four fingers of your right hand on the hip and pelvis area of the right foot. Repeat two or three times.

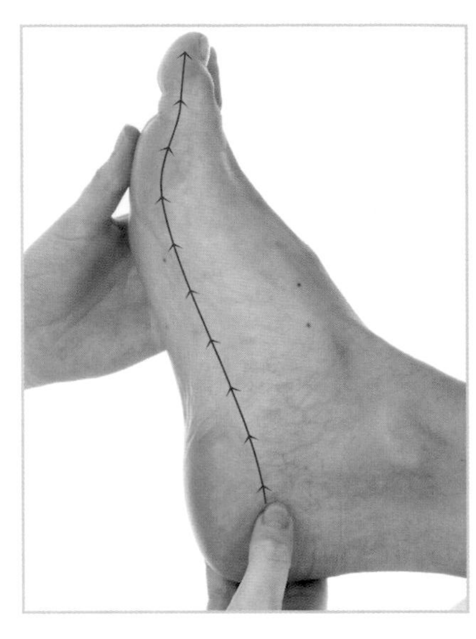

3 Use your right thumb to work up the spine area on the right foot (see page 134).

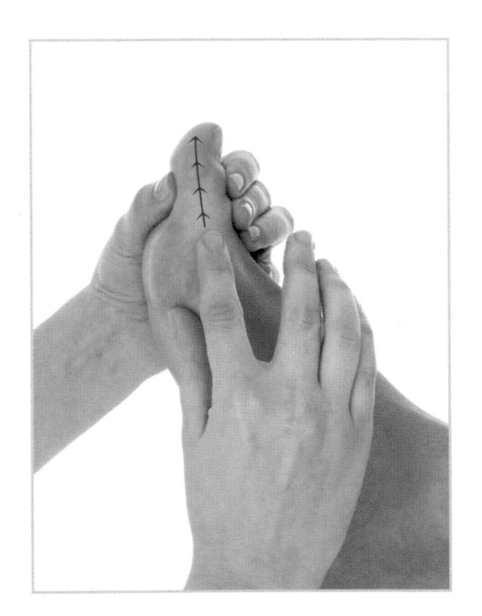

4 Use your right index finger to work up the fine area of the cervical spine on the right foot.

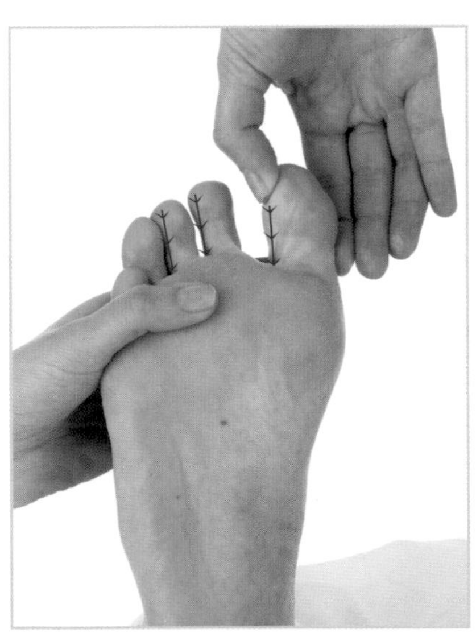

5 Use your right thumb to work down the side of neck area on the lateral sides of the first three toes of the right foot (see page 135).

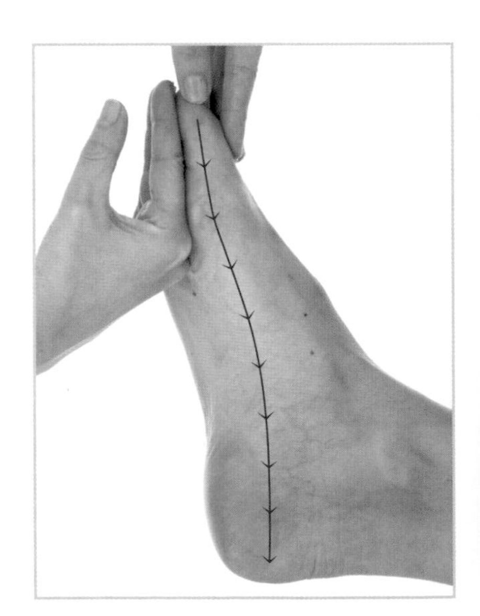

6 Work down the spine area of the right foot with your left thumb.

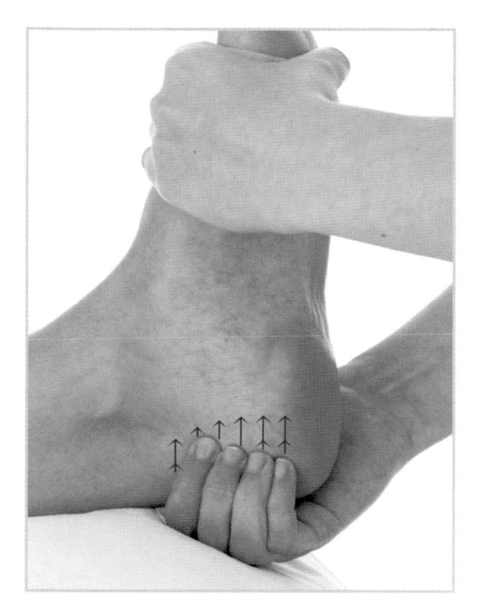

7 Use pressure from the four fingers of your right hand on the coccyx area of the left foot (see page 137). Repeat two or three times.

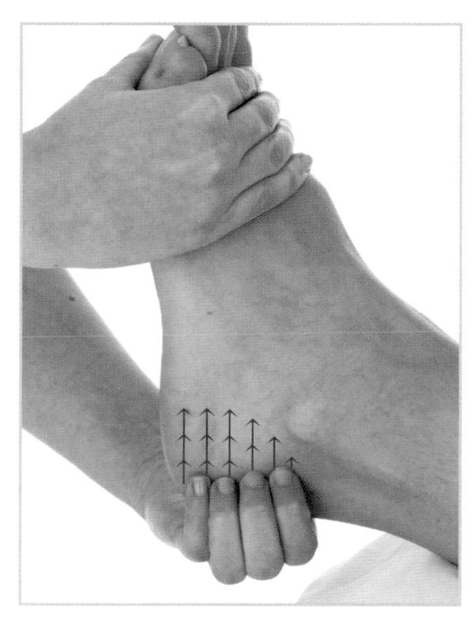

8 Use pressure from the four fingers of your left hand on the hip and pelvis area of the left foot. Repeat two or three times.

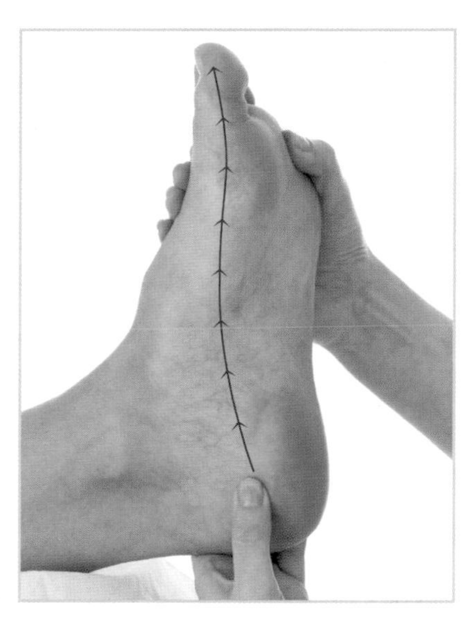

9 Use your left thumb to work up the spine area of the left foot (see page 137).

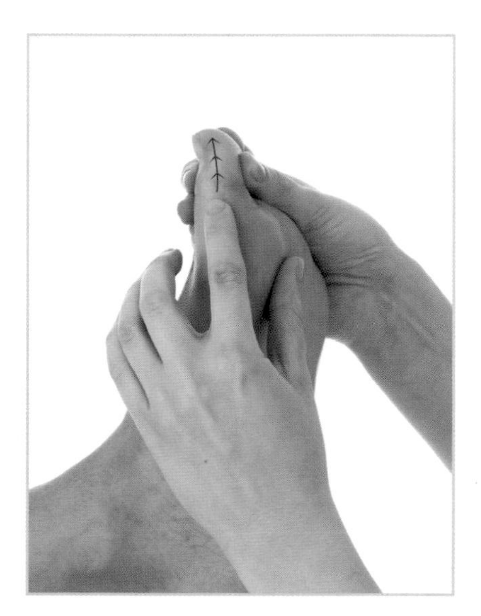

10 Use your right index finger to work up the fine area of the cervical spine on the left foot.

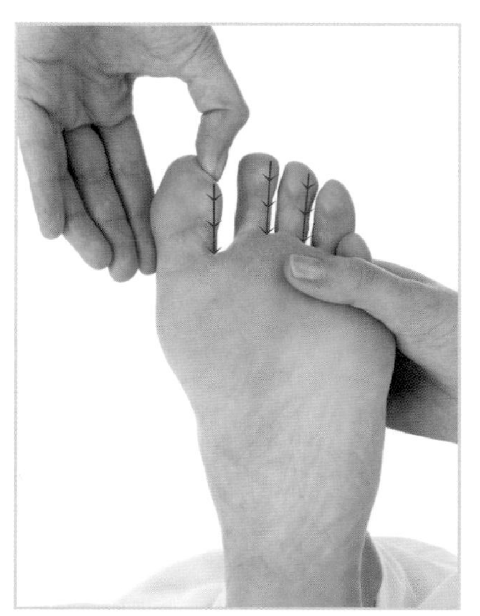

11 Use your right thumb to work down the side of neck area on the lateral sides of the first three toes of the left foot (see page 138).

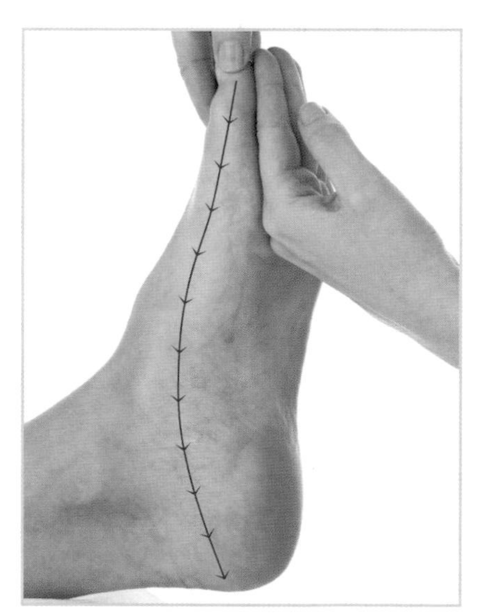

12 Work down the spine area of the right foot with your left thumb.

Labour

If you have been treating a woman during the course of her pregnancy, she may welcome the idea of receiving reflexology while she is actually giving birth as well. Women who have reflexology treatment during labour, whether at home or in hospital, seem to recover more quickly afterwards, as the body rebalances more easily.

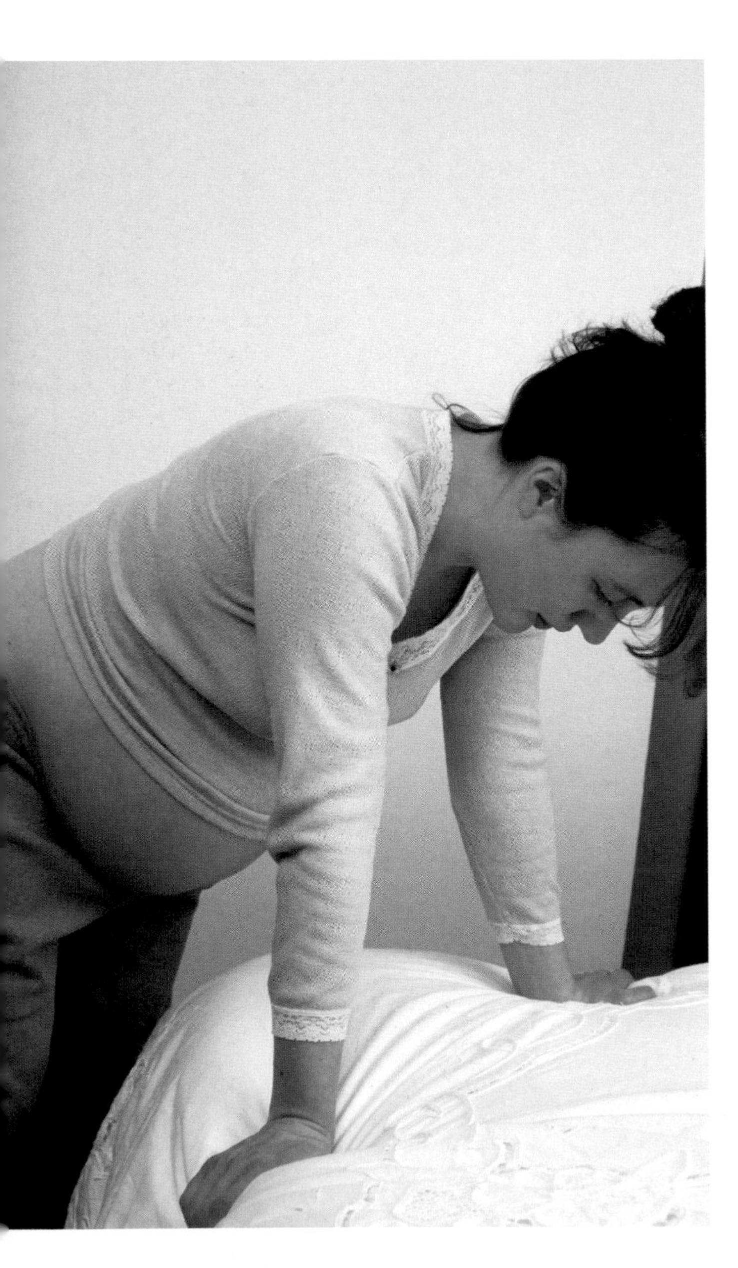

Over the years, I have treated many women right through their pregnancies and during labour. One particular patient had in the past endured long difficult labours as on all three occasions she produced very large babies. Another problem encountered during the previous births was that the placenta failed to detach itself from the uterus and had to be removed surgically.

Reflexology was used throughout the patient's fourth pregnancy and labour. The result was a very rapid labour with none of the difficulties that had been experienced on previous occasions.

There are several ways in which reflexology can be helpful during labour:

- Working the uterus will aid contractions and help the pain as the large horizontal and vertical uterine muscles move the baby down the birth canal and into the outside world.
- Working on the endocrine system – the pituitary and thyroid reflexes – encourages the production of hormones necessary during birth.
- Working the entire spinal area will help to stimulate nerve and muscle tone in the pelvic region.

Aim to treat the uterus, endocrine system and spinal areas for 10 minutes on each foot in every hour. You can also helping by encouraging the patient to keep active between sessions, walking round the room. Standing upright will help the contractions to move the baby lower into the pelvic cavity.

Labour Reflexology will stimulate the muscles and nerves and ease pain during the challenging experience of labour.

Areas to work for labour

The step-by-step sequence for leg and back pain in pregnancy (described on pages 212–213) is also particularly helpful during labour as it gives relief to the whole spinal area: the coccyx, hip and pelvis, spine, cervical spine and neck. Pay attention to the spinal stimulation point, as it treats the whole of the central nervous system and the vertebral column. The uterus, as well as the pituitary, hypothalamus and pineal regions, also benefit from stimulation during labour.

The spinal stimulation point

This reflex point is at the narrowest part of the foot on the medial side.

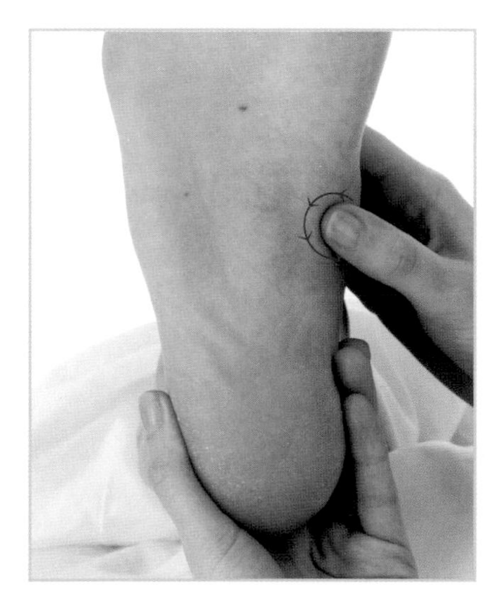

Use your right thumb to press down on the spinal stimulation point and rotate your thumb towards the spine for a count of five. Pause and repeat. Repeat on the left foot, using your right hand.

The uterus

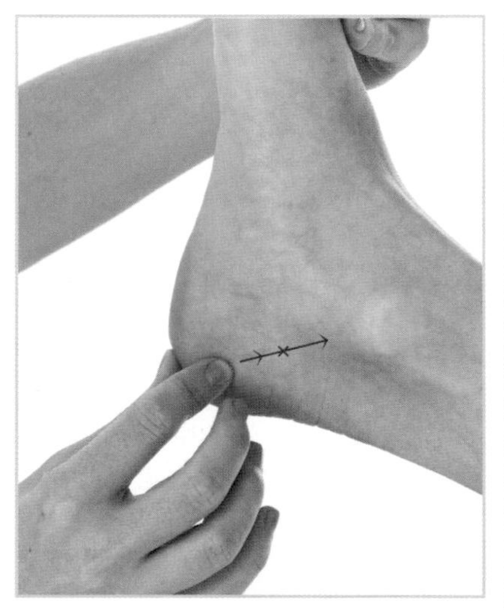

Use your right index finger to work in a straight line as shown on the uterus area of the right foot (see page 154). Repeat two or three times. Then repeat on the left foot, using your left finger.

The pituitary, hypothalamus and pineal areas

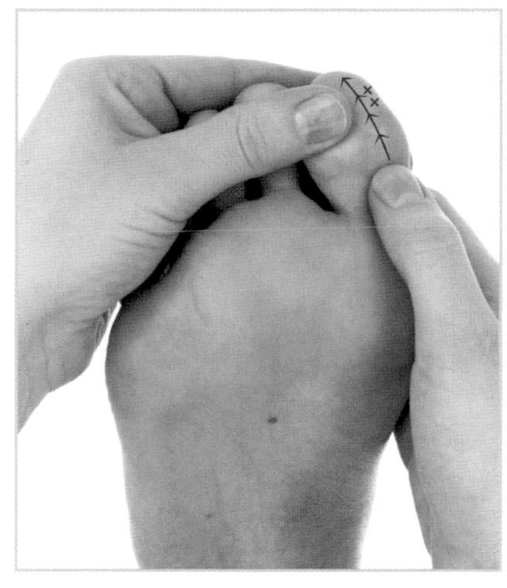

1 Use your right thumb to work the pituitary, hypothalamus and pineal areas of the right foot, working three times up the medial side of the big toe (see page 105).

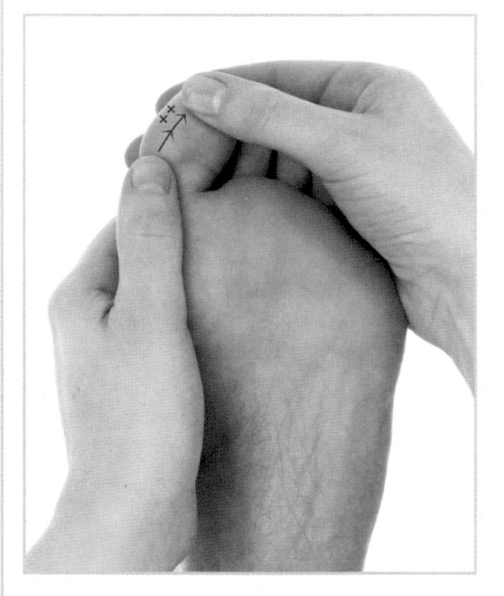

2 Use your left thumb to work the pituitary, hypothalamus and pineal areas of the left foot, working three times up the medial side of the big toe.

Menopause

The menopause affects women from about age 40 onwards and is a period of both physical and emotional adjustment. The classic symptoms of apprehension, sweating and palpitations are some of the more common discomforts.

Perhaps the main area to consider is the role of the glands during the menopausal years. Although the oestrogen production by the ovaries is greatly reduced during this time, signals continue to come from the pituitary and hypothalamus and this must create some biological confusion (see 'The endocrine system', pages 98–101).

The ovaries are not the only glands that produce sex hormones. The adrenal glands also manufacture oestrogens and androgens (male hormones), the latter being responsible for the sex drive in women as well as in men. The overall health of the adrenal glands will dictate whether they will be able to take over the production of hormones efficiently. Coffee in excess, alcohol, plus a stressful life, cause adrenal exhaustion.

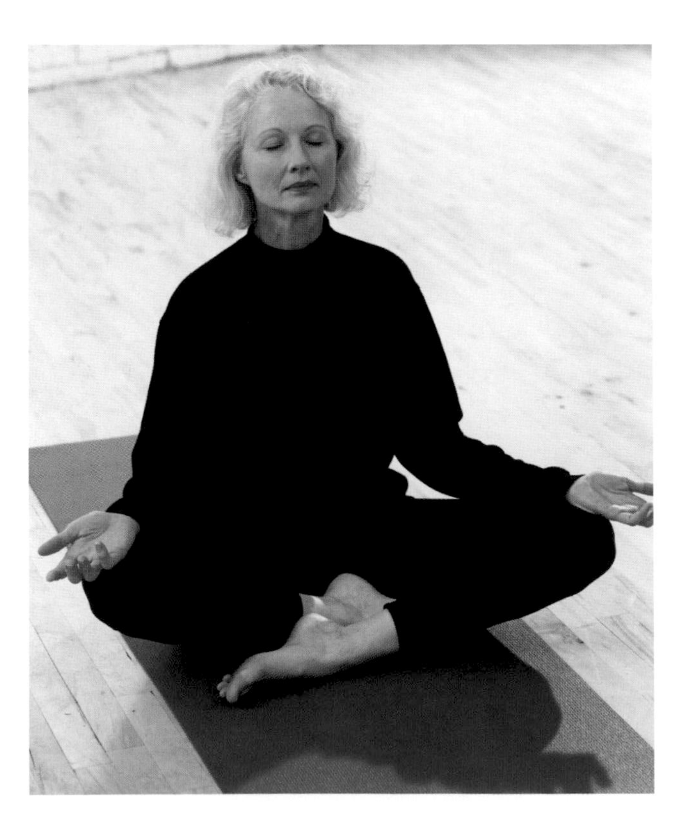

During her menstruating years a woman is less likely to suffer from coronary heart disease or osteoporosis, as the constant supply of oestrogen and progesterone protects against these problems. Once the ovaries reduce the supply of oestrogen, however, she becomes prone to circulation problems and brittle bones. The following tips will help to counteract these alterations:

- Maintain a highly nutritious diet with the lowest possible level of 'wasted calories'; avoid white sugar and white flour products in particular. Wholegrain bread, pasta and cereals are all to be recommended.
- Eat at least five pieces of fruit and three or more vegetables every day.
- Supplement the dietary intake with B vitamins, especially vitamin B6, and vitamins C, D and E. Also take sufficient minerals, particularly zinc, magnesium and calcium.
- Cut down on alcohol, avoiding it altogether if the menopausal symptoms are difficult.
- Stop smoking.

Mood swings are very common during the menopause, both due to changes in hormonal balance and to the need to adapt to and accept these changes. For some women, the cessation of their periods marks the beginning of 'old age', but for others the freedom from monthly discomfort, and a time of life when most children have fled the nest and become independent, marks a new beginning. Many women find that their post-menopausal years are the best years of their life.

As well as treating specific areas undergoing change during the menopause (see opposite), reflexology can be of great help in reducing the stress that is experienced by many women at this time.

Living through the menopause It is important for women going through the menopause to make time for themselves to relax and adjust to the changes that are taking place.

Areas to work for menopause

Most women find that treatment on the endocrine system (pituitary and thyroid glands) helps control hot flushes. I also recommend working on the spinal reflex area to stimulate the nerve and blood supply to the whole body. Other areas that benefit from treatment are the uterus, the ovaries and the liver.

The thyroid/neck area

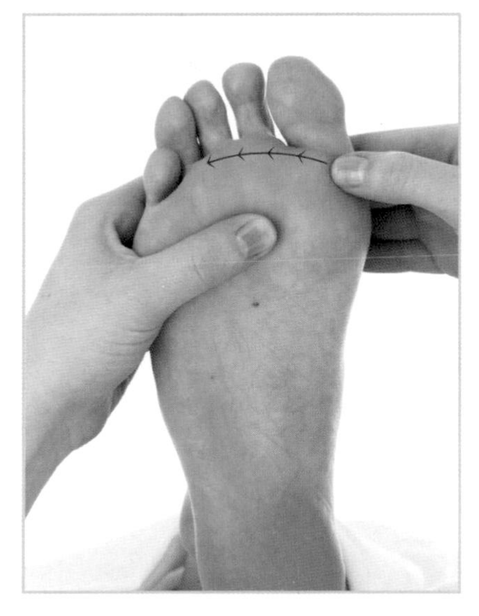

1 Use your right thumb to work across the thyroid/neck area at the base of the three toes on the right foot three times (see page 105).

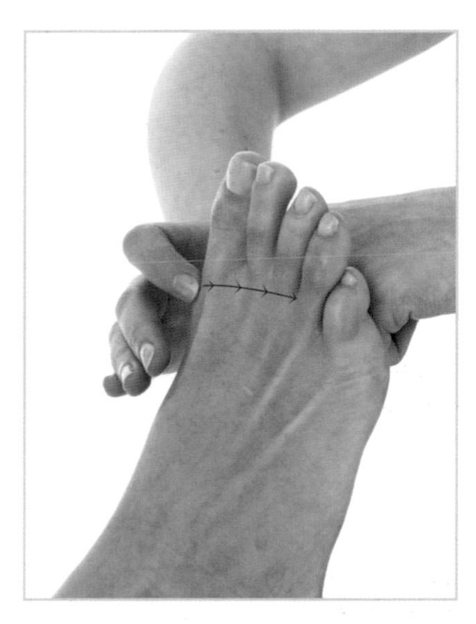

2 Support the right foot with your left fist and use the right index finger to work three times across the join of the toes on the dorsal side.

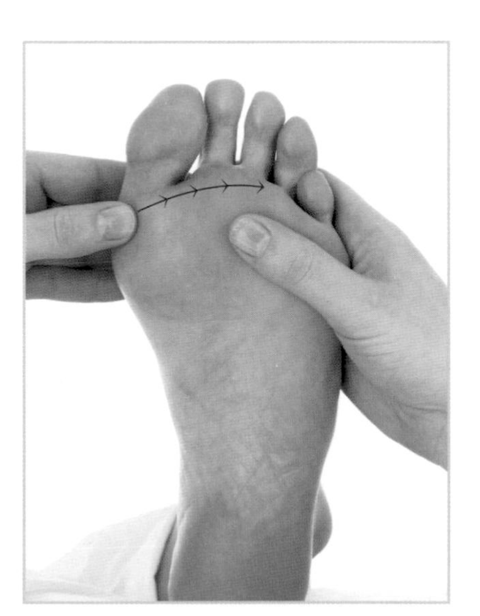

3 Use your left thumb to work three times across the thyroid/neck area at the base of the three toes on the left foot.

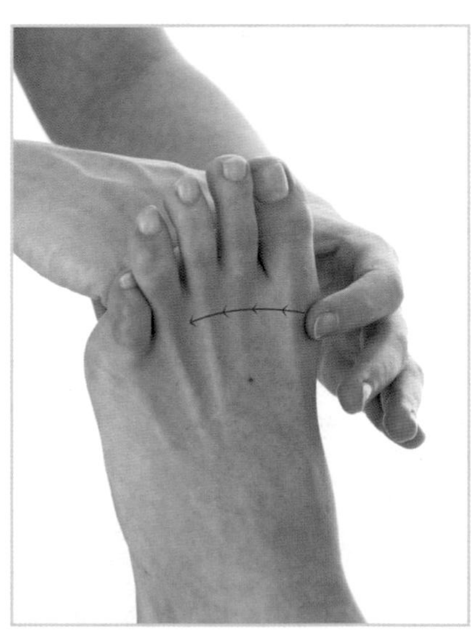

4 Support the left foot with your right fist and use the left index finger to work three times across the join of the toes on the dorsal side.

The pituitary, hypothalamus and pineal areas

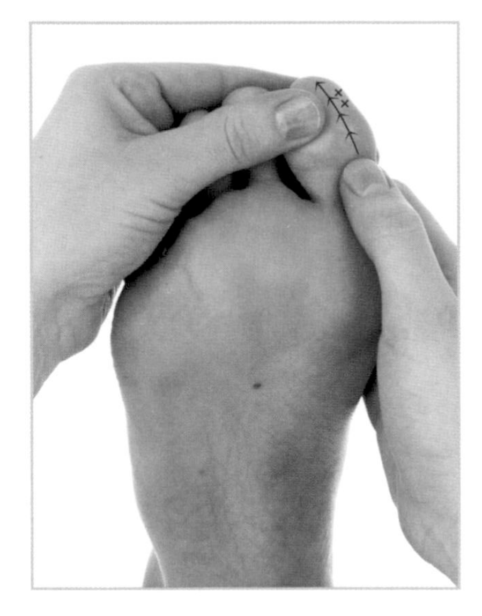

1 Use your right thumb to work the pituitary area of the right foot three times up the medial side of the big toe (see page 105).

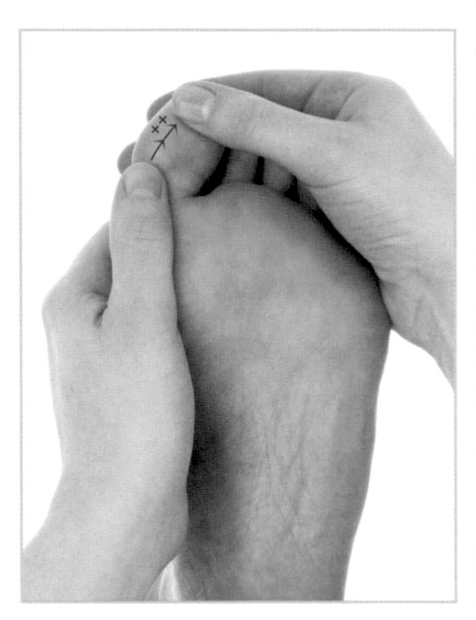

2 Use your left thumb to work the pituitary, hypothalamus and pineal areas of the left foot, working three times up the medial side of the big toe.

The uterus

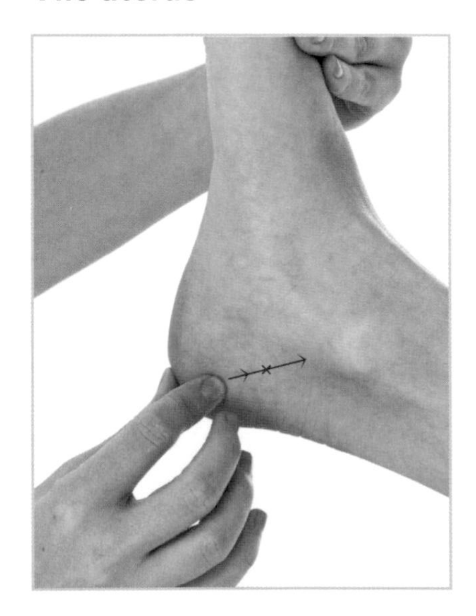

1 Use your right index finger to work in a straight line over the uterus area of the right foot (see page 154). Repeat two or three times.

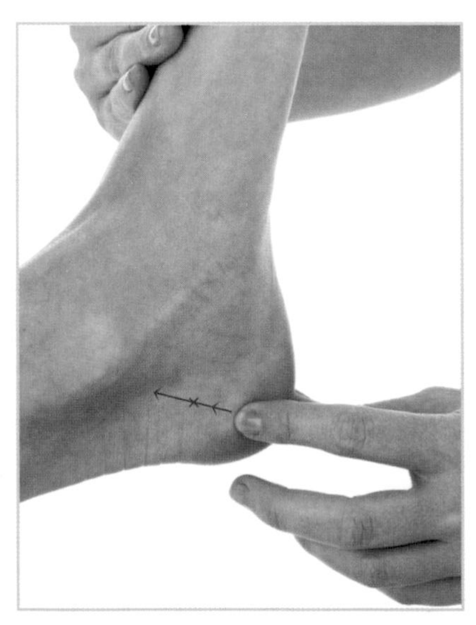

2 Use your left index finger to work in a straight line over the uterus area of the left foot. Repeat two or three times.

Ovaries

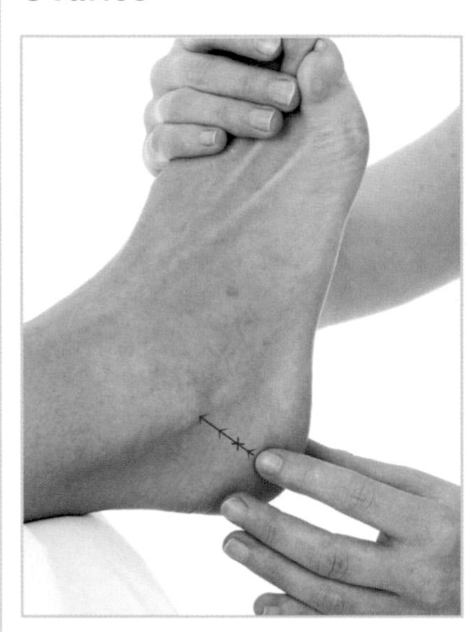

1 Use your left index finger to work over the ovary area on the right foot several times (see page 154). The cross indicates the exact position of the ovary.

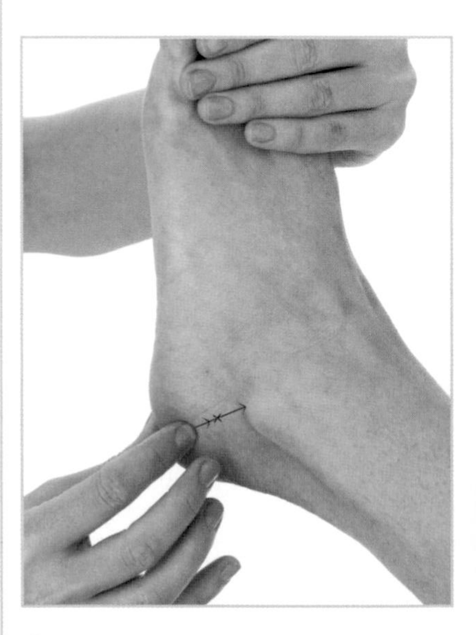

2 Use your right index finger to work over the ovary area on the left foot several times.

The spine

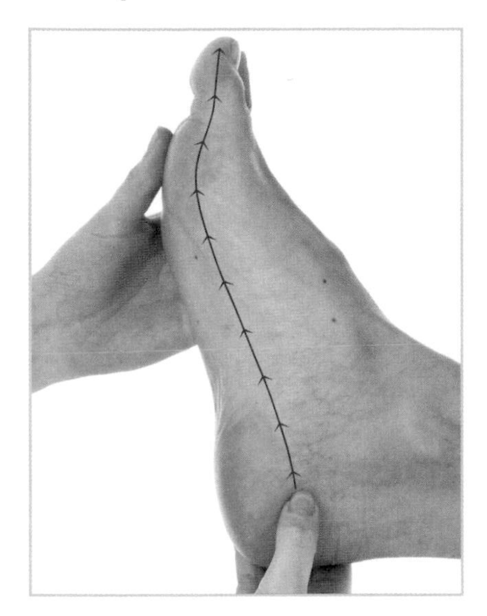

1 Use your right thumb to work up the spine area on the right foot (see page 134).

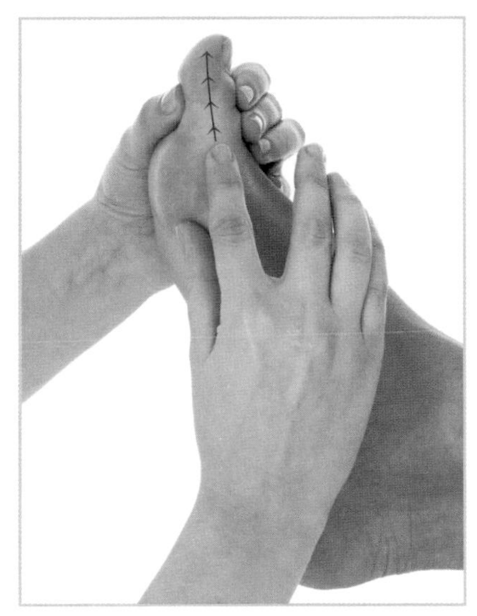

2 Use your right index finger to work up the fine area of the cervical spine on the right foot.

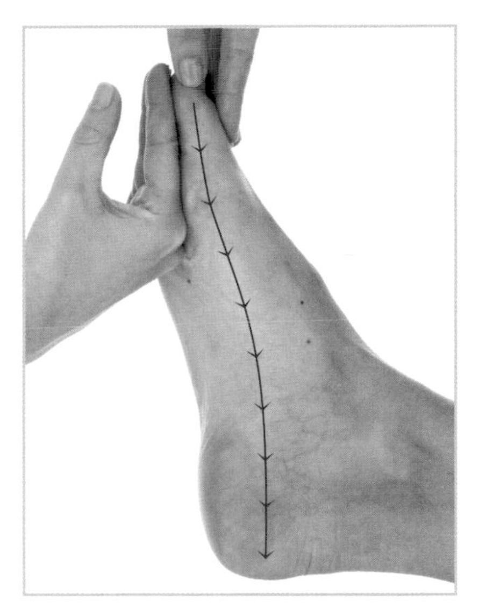

3 Work down the spine area on the right foot with your left thumb (see page 135). Then repeat Steps 1–3 on the left foot (see pages 137–138).

The liver

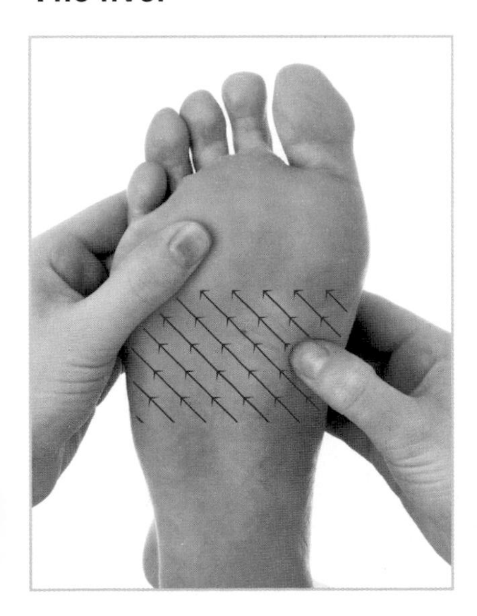

1 Use your right thumb to work out the liver area of the right foot in a criss-cross direction from the medial to the lateral edge (see page 79).

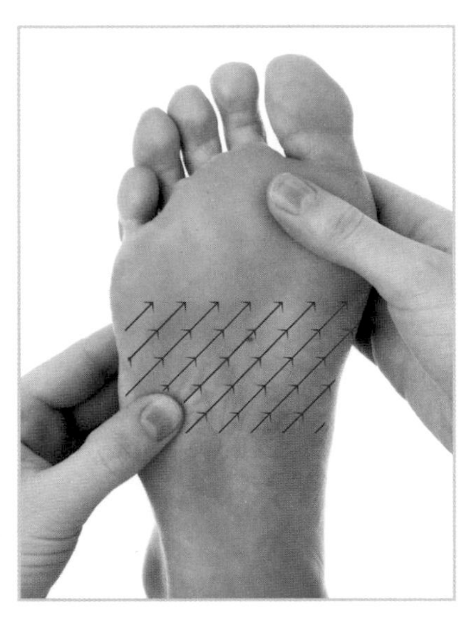

2 Use the left thumb to work the area in a criss-cross direction from the lateral to the medial edge.

Cancer

One in three people in the industrialized world will have cancer at some time in their lives. Indeed, as modern medicine overcomes more and more of the diseases that carried off our ancestors, it is increasingly likely that cancer will be responsible for the way that many of us will die.

The very word 'cancer' still fills most of us with dread, but increased understanding of how cancer is triggered and develops has given us the ability to reduce the risks. Different cancers have different causes, but there are contributing factors that increase risk in general, such as:

- **Smoking**: There is no doubt that smoking tobacco causes cancer. What many smokers fail to recognize is that smoking doesn't just threaten the throat and lungs; it encourages the growth of cancer in all parts of the body, including the mouth, stomach, intestines, prostate, pancreas, uterus and ovaries.
- **Obesity**: Being very overweight increases the risk of cancer, particularly cancers of the uterus, kidney, oesophagus, gall bladder, colon and rectum, and the breast in post-menopausal women. Researchers think that obesity encourages cancer growth by raising the level of sex hormones, in particular oestrogen (in both men and women), or protein-forming hormones like insulin. A link has also been shown between a high-fat diet and cancer, in particular colon cancer.
- **Environmental factors**: In most parts of the world we are constantly bombarded with pollution: traffic fumes, pesticides on foods, household chemicals. Threats also come from exposure to radioactive or chemical leakages and electromagnetic energy from power lines. Cancers have also been linked with x-rays and treatments such as hormone replacement therapy and drugs used to control cholesterol and aid fertility.
- **Stress**: There is no doubt that stress is linked with the development of cancer. This is simply because stress depletes our immune system, using up huge amounts of life-energy.
- **Genetic predisposition**: This is the one factor that is completely out of our control. Being aware of a familial propensity for a particular type of cancer, however, is an even more powerful motive for trying to reduce other risk factors.

Cancer seldom has a single cause. To give one example, risk factors for cervical cancer include: folic acid deficiency, smoking, a variety of sexual partners particularly in the teenage years when the cervix is immature, and excessive consumption of alcohol. Any one of these increases the chances, but bring them all together and the risk becomes very much higher.

What can we do to help ourselves?

We may not be able to do much to control pollution at a planetary level, and nothing at all about the genes we have inherited, but with a little effort we can do much to reduce those other risk factors:

- Eat a healthy diet, low in saturated fats and high in complex carbohydrates, with plenty of fresh fruit and vegetables and fluids, supplemented where necessary with vitamin and mineral supplements.
- Make time every day to exercise your body, whether it's a session in the gym, a swim, an aerobics class or just a brisk walk.
- Give up smoking. It is hard, but necessary.
- Look after your liver. It filters out toxins in your body, so don't overload it with alcohol or fats.
- Manage stress. Exercise is an excellent antidote, but look too at your outlook on life. Strive for optimism, try not to harbour grudges and don't bottle up feelings. Unexpressed emotions create havoc in our bodies.

How reflexology can help

Reflexology can be used to help cancer sufferers by aiding relaxation. The improvement in nerve stimulation and blood supply enhances the function of the immune system and keeps the hormonal system in balance. Reflexology can also help to protect against disease and a general 'maintenance treatment' on a regular basis will leave you feeling much better.

Areas to work for cancer

When treating cancer patients undergoing chemotherapy and/or radiotherapy, it is advisable not to treat for at least six days following each chemotherapy/radiotherapy session. Reflexology has a stimulating effect and could well give the patient more side-effects than necessary. Areas to work for cancer include the digestive system, the lymphatic system (spleen) and the urinary system (bladder and the ureter tube). Relaxation exercises are also highly beneficial (see pages 56–60).

The liver

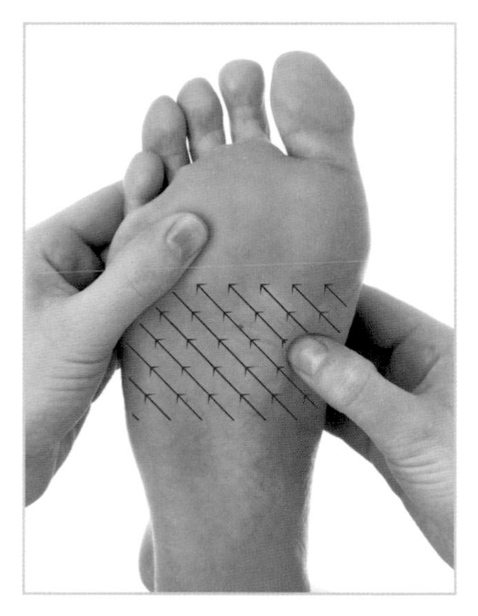

1 Use your right thumb to work out the liver area of the right foot in a criss-cross direction from the medial to the lateral edge (see page 79).

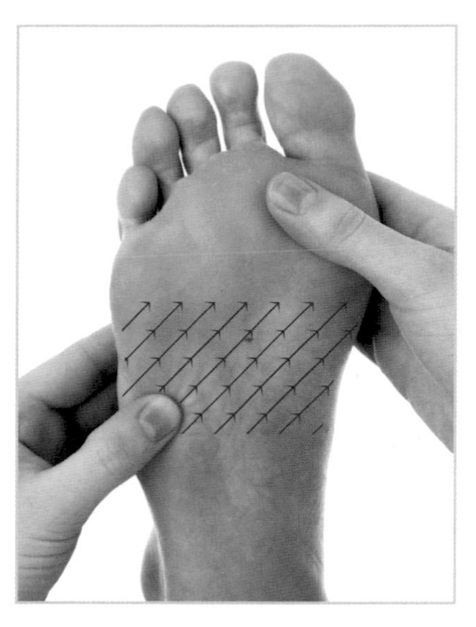

2 Use the left thumb to work the liver area in a criss-cross direction from the lateral to the medial edge.

The stomach

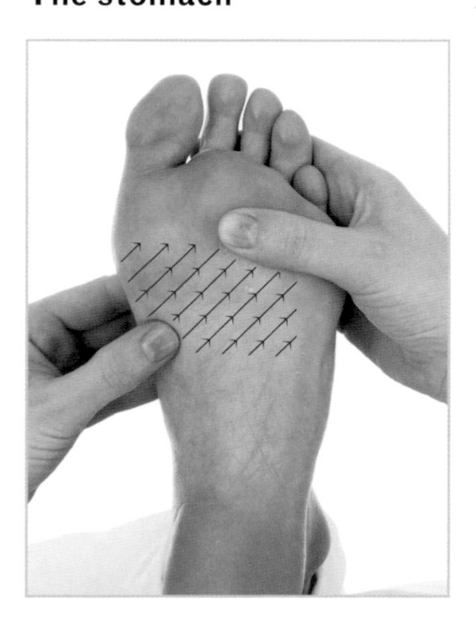

1 Use your left thumb to work the stomach area on the left foot in a criss-cross direction from medial to lateral (see page 79).

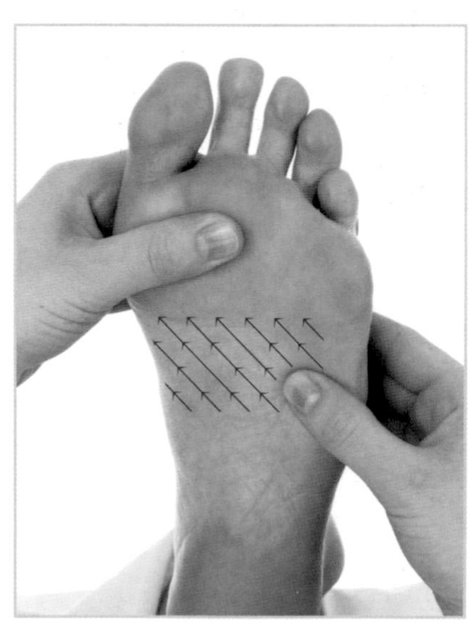

2 Use your right thumb to work the stomach area on the left foot from lateral to medial.

The intestinal area

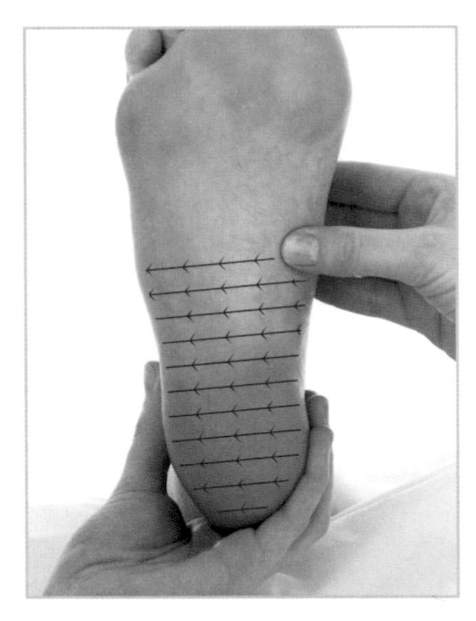

1 Use your right thumb to work the intestinal area of the right foot in straight lines across the foot from medial to lateral (see page 80).

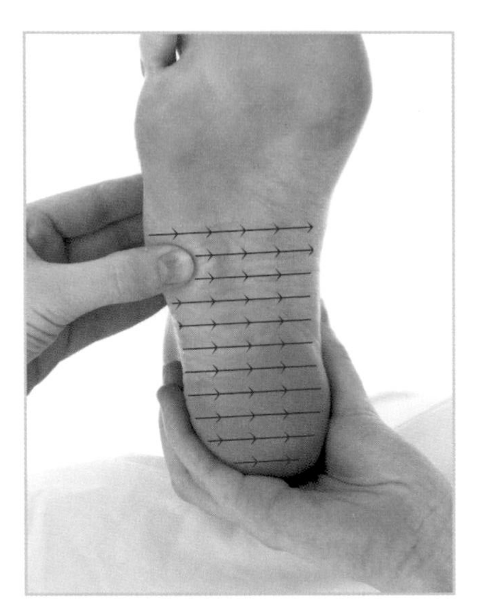

2 Use your left thumb to work the intestinal area of the right foot in straight lines from lateral to medial.

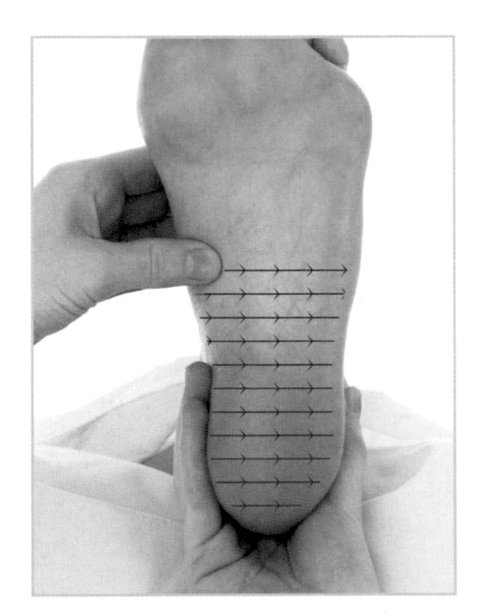

3 Use your left thumb to work the intestinal area of the left foot in straight lines across the foot from medial to lateral (see page 81).

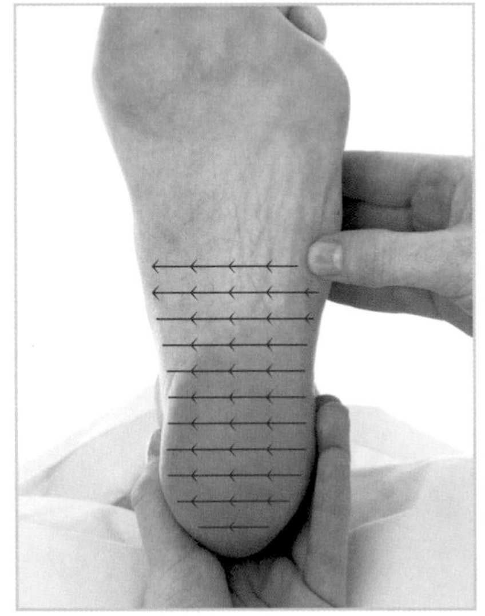

4 Use your right thumb to work the intestinal area of the left foot in straight lines from lateral to medial.

The spleen

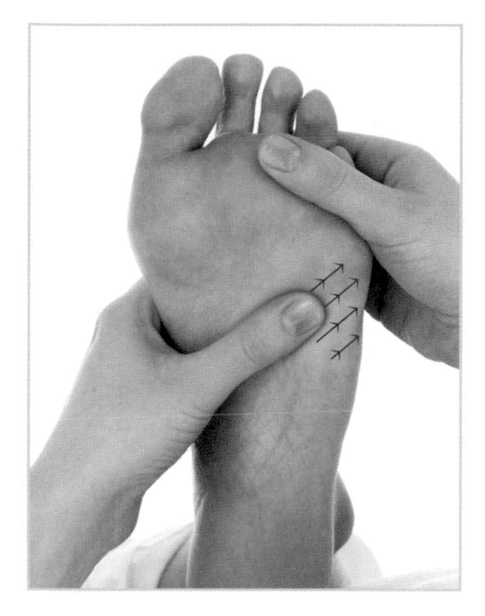

1 Use your left thumb to work the area of the spleen on the left foot, working from the medial to the lateral side of the foot.

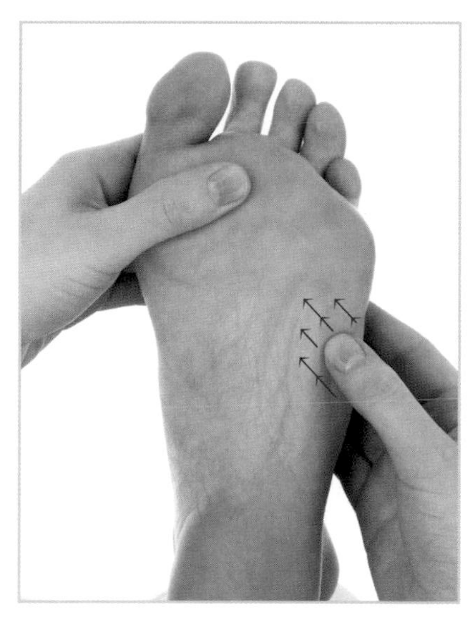

2 Use your right thumb to work the spleen area from the lateral to the medial side of the foot.

The bladder/ureter tube

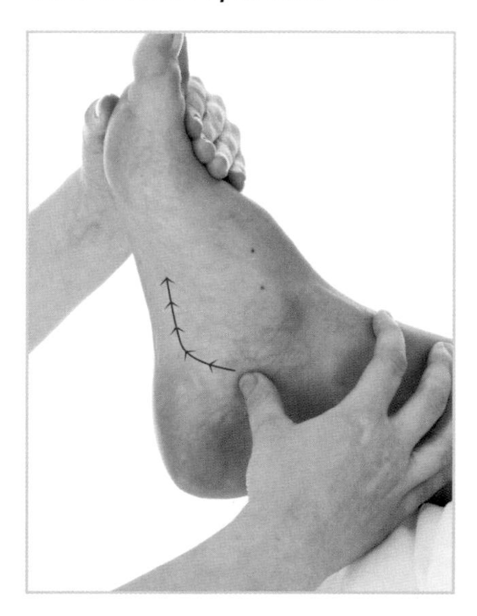

1 Use your right thumb to work on and over the bladder area on the right foot. Proceed up the medial side of the ligament line to work out the ureter tube (see page 145).

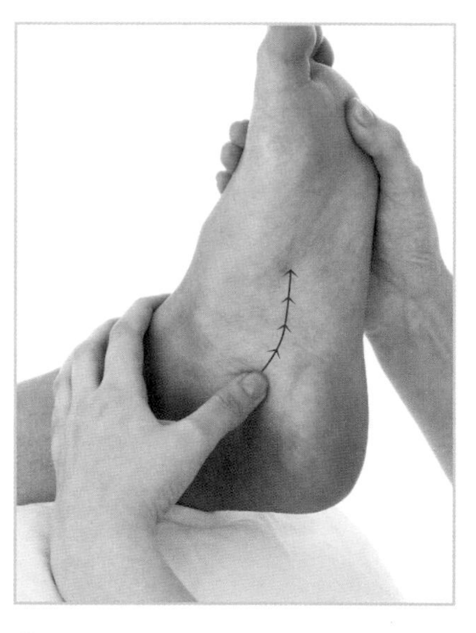

2 Use your left thumb to work on and over the bladder area on the left foot. Proceed up the medial side of the ligament line to work out the ureter tube.

TREATING PATIENTS WITH A SERIOUS ILLNESS

- Always use a light pressure when treating patients in a weakened state of health.
- Do not work for more than about 15 minutes on each foot.
- Concentrate on light relaxation exercises (see pages 54–60).
- Very sick patients often fall asleep during the treatment, which is beneficial. However, some do like to talk and communication with the therapist about their illness and any other anxieties that come to light is to be encouraged.

Heart disease

Heart attacks account for 39 per cent of all deaths in the UK, killing 117,000 people every year. Atherosclerosis, or hardening of the arteries, which eventually leads to coronary heart disease, is the major cause of death, particularly among men although the statistics on women are fast catching up. In fact, incidence of heart disease has reached almost epidemic proportions in the Western world.

'The circulatory system' (see pages 88–91) explains how the heart works and what can hinder its efficiency or lead to failure. While some people have a genetic predisposition to heart disease (which should be an extra warning to take precautions), most of the problems are linked to the way we live: an unhealthy diet, lack of exercise, unrelieved stress and smoking.

Swallowing doctors' pills may help but they are not the answer. If they were, the death rates from heart disease would not be so high. There are better and more effective ways to reduce the risk, but they take commitment and effort. You need to put energy into treating yourself kindly and taking responsibility for your illness.

What can we do to help ourselves?

- Stop smoking.
- Moderate alcohol intake.
- Eat a sensible diet (see below).
- Cut down on sugar. This increases concentrations of plasma, cholesterol and uric acid, all of which are involved in the development of atherosclerosis.
- Avoid an excess of stimulants, such as the caffeine in coffee, tea and cola drinks.
- Learn to relax.
- Take more exercise. The heart is a strong pump, it likes to be used and it will become stronger if it is exercised on a regular basis. Walking is ideal (brisk enough to make you perspire and be aware of your heart beating) and other aerobic exercise such as cycling and swimming is also highly recommended.

Helpful food

Most authorities agree that the level of plasma cholesterol is largely determined by the dietary intake of cholesterol, polyunsaturated fat and saturated fat. It is a good idea to reduce your intake of saturated fats (which are mostly derived from meat) and to be aware of the fat content of your diet. Fish oil, however, is beneficial, and a diet rich in fish oils is recommended.

Eat as natural and additive-free a diet as possible, and ensure you get plenty of fibre. This not only makes the digestive system perform its functions more effectively, but the type of fibre found in pectin, oat bran and psyllium seed also binds bile and cholesterol in the intestines, soaking up the fat content.

Onions have been proved to counteract the increased platelet aggregation seen after consumption of a high-fat meal, and have been shown to have anti-hypertensive and cholesterol-lowering effects. Garlic has similar effects and also thins the blood, leading to better flow through the arteries.

VITAMINS, MINERALS AND SUPPLEMENTS

The way most food is grown, transported, stored and cooked these days means that much of the vitamin content is lost before we eat it. Supplements may improve our dietary intake, although they should be treated as an addition and not as a substitute for a healthy diet.

- **Vitamin B**: Recent studies have revealed a link between vitamin B deficiency and the heart disease atherosclerosis.
- **Vitamin C**: This helps fat metabolism and boosts the health of arterial walls.

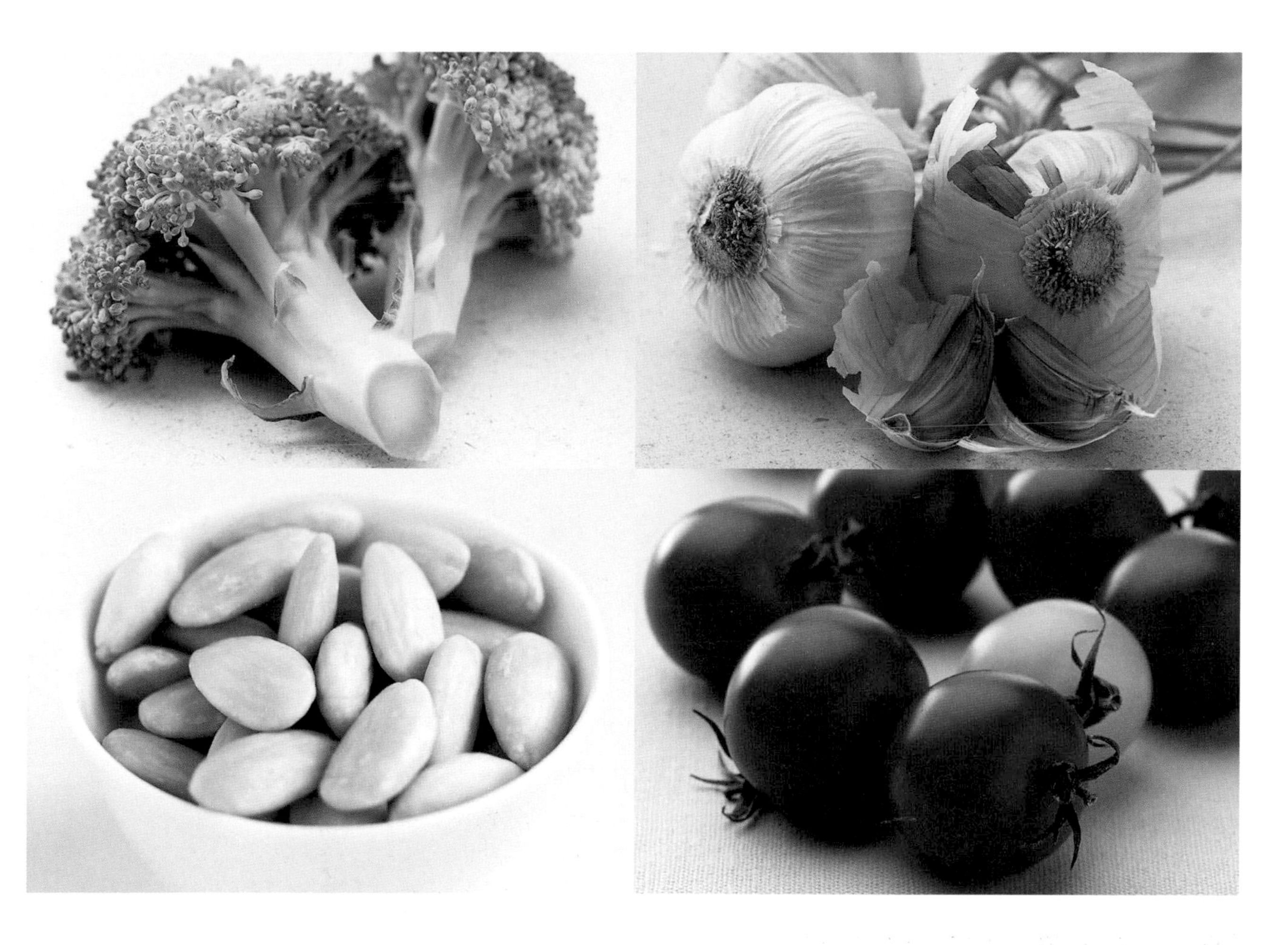

Foods to protect your heart Garlic helps prevent the formation of blood clots; tomatoes and broccoli are high in vitamin C; almonds are a good source of vitamin E.

- **Vitamin E**: A deficiency results in significantly higher levels of free radicals, which cause increased damage, particularly of the vascular endothelium. Supplemental vitamin E has been shown to inhibit the platelet-releasing action by which atheromatous plaque builds up in the arteries.
- **Carnitine**: This vitamin-like compound initiates the breakdown of fatty acids. If the heart does not receive an adequate supply of oxygen, as would be the case in sufferers from angina or following a heart attack, carnitine levels quickly decrease. Carnitine deficiency has been linked to diseases of the heart such as congestive heart failure and cardiac enlargement. Carnitine is available as a nutritional supplement.
- **Magnesium**: This mineral strengthens the heart muscle contractions. Magnesium has been found to be beneficial in the management of irregular heart beat, particularly bradycardia, and high blood pressure. A magnesium deficiency has been shown to produce spasms in the coronary arteries and is considered to be a cause of heart attacks in some cases.
- **Garlic, lecithin, vitamin E and ginkgo biloba** These all help the heart and assist the workings of the circulatory system.

How reflexology can help

For patients suffering from any form of cardiovascular disease, reflexology can be effective in improving the blood supply to the heart.

After someone suffers a heart attack, the heart muscle is damaged and needs time to heal. Most patients feel very anxious and fearful of a repeat occurrence after their discharge from hospital. Regular reflexology can help to repair the physical damage that has occurred and the one-to-one communication and support will also help the patient cope with the psychological effects during the convalescence period.

Areas to work for heart disease

The main areas to treat for angina, coronary heart disease, atherosclerosis and high or low blood pressure are the heart, the thoracic spine and the lungs. It is perfectly safe to treat on a daily basis if you have the opportunity so to do. As a reflexologist you will undoubtedly find sensitivity in the liver reflex when treating patients with coronary heart disease.

The thoracic spine

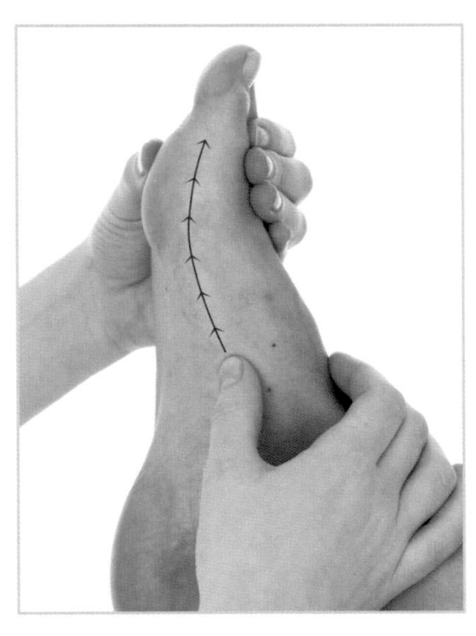

1 Use your right thumb to work up the line of the thoracic spine on the right foot.

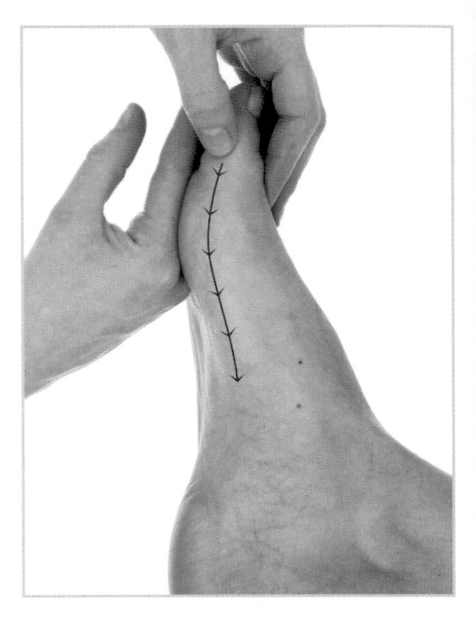

2 Use your left thumb to work down the line of the thoracic spine on the right foot.

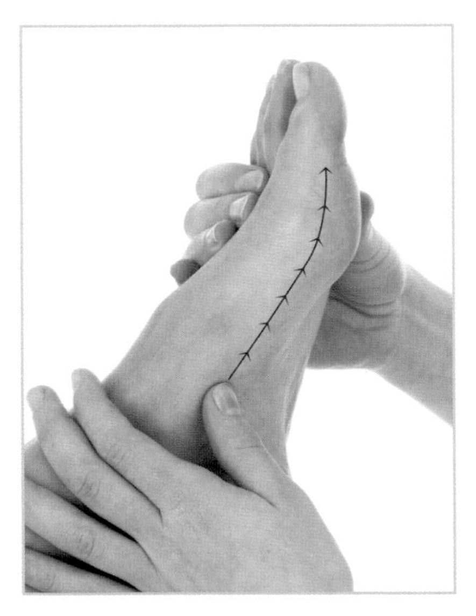

3 Use your left thumb to work up the line of the thoracic spine on the left foot.

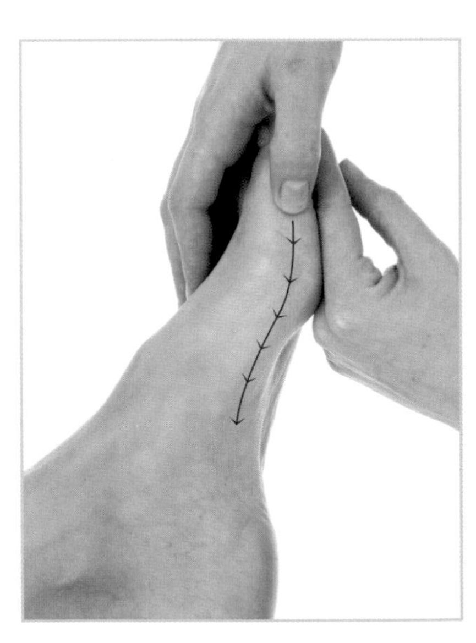

4 Use your right thumb to work down the line of the thoracic spine on the left foot.

The heart

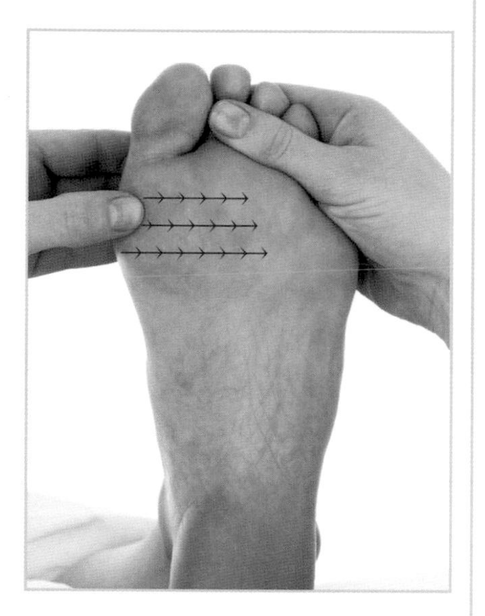

Use your left thumb to work in horizontal lines across the heart area on the left foot, from medial to lateral (see page 93). Note that the heart area is worked in one direction only as it is also worked out when the respiratory area is treated.

The lungs

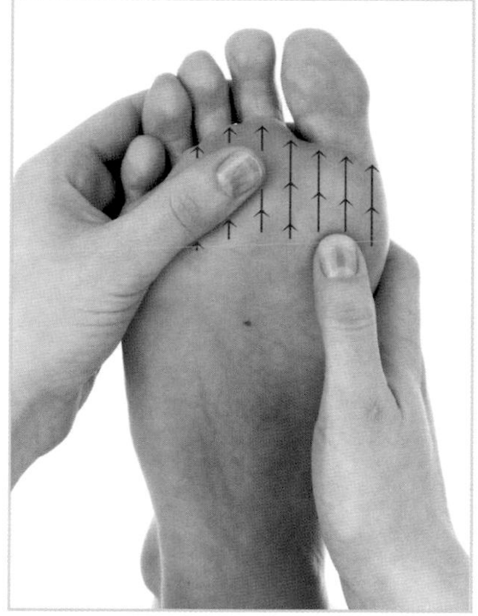

1 Use your right thumb to work up the lung area of the right foot in straight lines, from medial to lateral (see page 86).

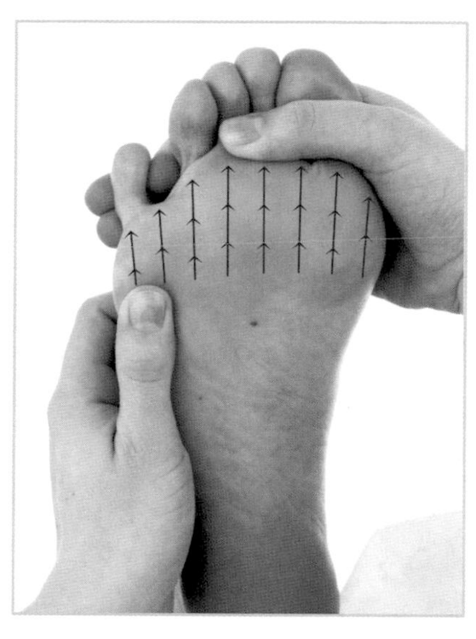

2 Use your left thumb to work up the lung area of the right foot in straight lines from lateral to medial. Separate each toe as you proceed.

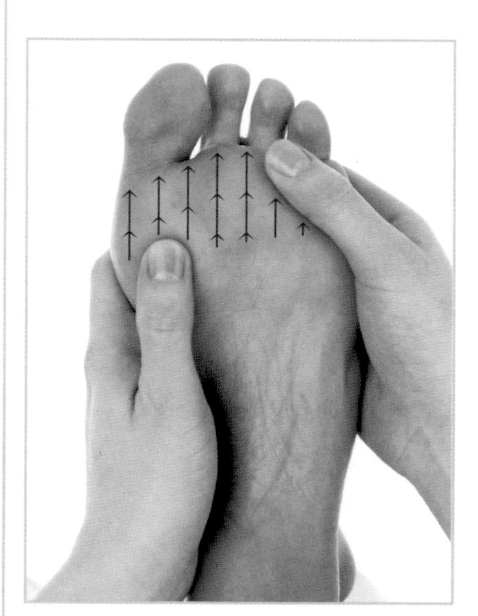

3 Use your left thumb to work up the lung area of the left foot in straight lines, from medial to lateral (see page 87).

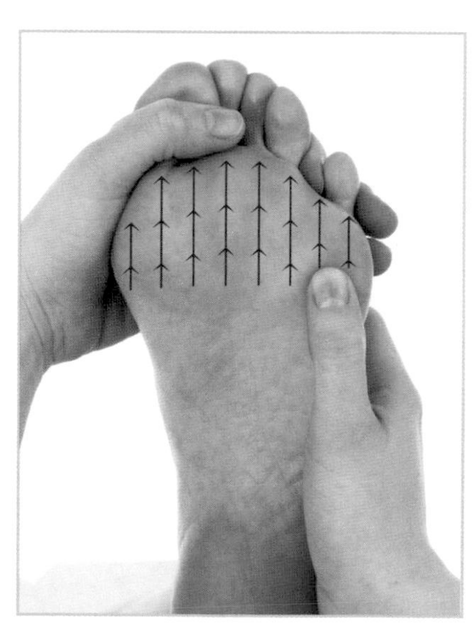

4 Use your right thumb to work up the lung area of the left foot in straight lines from lateral to medial. Separate each toe as you proceed.

Helping the terminally ill

Reflexology has many benefits to offer the terminally ill. It can help with pain relief and is also useful for encouraging general relaxation and helping to relieve anxiety.

Many reflexology practitioners work in hospices these days and their presence is greatly respected by the medical profession. Patients enjoy the treatment sessions and usually ask for a return visit, and, after all, if someone only has a very short time to live then it really is up to them to decide for themselves if reflexology gives them relief and a feeling of wellbeing.

A short, light treatment can be given daily, if requested. You should always use a light pressure when working on the feet of a terminally ill patient.

Areas to work for the terminally ill

Work on all the relaxation techniques, particularly the diaphragm relaxation, which aids respiration. The undergrip and overgrip relaxations are also shown here, but in fact any of the relaxation techniques will be effective. Working the pituitary gland will stimulate the release of endorphins ('feel-good hormones'), producing a sense of wellbeing and lessening pain.

Overgrip

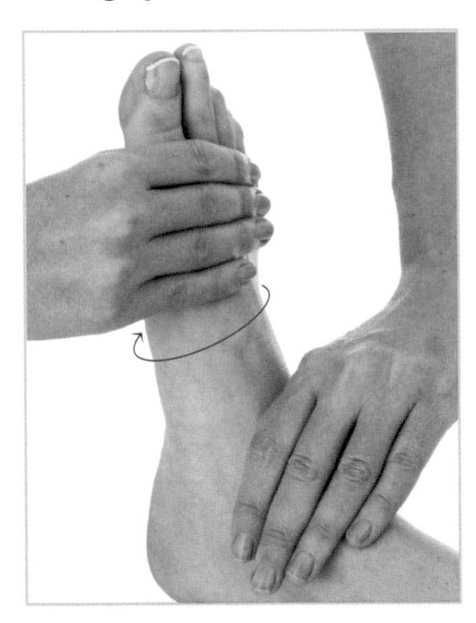

1 Place your left hand over the top of the right ankle, making sure that the thumb of your left hand is on the lateral edge of the foot. Turn the foot in an inward direction, using a light, circling movement (see page 58).

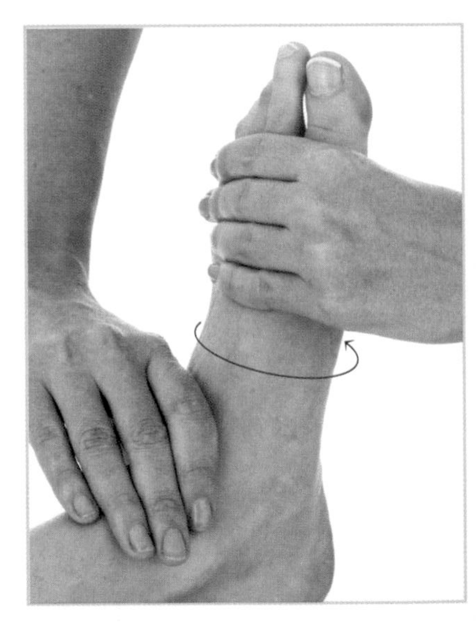

2 Reverse the procedure, placing your right hand over the top of the left ankle and rotating the foot inwards as before.

Undergrip

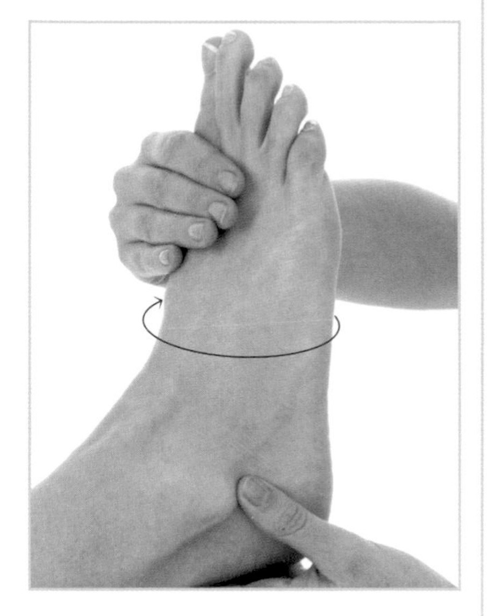

1 Place your left hand under the right ankle, with your thumb on the lateral edge of the foot. Turn the foot in an inward direction, using a light, circling movement (see page 57).

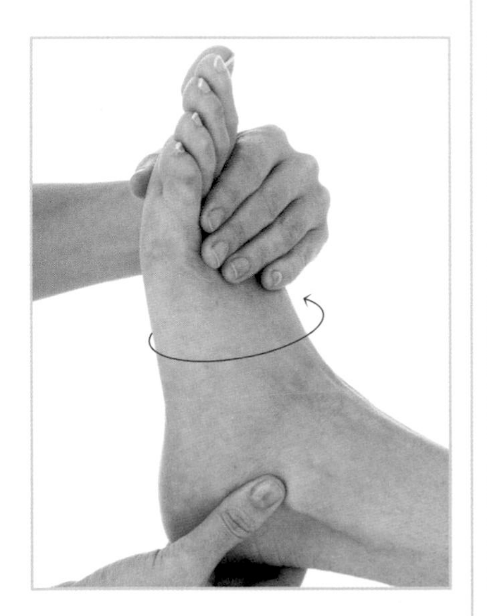

2 Repeat the same exercise, this time placing your right hand under the left ankle and then turning the foot inwards with your left hand (see page 58).

Diaphragm relaxation

This is a great relaxant to the diaphragm muscle, and produces nice, slow, rhythmic breathing, almost putting the body into 'sleeping mode'. It is especially beneficial for patients in pain.

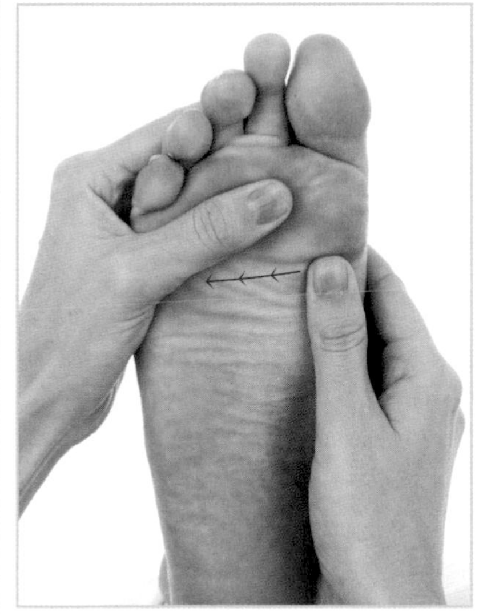

1 Place your right thumb on the start of the diaphragm line on the right foot. As you move it to the lateral edge, bend the toes down towards your thumb (see page 55).

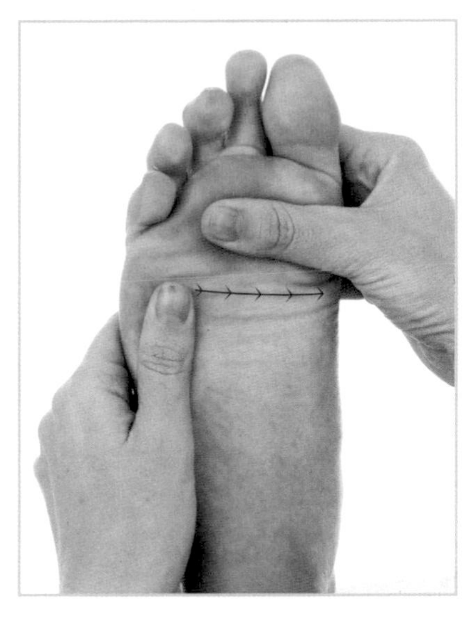

2 Place your left thumb on the diaphragm line. As you move it to the medial edge, bend the toes downwards towards your thumb.

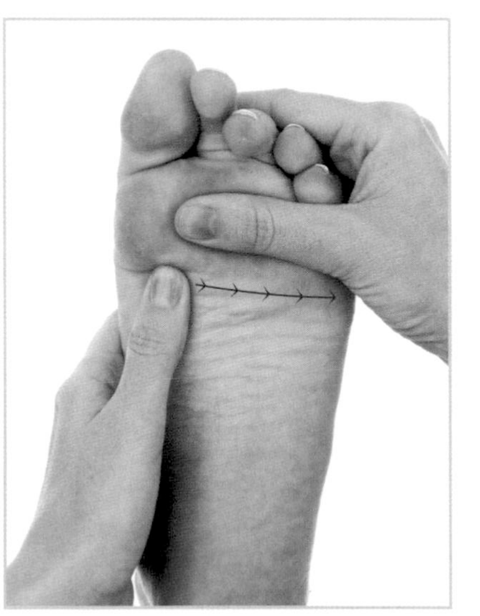

3 Place your left thumb on the start of the diaphragm line on the left foot. As you move it to the lateral edge, bend the toes downwards towards your thumb.

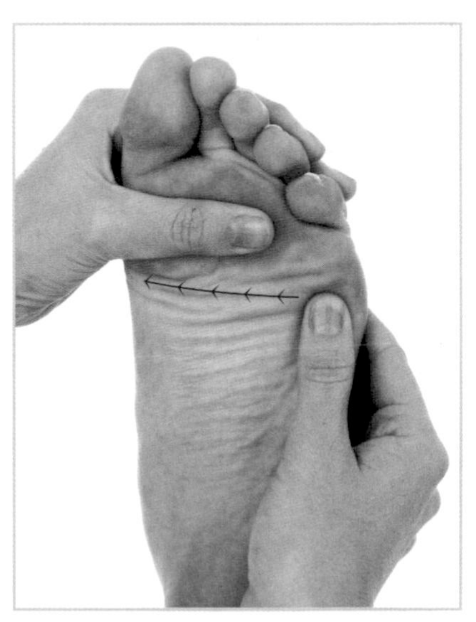

4 Place your right thumb on the diaphragm line of the left foot as indicated. As you move it to the medial edge, bend the toes downwards towards your thumb.

Reflexology for babies

Babies enjoy the calming and relaxing effects of reflexology just as much as adults do. Treatment has a beneficial effect on babies who had a difficult birth and can also help with cases of allergic reactions such as eczema and digestive upsets.

Working a baby's feet

The working out of the reflexes in a young child's foot is simple as you will notice that, until they are about four or five years old, there is little arch on the underside of the foot. In fact, a baby's foot really resembles an oval. Because of this, you just need to work over the complete surface of the foot, starting at the heel and working up the entire area to where the toes begin, using tiny, forward-creeping movements.

An all-important area to work for babies is the inside of both feet, which is the reflex area for the spine. It reaches right up to the top of the big toe, which is the reflex area for the brain.

How reflexology can help

As well as providing a pleasant form of relaxation for a baby and benefiting the baby's general state of health and wellbeing, reflexology is particularly helpful in alleviating problems stemming from birth trauma and easing discomfort associated with wind. It can also provide a stress-free way of helping to overcome symptoms relating to infant allergies.

Colic

Colic is a distressing condition that affects many babies in the first three months of life. Evening colic, when the baby cries and seems to be full of wind every evening, is especially difficult for all the family. The more the crying continues the more air is taken into the digestive system and so a vicious circle begins.

Reflexology will certainly help the digestive system, improving circulation to the digestive and intestinal areas and easing episodes of wind and pain. Try working on the entire surface of the baby's feet during these restless periods. Do not be surprised if you hear a lot of rumbling and gurgling in the abdominal area; this is a sign of increased muscular activity in the stomach and bowel, which should reduce the pain of colic. Most practitioners will be happy to teach parents how to use a forward-creeping movement to treat colic in their babies.

Plantar (0–3)

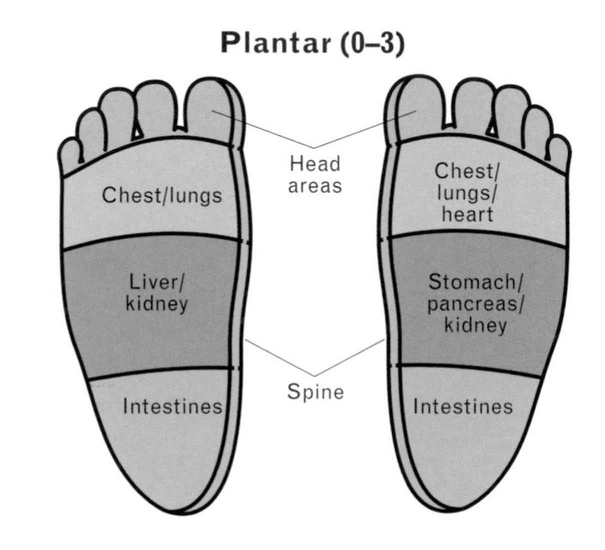

Plantar (3–5)

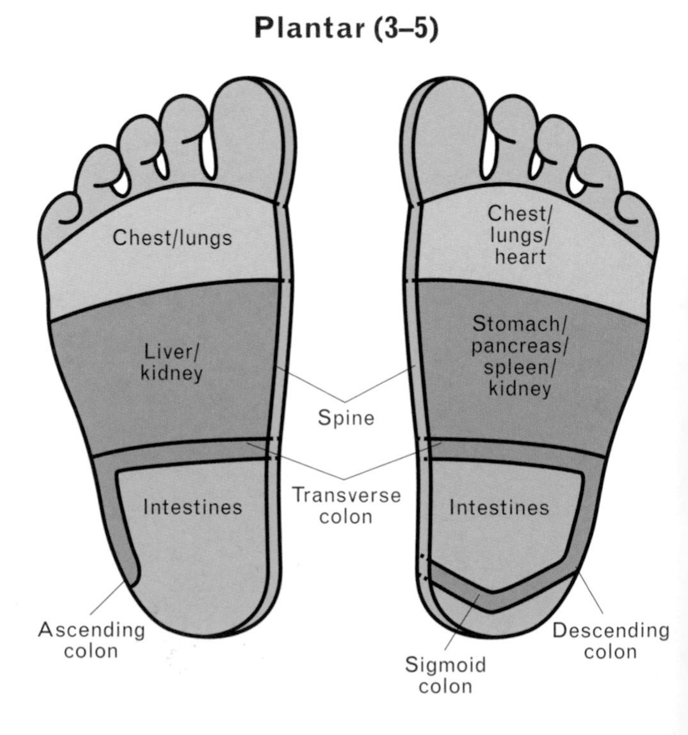

Working on tiny feet Babies rarely keep their feet still, but even a few minutes of reflexology will calm a baby with colic or one who is having trouble settling down to sleep.

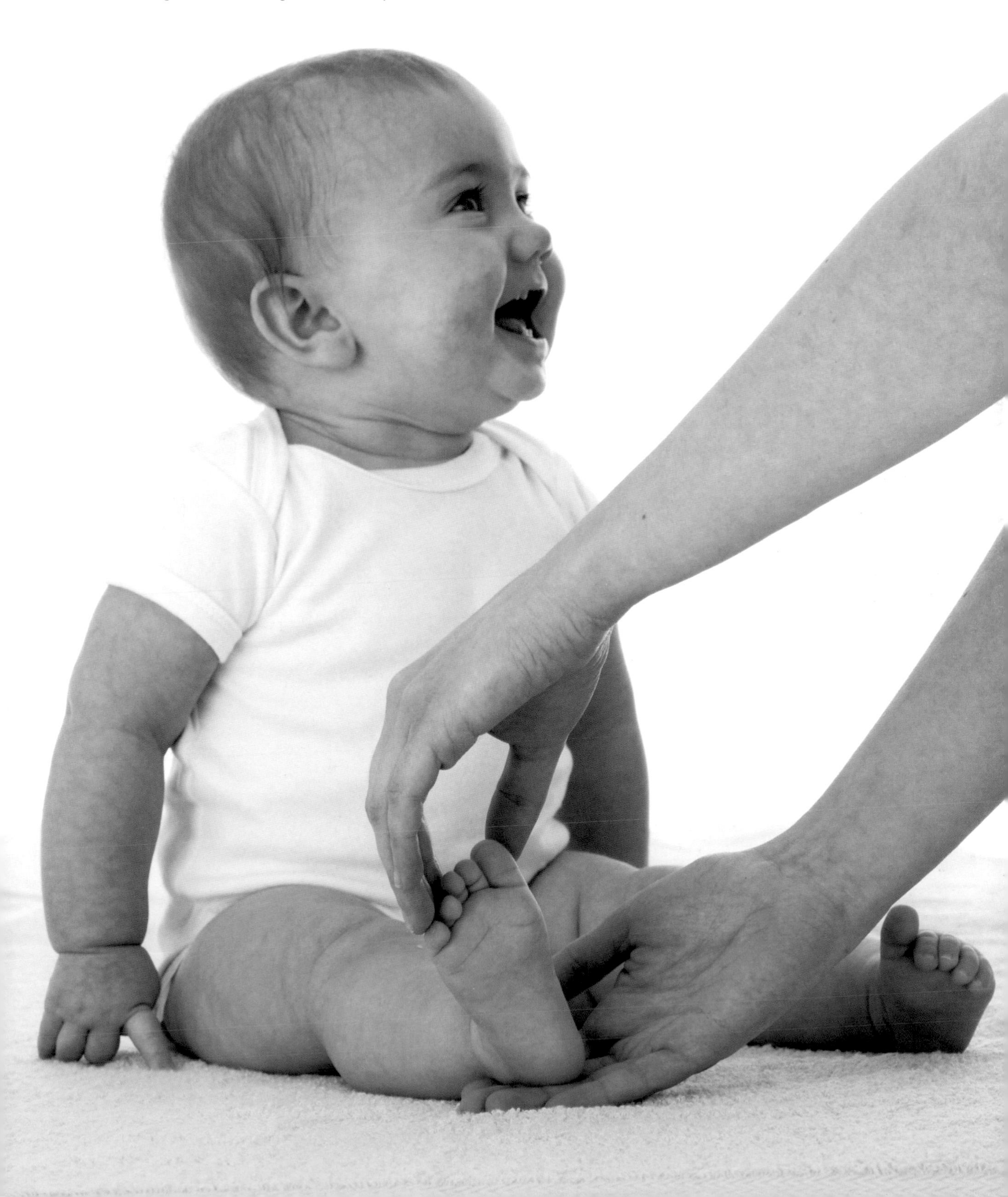

BREASTFEEDING AND ALLERGY

Not only does breastfeeding help to build strong digestive and immune systems, but there is now evidence that long-term breastfeeding actually helps to prevent cancer.

The breastfeeding mother should make absolutely sure that her diet is as natural as possible, with plenty of carbohydrates in the form of rice, pasta, wholewheat bread and potatoes. A vegetarian diet is preferable if the baby is suffering from eczema – very few vegetables, fruits and pulses cause allergies. A good intake of calcium is also necessary, preferably in the form of a supplement rather than large quantities of milk and cheese, in case the baby is allergic to dairy products.

Remember, it is not necessary to drink lots of milk to produce breast milk, just a lot of fluid. Drink juices, preferably apple, grape and mango because orange juice can be the cause of allergic reactions.

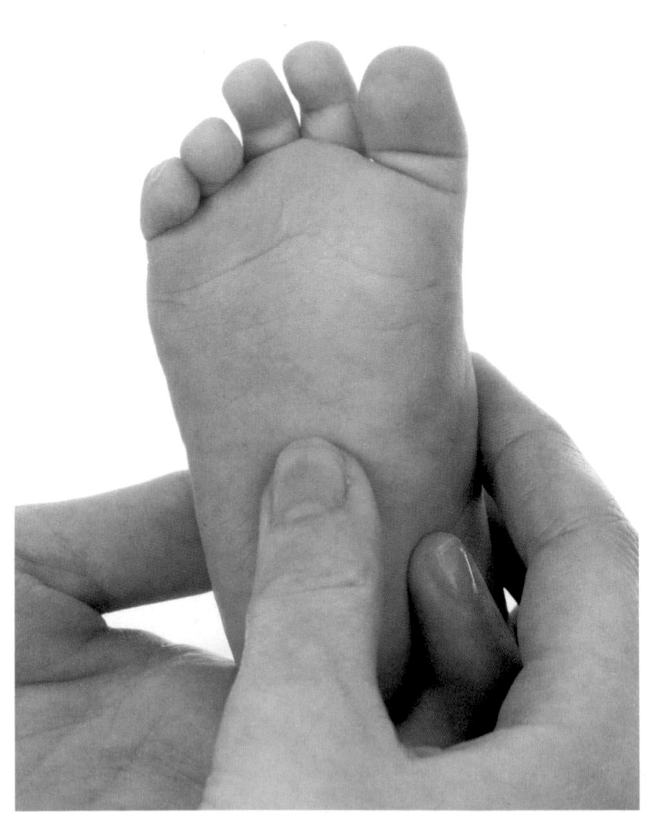

Birth traumas

Incessant crying or difficulties in establishing good feeding or sleeping habits can often be the result of a baby's hazardous journey into the world. Although the birth canal is relatively short, the journey from the uterus to the outside world is, in some ways, the most traumatic transition we ever make. Treating the spinal area is of major benefit to those babies who suffered a difficult birth, such as a prolonged labour which may have resulted in a forceps birth.

Allergies and eczema

An allergy is not an illness; it is a symptom of a condition and an indication that something is wrong. We need to pay heed to symptoms such as eczema and take action to do something about whatever is causing them rather than just treating them superficially.

Babies are sometimes born with an allergic reaction to foods and have outbreaks of eczema, which is both unsightly and distressing to the baby, as well as the parent. Eczema should be regarded as a warning signal from the body that certain foods are causing a stress on the baby's delicate digestive system. 'Cradle cap' is another sign of possible allergy.

Sometimes the very food that the mother craved during pregnancy was the food that, because it was eaten or drunk in excess, caused the allergic reaction in the baby. The list of allergens is endless, but frequent culprits include fizzy drinks containing artificial sweeteners or colourings in sweets and cakes.

To ease the itching, keep the baby's skin well oiled with a light olive oil, rather than using medicated creams.

Weaning

When it comes to weaning a baby, it is advisable to follow the same dietary rules that apply to the breastfeeding mother (see box). You should avoid introducing any foods from the cow into the baby's diet until the child has his or her first grinding teeth, which will be towards the end of the second year. By this time the digestive system will have become mature and there will be far less likelihood of an allergic reaction.

Reflexology for babies As a baby's foot is oval in shape and lacks an arch, treatment involves simply working over the whole foot surface from the heel to the start of the toes.

Areas to work

Digestive system

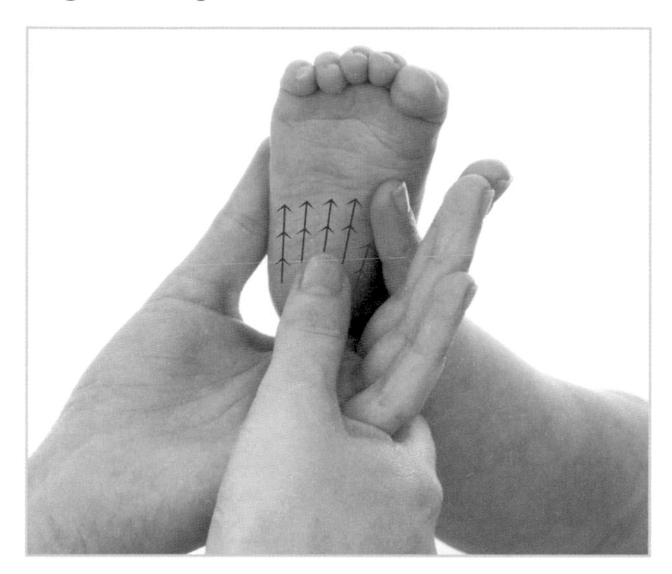

1 Supporting the baby's right foot with your left hand, use your right thumb to work over the entire heel area. Do this gently 2 or 3 times.

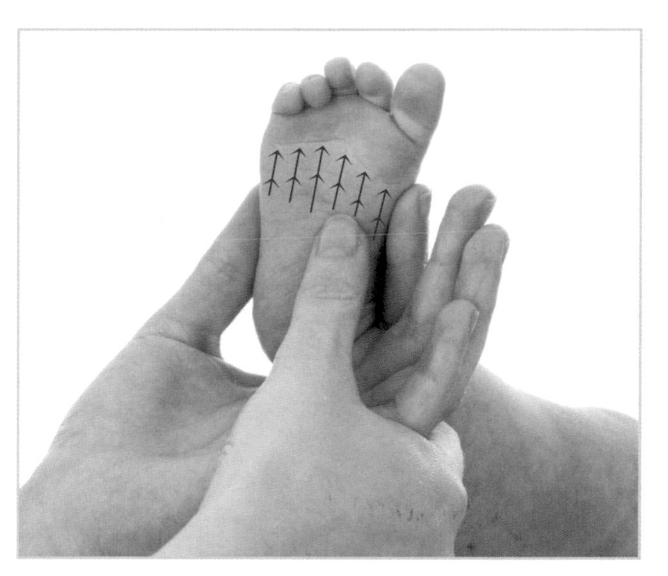

2 Still maintaining only gentle pressure, move up to work across the middle area of the foot, from the inside to the outside edge. Repeat both steps on the left foot.

Head and neck area

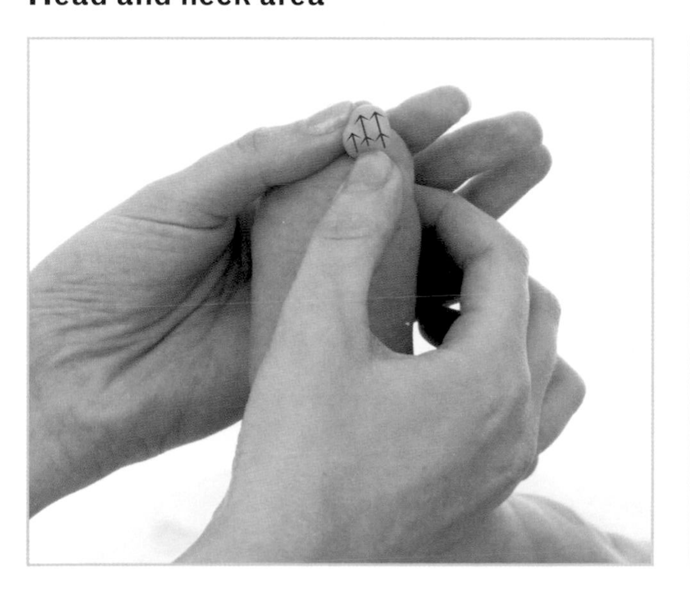

Supporting the top of the right foot with your left thumb, apply gentle pressure to the general area beneath and over the toes. Repeat on the left foot.

The spine

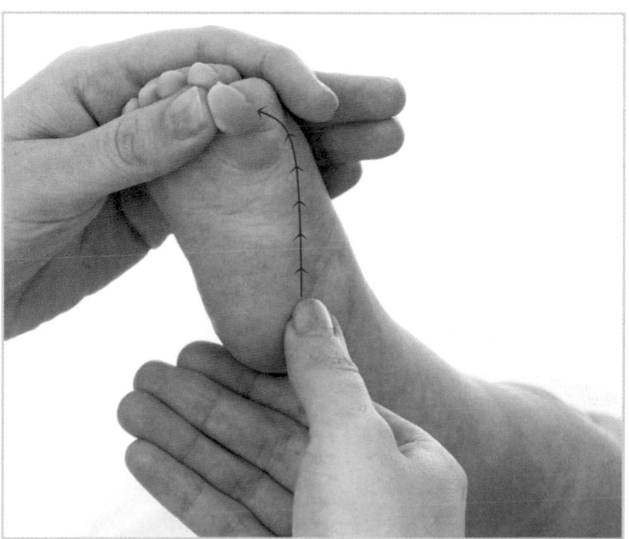

Support the right foot with your left hand as shown and work the spine reflexes along the side of the foot up to the top of the big toe. Repeat on the left foot.

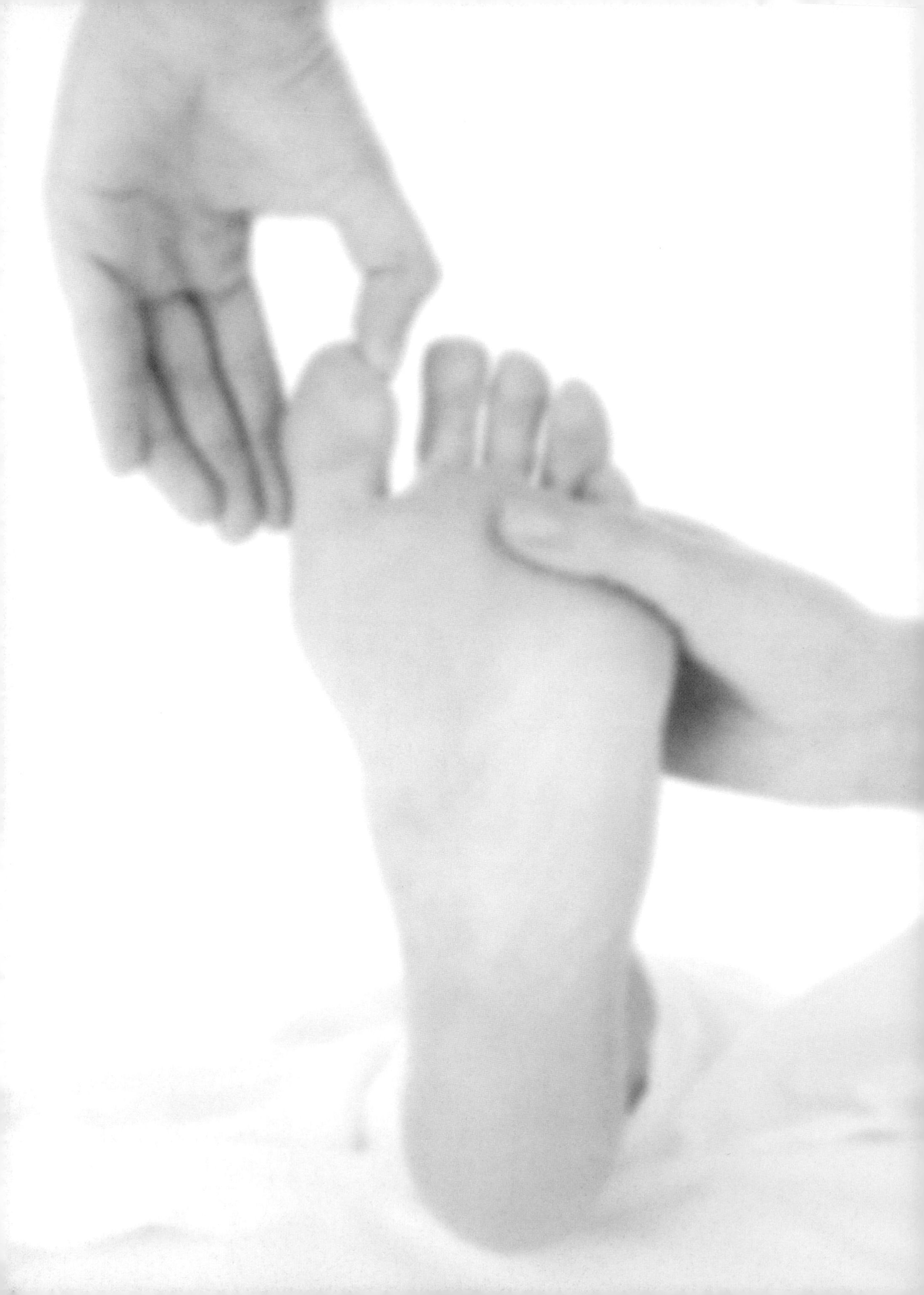

A reflexology practice

Once you have put in the hard work in training to achieve your qualification as a reflexologist, the next hurdle is to promote yourself and start building a practice. Interest in many complementary therapies is growing, but you will need to be your own ambassador and spread the word, both about the advantages of reflexology and what you personally can offer. Once you have treated a few patients, recommendations will start to come your way and you will start building a clientele.

Setting up a business

Becoming qualified as a reflexologist will have taken time and a lot of hard work, and perhaps considerable expense. The time has now come to put all you have learnt to work and to set yourself up as a practising reflexologist.

Researching the basics

Before you embarked on the training you will probably have looked into what is already being offered in your area and be reasonably confident that there are opportunities for a reflexology practice. If you are new to the area, you will need to do some homework.

Find out what fees practitioners are charging for complementary therapies generally in your area. Check out local massage therapists and aromatherapists, as well as any other reflexologists. Estimate what your regular outgoings will be. For example, if you are setting up business working from your own home you may be able to charge less than if you are working in a therapy centre, for which you are going to have to pay rent for a room in which to work.

Your working day

Make a decision on how many hours your lifestyle allows you to work and the times in the day that are convenient. A mother with children at school will find it easier to work during school hours and evenings, whereas a single person may prefer to offer more flexible hours or be able to travel further afield.

You should reserve an hour for each treatment session. This will give you time to communicate with your patients without rushing them, and also allows for a short pause between patients.

Equipment

Your main purchase will be some form of massage couch or reflex stool for your patients and perhaps a therapist's adjustable stool for you to sit on (see 'Preparation', page 40). What you choose depends on your planned mode of working, particularly on whether you aim to do home visits or will be working solely from a base. Bear in mind that even a portable massage couch is still very heavy if you are going to be taking it in and out of your car and into people's homes. In this instance a portable reflex stool may be more suitable.

You will also need a cover for your couch or stool, towels, foot creams or powders, and perhaps some form of uniform to wear when you work.

Record-keeping

You will need to keep adequate records of each patient that you treat (see 'Taking a case history', pages 42–43). Whether you opt for keeping manual files or computerize this information is up to you, but choose a method that is secure (you will be holding confidential data) and easy to maintain. Your records should help you run your practice, not become a paperwork (or virtual paperwork) monster.

Book-keeping

At the end of each financial year you will need to provide complete information on all your income and expenditure, so that your tax can be calculated.

Fees received for treatments are straightforward on the income side, but some people just starting up in business, or who do it on a very part-time basis, are not always so precise about the costs they incur. Expenses relating to your practice will be tax deductible but it is essential to keep records and receipts of them. They includes obvious items such as:

- Rental of premises
- Equipment, such as a stool or couch
- Foot balms or powders
- Stationery
- Advertising costs
- Insurance premiums.

They also include costs that you might overlook, such as:

- Car expenses (if you are working as a mobile practitioner)
- Postage and telephone
- Costs of further, advanced courses once you are qualified and in business.

Whether you do manual book-keeping or use an accounting system on your computer is simply a matter of personal preference.

Insurance

Become a member of one of the reflexology associations, which will deal with insurance for you. It is essential to be insured for professional indemnity and public liability.

Promotion

Marketing is essential for the success of your reflexology practice, especially when you are just starting out, because this is a business that is extremely customer-orientated. You need to let people know that you are there and tell them how you can help them. See over the page for a range of different ideas on spreading the word to potential patients.

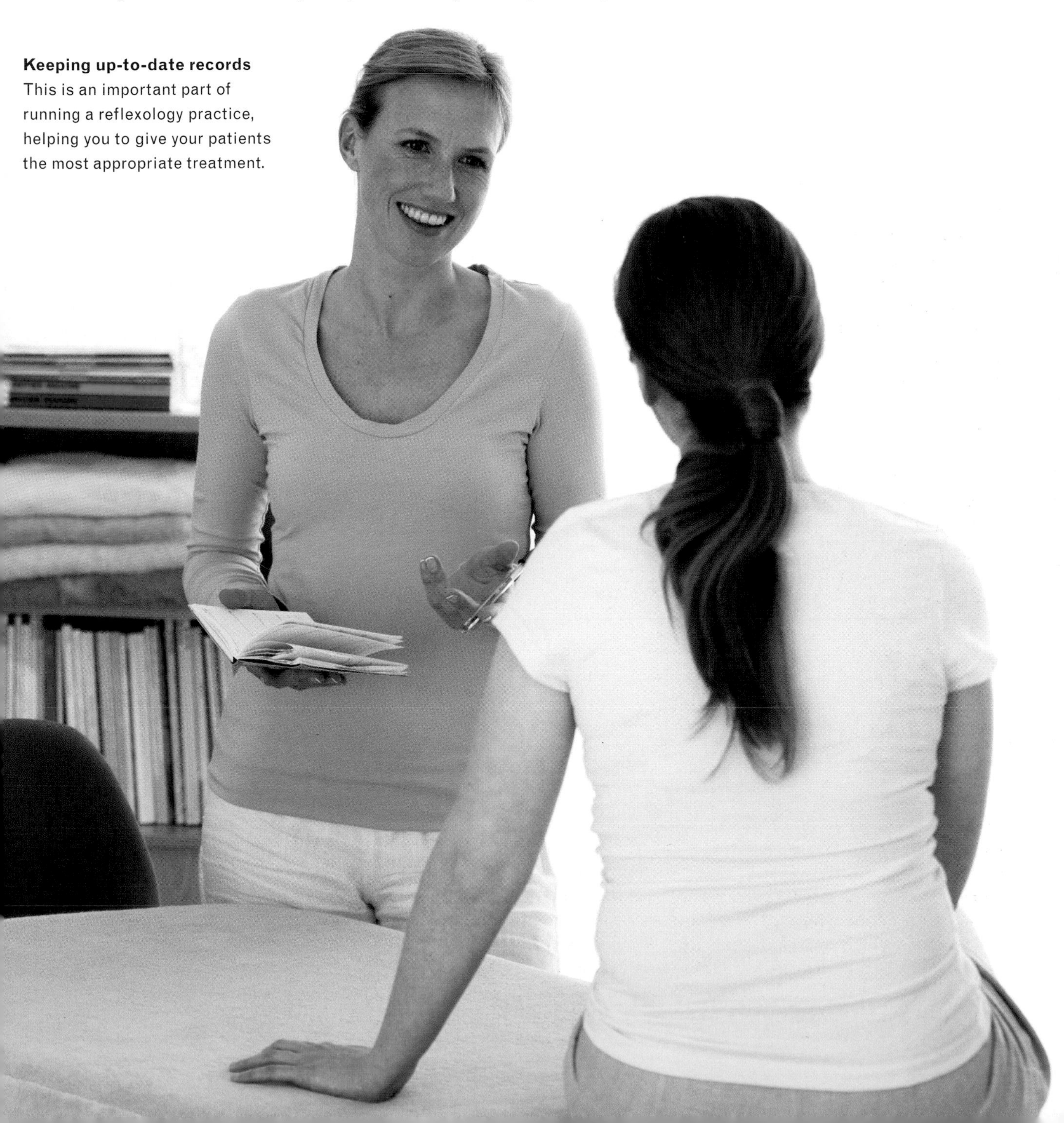

Keeping up-to-date records
This is an important part of running a reflexology practice, helping you to give your patients the most appropriate treatment.

Getting patients

Word of mouth will ultimately be your most successful way of getting new patients, but at the very beginning it can seem daunting to know just where to begin. How do you get started and find those very first few patients?

To get your name and practice known, look for organizations and health centres that are likely to be receptive to what you have to offer.

Local organizations

Find out what goes on in your area in the way of women's clubs, mother and baby groups and so on. Your local town hall or library will usually have a list of names and addresses of associations and details of when and where they meet. And don't forget your local sports centre.

If you feel that you could give an informal talk, you could write to these groups offering to talk to them on the history, development and benefits of reflexology. Many clubs and groups welcome speakers on interesting topics, and this is a powerful way of introducing people to reflexology and allowing them to experience a sample treatment. Most practitioners find that they usually get at least one new patient from each talk. For some hints on how to give a talk, see page 240.

Ann Jones MBSR

Reflexology practitioner

Reflexology can help to relieve all the stress-related conditions of today's busy world and is particularly useful in treating migraine, asthma, digestive conditions, skeletal dysfunctions, arthritis, menstrual and menopausal problems.

Telephone for an appointment

01234 567890

Sample flyer Use the initials applicable to your training school and mention membership of any relevant society; for example MBSR (Member of the British School of Reflexology) and AOR (Association of Reflexologists).

Hotels and leisure centres

Many hotels and leisure centres are beginning to incorporate complementary therapies into their spas and beauty services. It would be well worth writing to the manager of suitable hotels and centres enquiring whether they would be interested in offering reflexology as a treatment. The hotel will usually give you a percentage of the fee charged to the client. Working for, say, one full day a week in a hotel or spa is a great way to get started.

Local commercial companies

Retail outlets and medium- and large-sized offices are finding it is cost-effective to offer treatments such as reflexology to their staff. Such therapies decrease levels of stress-related illnesses, increase staff wellbeing and reduce absenteeism. Write a professional letter to the personnel manager or human resources department of potentially suitable companies, giving details of your qualifications. If you do not get a response, it is worth making a telephone call to see if you can get an interview.

When visiting an organization to talk about potential business, present yourself in the most professional way that you can: dress smartly, and go armed with business cards giving your contact details and qualifications and some informative leaflets about the history and development of reflexology. (You may be able to produce a professional-looking leaflet on your own computer without having to go to the expense of using a printing company – see left for an example.)

Health centres, clinics and residential homes

Some family doctors and local clinics are happy to promote the benefits of reflexology. Contact the practice manager and, if he or she is amenable, ask to place a flyer or some cards in the reception area.

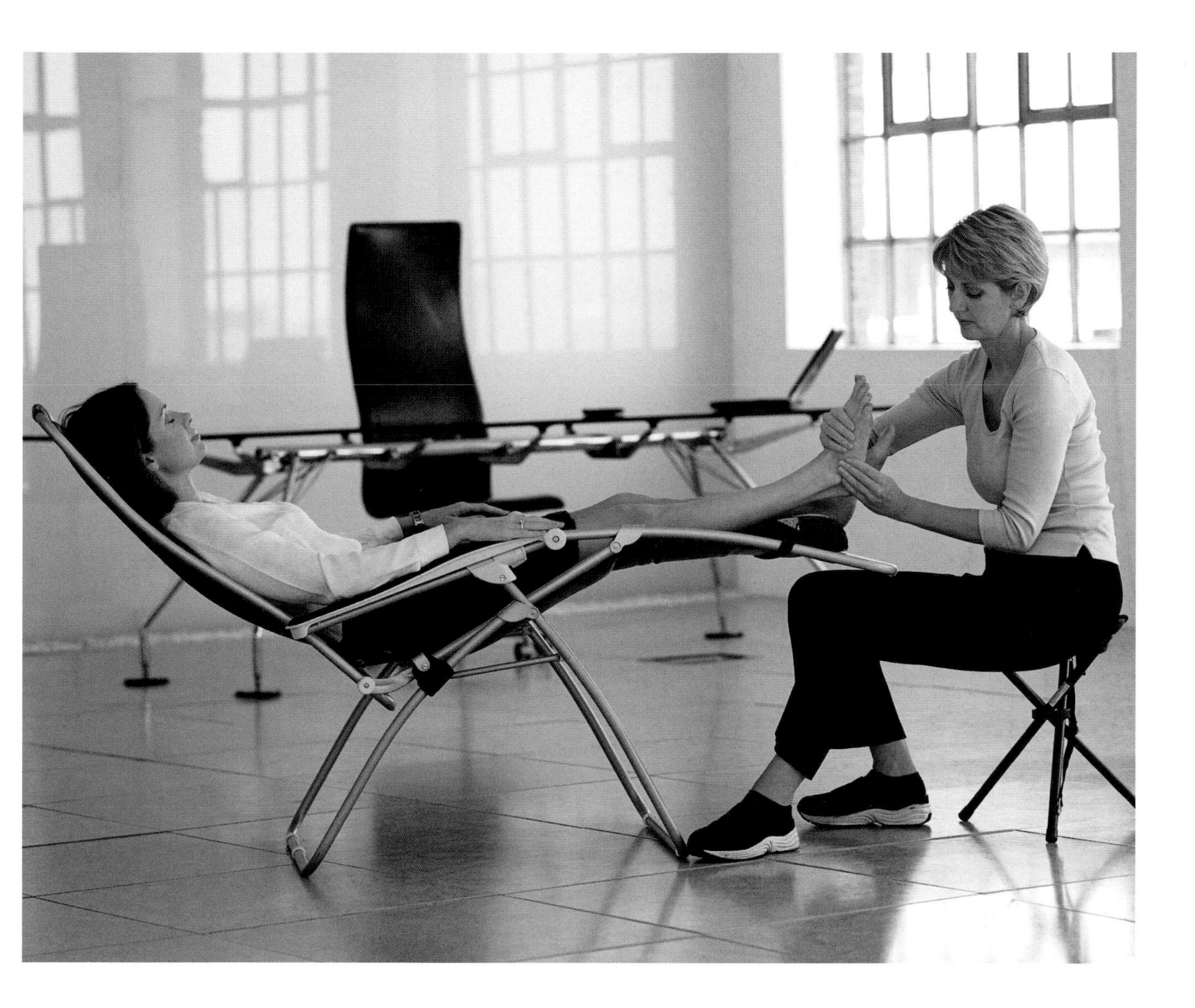

Many care homes are happy to introduce reflexology to their residents. Although the fee which you will receive will be less than what you would get on a one-to-one basis in your own practice, if you are able to treat four or five elderly people in one visit the visit will be an efficient use of your time. It may also turn out to be regular work, which is always worth having.

Other promotional ideas

- Organize a leaflet drop, delivering leaflets through a few hundred doors in your locality.
- Advertise in local papers and telephone directories.
- Put up flyers on noticeboards in your local library, church hall and supermarket.
- Contact your local radio station to see if they would be interested in an interview.

Finding clients Hotels, leisure centres and businesses may be interested in engaging you to provide treatment sessions on their premises.

- Hold an 'open house' and invite as many friends and business associates as possible to join you for an evening of reflexology demonstrations and a short talk on its benefits. A glass of wine and some snacks will help to enhance the enjoyment of the evening.

It does take time and effort to promote a practice but once you have treated just a handful of patients for various health conditions successfully, you will find that personal recommendations, which really are the best form of advertising, will soon follow.

How to give a talk

Speaking to an audience may seem alarming if you have never done it before, but remember that you are talking about something you know about and the people listening are eager to hear what you have to say. You can use a variety of visual aids and demonstrating techniques to make the talk even more interesting.

Constructing your talk

Begin by writing out what you want to say, covering all the subject areas in turn. Start with the history of reflexology – people are very interested in learning where the science originated. Information on the history can be found in 'A history of reflexology', pages 12–15.

Give a simple explanation of how perfectly the feet reflect the body, the right foot representing the right side of the body; the left foot, the left side.

Explain how there are reflexes in the feet to every organ, structure and function of the human body. Point out examples of how the reflex areas mirror the body's layout: the toes reflect the sinus areas; below the thyroid area (where the first three toes join the feet) lie the lung and breast areas, just as in the body; the middle of the feet are associated with the digestive organs in the middle of the body; the base of the feet reflect the intestines and pelvis; and the inside edge of the feet reflects the spine.

Next explain how, when there is a problem in the body, the associated reflex area will reveal a sensitivity when pressure is applied. The treatment is to work on and through these sensitivities with an alternating pressure of the thumb and index fingers, making contact with these reflexes, which are just the size of pinheads. This pressure stimulates an energy through the body that improves nerve and blood supply, increases circulation to sluggish areas, reduces pain and normalizes bodily functioning.

Then cover the types of conditions that can be relieved by reflexology. You might mention in particular migraine, asthma, all forms of skeletal problems, in particular back pain, infertility, menstrual and menopausal disorders and digestive disturbances. Most of the people in the audience will have suffered from one or more of these at one time or another.

End your talk by giving just one good case history (not using the patient's real name, of course). By the time you feel confident about giving a talk you will no doubt have had some good results with several patients, and maybe one in particular will have struck you as an especially convincing example of the power of reflexology. That is the one your audience would like to hear about.

PROFESSIONAL POLISH

- Read over your first draft and check you have not repeated yourself or left out anything vital, that what you say follows a logical sequence and is expressed in a clear and interesting way.
- Read your talk out loud at a measured but conversational pace and time yourself. You may have been given an indication of how long you should talk; if not, ask. Remember to allow plenty of time for a demonstration and answering questions.
- When your talk is in good shape, keep on reading it over and over again until you have absorbed the information; the preparation process is really just like learning a script for a play.
- Visual aids will help your talk. They do not need to be very high-tech. Simply go armed with a large foot chart that can be placed on a stand where it can be viewed by all, and use a pointer to identify the areas you are describing.

Delivering your talk

Because you have thoroughly absorbed everything that you want to say and how to say it, all you need to take is a small card with subject headings as a prompt. It is

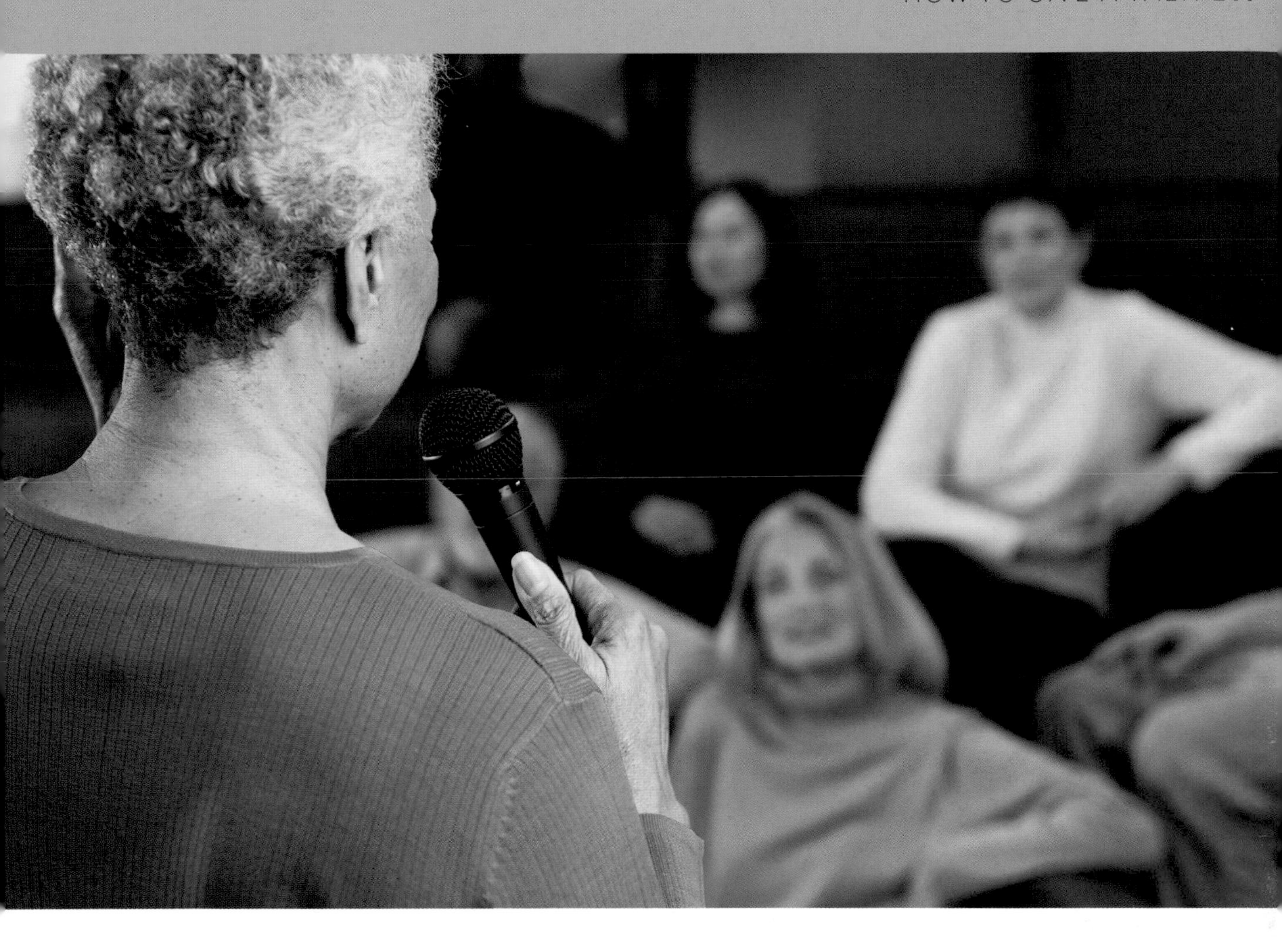

Looking professional Prepare your talk as thoroughly as possible so that you can engage with the audience as you speak rather than leafing through piles of notes.

off-putting to see a lecturer wade through reams of paper while talking, and not necessary.

Always start by introducing yourself: 'I am Jane Brown and I qualified as a reflexology practitioner in 2008. I'd now like to spend a little time introducing you to the fascinating science of reflexology.'

Leave plenty of time at the end of your lecture to give a short demonstration on one or two people. Ask for volunteers from the audience: you will have no trouble in creating an interest here. To finish off, ask your audience if they have any questions.

Be sure to produce a factsheet and clip your business card to it. People like to have something to take away from a talk and they will then have your name and telephone number and some interesting basic information about reflexology should they want to use your services in the future.

Notes for reflexology talk

- *Introduce myself*
- *Talk on the history of reflexology*
- *Use visual aid (foot chart) in describing the relationship between the feet and body*
- *Describe how reflexology works (energy; aids the body in healing itself)*
- *Cover the types of medical conditions that reflexology can help*
- *Mrs Smith's back pain as a case history*
- *Leave time for a demonstration*
- *Questions and answers*

Sample reminder card A few headings on a card should be enough to remind you of your prepared topics.

First aid

In a caring profession such as reflexology, it is essential to have a basic knowledge of first aid. Patients will expect you to be able to handle minor problems and if a medical emergency arises you should be able to cope in a professional way.

Being a competent first-aider means that you can provide initial assistance if a problem presents itself during one of your sessions. You should be able to assess a situation when it arises, identifying the problem and taking the necessary action. This may involve removing someone from danger or contacting the medical services to arrange an admission to hospital. You should also be able to deal calmly and competently with more minor events, such as a person who has fainted or has a panic attack, taking the appropriate action and providing reassurance. You must always have an adequate first-aid box available (see page 244); remember that anything that you use should be replaced as soon as possible so that it is always up to date.

A few examples of situations in which your first-aid skills may be needed are described below.

A foreign body in the eye

Wash the eye with cold water. If you have a medicine dropper then fill this with sterile water and apply drops to the eye starting from the inside edge. This will usually wash out the irritant, but if there appears to be a more serious problem or the condition persists, cover the eye with a sterile pad and get the person to the accident and emergency department of a hospital.

GETTINGTRAINING

There are many short first-aid courses available. You should attend a course locally and gain your Certificate of Competence, which should then be displayed on the wall of the room in which you work. It will be necessary from time to time to upgrade your qualification.

Fainting attack

Fainting can have many causes, including emotional shock or a severe drop in blood sugar levels (either in someone with diabetes or from lack of food). It could also be due to what is known as a 'silent heart attack': not all heart attacks announce themselves with severe pains in the chest.

Regardless of the possible cause, never place the head between the legs of the patient. This used to be the recommended treatment, but doing so severely restricts the blood flow to the diaphragm and consequently circulation to the heart, which must be avoided in the case of a heart condition.

Loosen all clothing, in particular belts around the waist and tight collars and ties. Place the patient in the recovery position (see opposite), which means lying them on their side with the uppermost leg bent towards the chin. Support the head with a pillow and cover the person with a blanket.

If the patient is unconscious and not breathing, use mouth-to-mouth resuscitation, which will have been a part of your first-aid course. Get somebody to summon an ambulance while you concentrate on aiding the unconscious person.

If the patient beings to feel slightly dizzy while lying on the therapy table you can raise their legs, supporting the legs with pillows and towels (see the picture on page 244).

Panic attack

Place a paper bag over the nose and mouth of the affected person and get them to breathe deeply for a few breaths at a time (but not continuously). Inhaling the carbon dioxide of exhaled air has a calming effect. Reassurance is essential and in most cases the situation is relieved quite rapidly. If distress continues, call for medical assistance.

Asthmatic attack

When these attacks occur, the person is usually in a distressed nervous state, with very laboured breathing. They are usually pale and in some very serious states

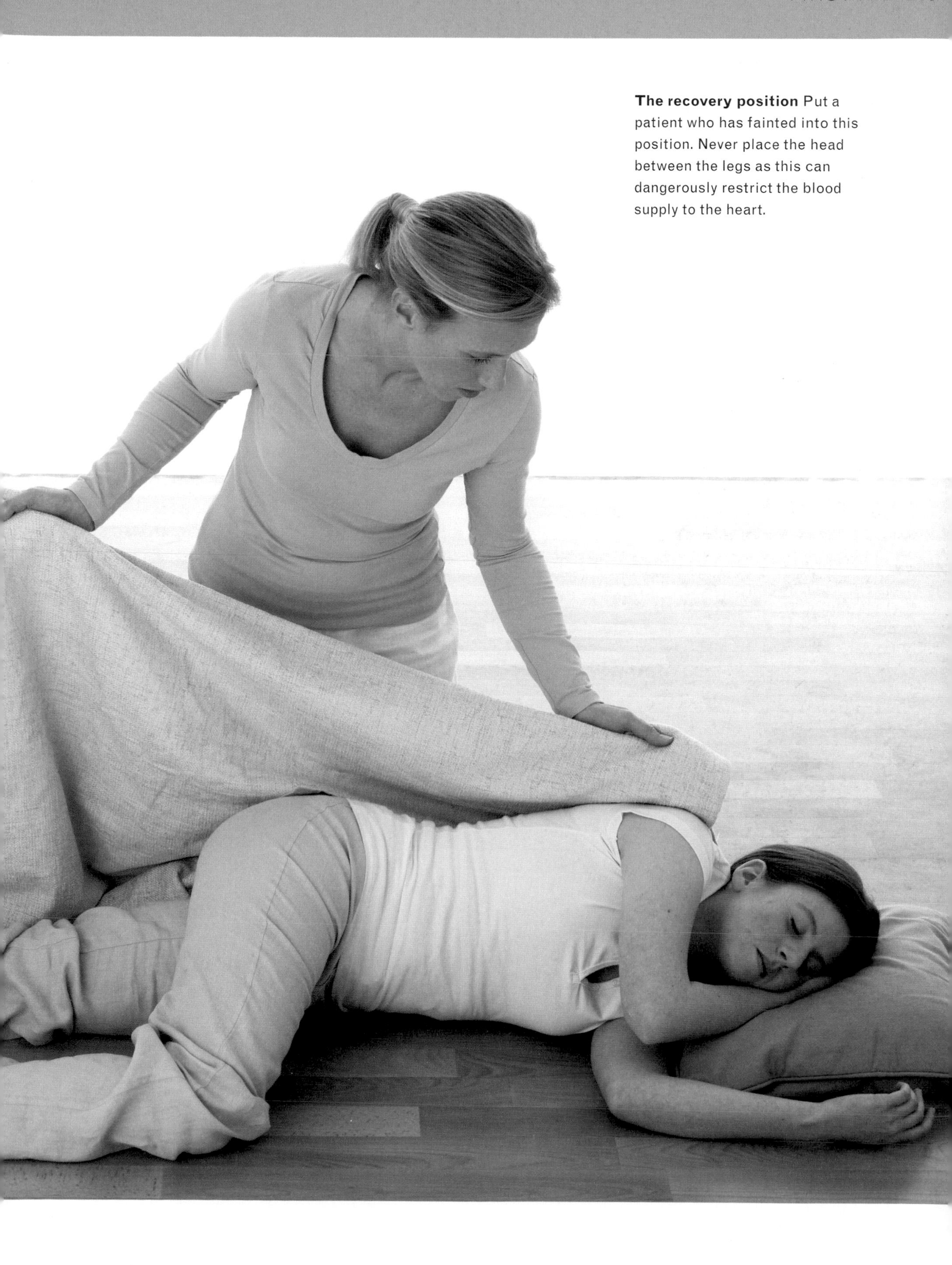

The recovery position Put a patient who has fainted into this position. Never place the head between the legs as this can dangerously restrict the blood supply to the heart.

there is a 'blue tinge' to their lips and under their eyes (this warrants urgent medical attention). These symptoms are caused by the inability to breathe in and by difficulties in the exhalation of waste gases.

Always have the person placed in a sitting position, preferably leaning forwards onto several pillows. If they have their asthma medication available then encourage them to use this. If their breathing improves within a short time then the emergency will have passed.

Should the laboured breathing continue beyond a few minutes, it will be necessary to call an ambulance immediately so that the person can be treated in the nearest hospital.

Cuts, wounds or stings

Clean a minor cut with water to which a mild antiseptic has been added and apply a sterile pad. An insect sting is usually just a momentary annoyance and the pain can be lessened if the area is quickly covered with an antihistamine cream; a cold compress will also reduce any swelling. However, do check that the person does not have an allergy to stings.

Minor burns or scalds

Always cool down the scald by immediately immersing or liberally dousing the area under running cold water for about 10 minutes. Cover with a sterile dressing. As burnt or scalded areas tend to swell, remove the patient's rings or watch if necessary.

Sudden chest pain

People who suffer from heart attacks usually experience a crushing pain in the centre of the chest which radiates down the left arm and often up into the lower jaw. Sometimes they feel pain in the upper part of the back, and there may be associated nausea, dizziness, profuse sweating and faintness.

In the case of an angina attack, again there will be symptoms such as pain in the chest and the skin may look ashen; a general weakness may occur, accompanied by shortness of breath.

Should you be involved in a situation where someone experiences symptoms such as these, immediate medical attention will be required. Call for an ambulance without delay, and while you are waiting for it use the lifesaving techniques you learned during your first-aid course.

FIRST-AID BOX

Your first-aid kit should include the following:

- Antiseptic cream, antiseptic solution and sterilization wipes
- Plasters, bandages and sterile dressings
- A sling
- Safety pins and adhesive tape
- Scissors and tweezers

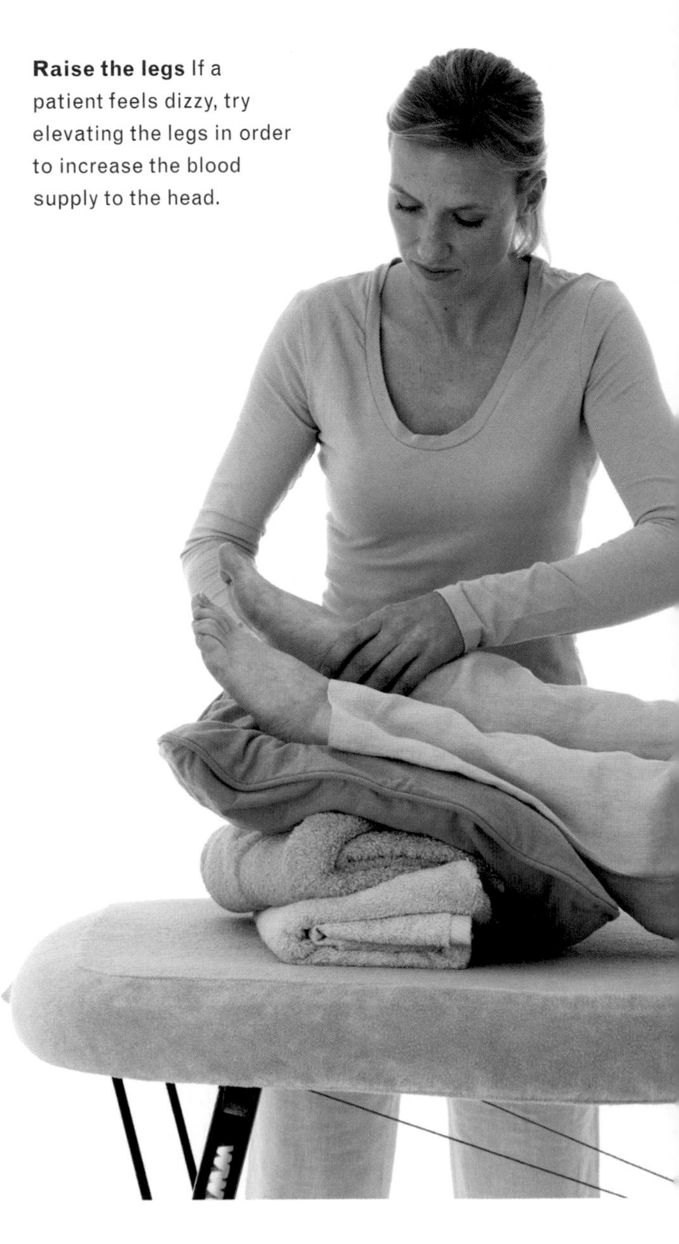

Raise the legs If a patient feels dizzy, try elevating the legs in order to increase the blood supply to the head.

Other complementary therapies

While orthodox medicine and modern drugs have an important role to play in the treatment of illness, complementary medicines offer alternatives. These are supportive of modern medicine and help strengthen the body's natural ability to recover from illness and injury at both a physical and psychological level.

Complementary therapies can help in a wide range of acute and chronic conditions, providing safe, natural and effective treatments to help prevent ill-health and also preventative measures to maintain good health. What they have in common is that the aim is to treat the whole person. This holistic approach takes into account not just the manifesting illness but an individual's overall physical, emotional and mental health. Complementary therapies offer a method of alternative treatment that adopts a gentle approach to healing the body, mind and spirit. A few therapies that can be used together with reflexology are described below.

Traditional Chinese medicine

This approach views health and disease quite differently from Western medicine. According to traditional Chinese medicine, illness is a disharmony of the whole body and treatment aims to restore harmony. This can be achieved by various therapies, which can include acupuncture, herbal medicines, massage, exercise and meditation. Chinese herbal medicines are derived from natural sources, with the herbs being first boiled and the liquid then drunk or made into tablets or powders.

Acupuncture aims to restore the body to a state of health and balance by regulating the flow of energy (*chi*) along the meridians, the invisible pathways along which energy is said to flow around the body. Fine long needles are inserted into the skin at specific points on the meridians that affect a particular organ or function. Like reflexology, acupuncture works on one area of the body in order to affect another and, although it follows the Chinese meridian map rather than reflexology's zones, most of the principles are similar. In fact, reflexology has been described as 'acupuncture without the use of needles' (see page 12). Acupressure is an aspect of acupuncture in which the pressure points on the meridian are stimulated without needles.

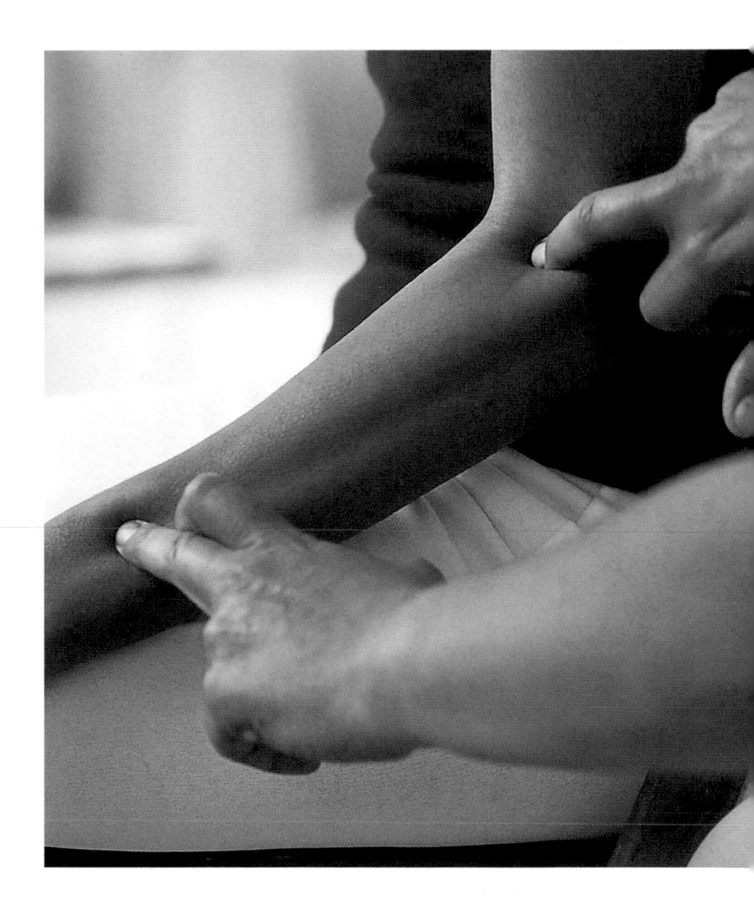

Acupressure In this ancient Chinese therapy, pressure points along the meridians, or energy pathways, are stimulated in order to heal different parts of the body.

Practitioners in China have been using acupuncture and acupressure for thousands of years, in order to treat a variety of diseases including depression, musculoskeletal problems, high blood pressure, menstrual and menopausal symptoms, headaches and allergies.

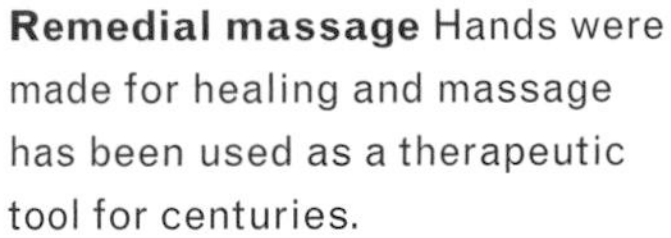

Remedial massage Hands were made for healing and massage has been used as a therapeutic tool for centuries.

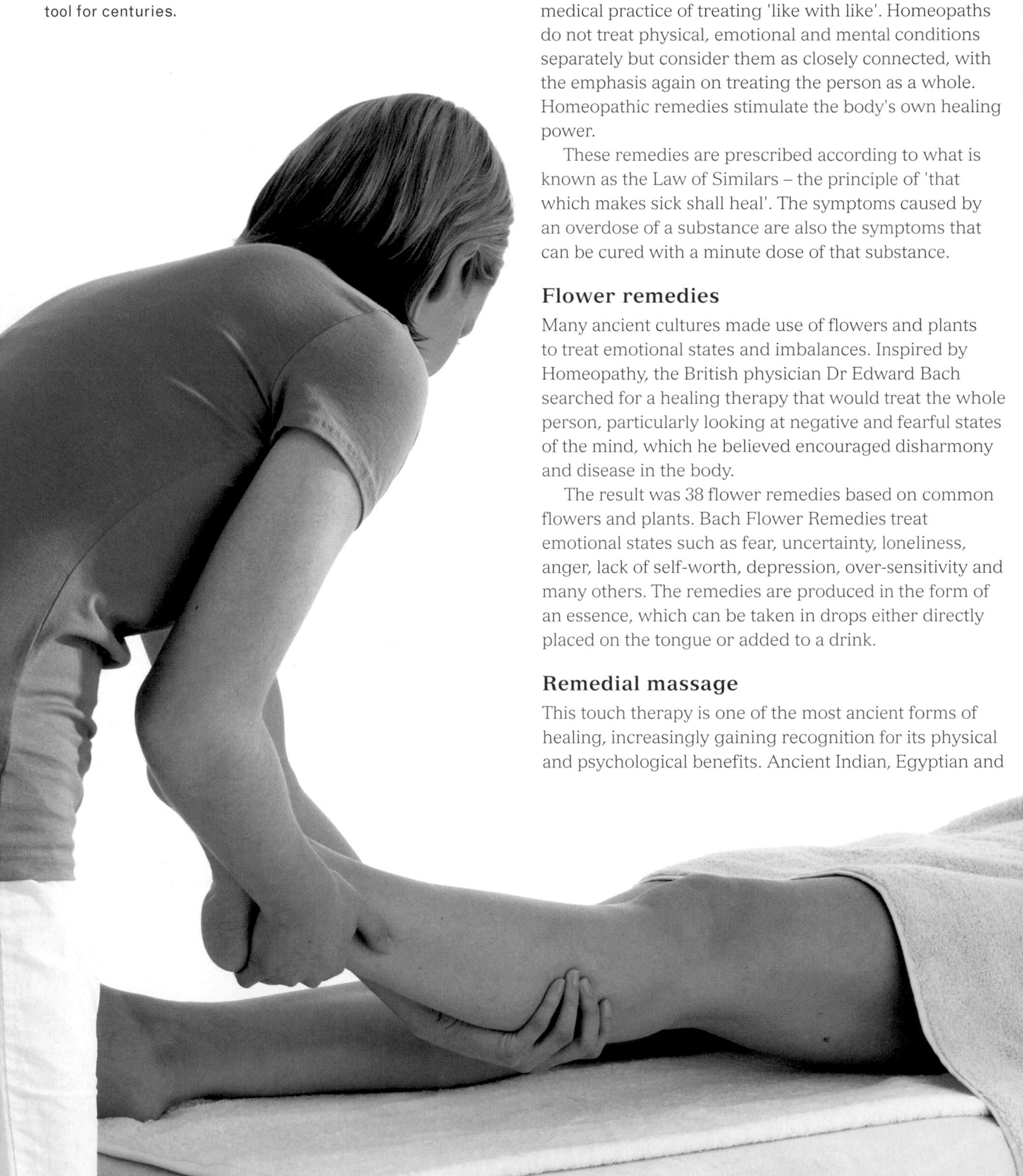

Homeopathy

Derived from the Greek words homo and pathos meaning 'similar' and 'suffering', Homeopathy involves the medical practice of treating 'like with like'. Homeopaths do not treat physical, emotional and mental conditions separately but consider them as closely connected, with the emphasis again on treating the person as a whole. Homeopathic remedies stimulate the body's own healing power.

These remedies are prescribed according to what is known as the Law of Similars – the principle of 'that which makes sick shall heal'. The symptoms caused by an overdose of a substance are also the symptoms that can be cured with a minute dose of that substance.

Flower remedies

Many ancient cultures made use of flowers and plants to treat emotional states and imbalances. Inspired by Homeopathy, the British physician Dr Edward Bach searched for a healing therapy that would treat the whole person, particularly looking at negative and fearful states of the mind, which he believed encouraged disharmony and disease in the body.

The result was 38 flower remedies based on common flowers and plants. Bach Flower Remedies treat emotional states such as fear, uncertainty, loneliness, anger, lack of self-worth, depression, over-sensitivity and many others. The remedies are produced in the form of an essence, which can be taken in drops either directly placed on the tongue or added to a drink.

Remedial massage

This touch therapy is one of the most ancient forms of healing, increasingly gaining recognition for its physical and psychological benefits. Ancient Indian, Egyptian and

Chinese manuscripts refer to the use of massage to heal and prevent disease and injuries as far back as 2700 BCE.

As a healing therapy, massage relieves muscular aches and pains, eases stress and tension and improves the circulation. Oil is usually applied to the body, and the main target areas, where most stress and tension occur, are in the neck, shoulders and spine. Massage creates a sense of wellbeing, boosts the immune system, mobilizes stiff joints and generally restores balance to the body.

Reiki

A Japanese word meaning 'universal life energy', reiki is a natural healing method that seeks to restore and rebalance energy in the body. Dr Mikao Usui, who was a Japanese professor of theology in the 19th century, developed this form of relaxation and healing from ancient Buddhist teachings.

In reiki, practitioners channel universal life energy (or *ki*, which corresponds to the *chi* of Chinese medicine, see page 245) through their hands into the recipient, encouraging the unblocking of energy pathways for the purpose of healing the body, mind and spirit. The practitioner's hands are placed in a sequence of positions over the patient's body. Some people experience a deep warmth or tingling, accompanied by a great sense of emotional relaxation. Specific conditions treated include menstrual and menopausal problems, cystitis, headaches, sinusitis, eczema, arthritis, back pain, sciatica, stress, anxiety, depression and insomnia.

Nutritional therapy

We are what we eat, and good nutrition is essential for good physical and emotional health. Practitioners aim to help bodily ailments by examining the diet of the individual and encouraging the use of supplements as well as suggesting changes to the patient's diet in an attempt to improve general health. Nutritionists are trained to detect deficiencies, food intolerances and allergies as a part of a programme that helps the body to eliminate toxins and promotes health and healing. An organic diet is often recommended in order to avoid ingesting the disease-causing chemicals that are now used so freely in the cultivation and storage of foods.

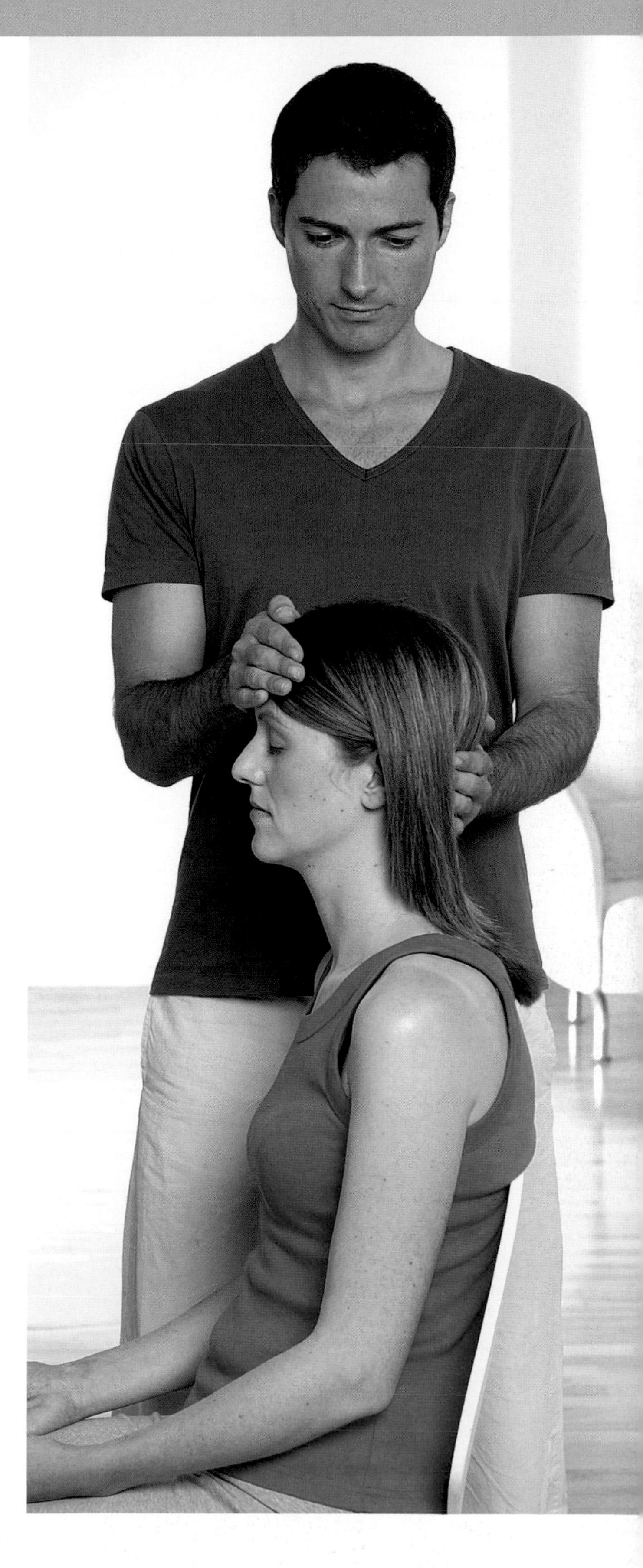

Power of reiki Practitioners of reiki channel healing energy through their hands and into the body of the receiver.

Glossary

Adrenal glands – two triangular endocrine glands positioned one on top of each kidney. They produce the hormones adrenaline and noradrenaline.

Analgesia – the loss or reduction of sensitivity to pain. It can be produced by use of analgesic drugs.

Angina – a suffocating, constricting chest pain.

Area of assistance – in reflexology, this term is used to mean an area or system of the body that is instrumental in helping to remedy dysfunctions in other parts of the body, even though the area in question may seem to have no particular relationship to the illness.

Atherosclerosis – an arterial disease in which fatty plaques develop, obstructing blood flow.

Blood pressure – the pressure blood exerts against the walls of blood vessels. Systolic pressure relates to the force exerted when the heart's ventricles contract; diastolic to the pressure when the heart relaxes.

Calcaneus – heel bone; the large bone in the tarsus of the foot that forms the projection of the heel behind the foot.

Cervical – relating to the neck, both at the base of the head and the entrance to the uterus.

Chakras – regions of the body where maximum energy gathers.

Coccyx – the four fused bones (coccygeal vertebrae) that form the tail end of the spine.

Congestion – an accumulation of blood/fluids in the tissues of the body.

Creeping – a reflexology technique, in which thumb or fingers move forward in a slow, bending movement.

Cuneiform – the three bones in the tarsus.

Detoxification – removal of toxic substances (one of the functions of the liver).

Diabetes – a disorder of carbohydrate metabolism due to malfunction of the pancreas.

Dorsal – relating to the back; on the foot, the upper part (*see also* Plantar).

Elimination – excretion of metabolic wastes from the body.

Endocrine system – the body system that produces hormones.

Endorphins – a group of chemical compounds found in the brain and having pain-relieving properties.

Energy field – a stimulating energy surrounding all living things.

Foot map – chart depicting the relationship between the feet and body parts.

Guidelines – lines dividing the feet into specific areas equated to body areas.

Healing crisis – a situation arising during the healing when symptoms temporarily become exacerbated.

Holistic – pertaining to treating the whole person, in body, mind and spirit.

Hooking out – a reflexology technique by which pressure is applied to a reflex point and the thumb then drawn back (resembling a hooking movement).

Hormone – chemical substance that is secreted by the endocrine glands to trigger a specific effect on another part of the body.

Hyperkeratosis – thickening and roughening of the outer, horny layer of the skin. It may be an inherited disorder affecting the palms and soles.

Hypertension – high blood pressure.

Hypotension – low blood pressure.

Immune system – the body's defence against disease.

Lateral – relating to the side; on the foot or hand, the outer edge (*see also* Medial).

Lateral longitudinal arch – the shallow, outer arch of the foot, aligned with the fourth and fifth toes.

Longitudinal arch – the highest and most important arch of the foot.

Lumbar – relating to the loin or lower back (lumbar vertebrae).

Lymphatic system – network of vessels carrying lymph (a clear fluid derived from blood) and drained by lymphatic vessels.

Medial – relating to the centre; on the foot or hand, the inner edge (*see also* Lateral).

Medial longitudinal arch – arch of the foot made up by the calcaneus, the talus, the navicular and the cuneiform.

Metatarsals – the bones of the feet.

Navicular – a boat-shaped bone of the ankle.

Neuralgia – severe burning or stabbing pain, often following the course of a nerve.

Oedema – excessive accumulation of body fluid in the tissues, causing swelling.

Osteoarthritis – degenerative disease of the joints, resulting from wear of the cartilage.

Overgrip – a rotating movement to relax the foot, with the foot supported from above.

Parasympathetic nervous system – the part of the nervous system concerned with conserving and restoring energy.

Phalanges – the small bones of the fingers and toes.

Pituitary gland – pea-sized gland in the centre of the brain that orchestrates the entire hormonal system.

Placebo – an inactive medicine that may help symptoms because of the patient's belief in its powers.

Plantar – relating to the sole of the foot (*see also* Dorsal).

Plexus – a concentration of nerves or blood vessels. The solar plexus is an important group of sympathetic nerves and ganglia high in the back of the abdomen.

Randomized controlled study – a comparison of the outcome between two or more groups of patients undertaking different forms of treatment.

Reflex – automatic or involuntary action brought about by relatively simple nervous circuits.

Reflex point – minute area of nerve endings in the feet/hands that influence a change in the functioning of the body.

Rheumatoid arthritis – disease of the synovial lining of the joints, causing pain, swelling and stiffness.

Sacral vertebrae – the five fused vertebrae (forming the sacrum) at the base of the spine, above the coccyx.

Sciatic nerve – the major nerve of the legs, which has the thickest diameter of all nerves in the body.

Sensitivity – a moderately painful sensation when pressure is applied to a reflex.

Solar plexus – *see* Plexus.

Spinal friction – reflexology technique of vigorous movement applied along the medial edge of the foot, reflecting the spinal reflexes.

Sympathetic nervous system – the part of the nervous system concerned with motor function.

Talus – the ankle bone.

Tarsals – the bones of the ankle and the foot.

Thoracic – relating to the 12 bones of the thoracic spine, to which the ribs are attached.

Transverse arch – the arch across the sole of the foot.

Undergrip – a rotating movement to relax the foot, with the foot supported from below.

Vascular system – a circulatory system for bodily fluids; the cardiovascular system comprises the heart and the network of blood vessels.

Zone therapy – the therapy based on the lines of energy that run through the body from the feet/hands to the brain; the foundation of reflexology.

Index

Acknowledgements

The author would like to thank her editor, Gill Paul, for all her professional input to the book and for her enthusiasm for reflexology. Thanks also to Katarina Tilley, and to Jessica Cowie, Fiona Robertson and Leigh Jones at Hamlyn.

For more information about reflexology, please visit Ann Gillanders' website www.footreflexology.com or email her at ann@footreflexology.com.

Special Photography:
© Octopus Publishing Group Limited/Ruth Jenkinson
Models Amanda Grant, Sam Whyman and Michelle Liebetrau at Modelplan

Other Photography:
Alamy/Bubbles Photolibrary 208; /Jennie Hart 214.
Art Archive/Ragab Papyrus Institute Cairo 13.
Corbis/ Michael A. Keller 84; /Ingolf Hatz/zefa 146; /Alan Schein/zefa 195; /Image Source 239.
Digital Vision 191.
Getty Images/Sylvain Grandadam 15.
Octopus Publishing Group 21; /Frank Adam 225 bottom left; /Paul Bricknell 17, 150; /Frazer Cunningham 19; /Randy Faris 241; /Jeremy Hopley 192 top right; /Ruth Jenkinson 23, 65; /William Lingwood 192 top left, 225 top left, 225 top right, 225 bottom right; /Lis Parsons 192 bottom left; /Peter Pugh-Cook 192 bottom right; /William Reavell 75; /Russell Sadur 96, 149, 197; /Gareth Sambidge 77; /Niki Sianni 131 top right; /Ian Wallace 245.
Photodisc 103, 131 top left, 142, 143, 216.
Science Photo Library/Greg Schaler 18.

The publisher would like to thank Katarina Tilley, Poppy Gillioz and Cate Barr. Thanks also to Bonnie Fraser of Alternative Products Limited for supplying the Starlight massage table and the therapist's stool used in the photography.

Executive Editor Jessica Cowie
Project Editor Fiona Robertson
Executive Art Editor Leigh Jones
Designer Peter Gerrish
Illustrators Susan Tyler and Kate Nardoni
Picture Researcher Jennifer Veall
Production Controller Simone Nauerth